Patient Teaching Manual 2

Patient Teaching
Manual 2

Springhouse Corporation
Springhouse, Pennsylvania

73205

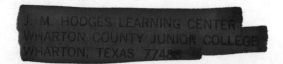

Publisher: Keith Lassner
Editor: Regina Daley Ford
Clinical Editors: Cindy Boyer, RN, BSN, MSN; Marlene Ciranowicz, RN, BSN, MSN; Mary Chapman Gyetvan, RN, BSEd; Susan Krupnick, RN, MSN, CCRN, CEN, CS; Susan Weiner, RN, MSN; Nina P. Welsh, RN
Drug Information Manager: Larry Neil Gever, RPh, PharmD
Art Director: John Hubbard
Editorial Services Manager: David Moreau
Senior Production Manager: Deborah C. Meiris

The clinical procedures described and recommended in this publication are based on research and consultation with nursing, medical, and legal authorities. To the best of our knowledge, these procedures reflect currently accepted practice; nevertheless, they can't be considered absolute and universal recommendations. For individual application, all recommendations must be considered in light of the patient's clinical condition and, before administration of new or infrequently used drugs, in light of latest package-insert information. The authors and the publisher disclaim responsibility for any adverse effects resulting directly or indirectly from the suggested procedures, from any undetected errors, or from the reader's misunderstanding of the text.

Some of the material in this book was adapted from the following Springhouse series: Nurse's Reference Library, Nursing Now, Nurse's Clinical Library, Nursing Photobook, and New Nursing Skillbook.

Library of Congress Cataloging-in-Publication Data
Main entry under title:

Patient teaching manual.

   Includes bibliographies and index.
   1. Patient education—Handbooks, manuals, etc.
I. Ford, Regina Daley.   II. Springhouse Corporation.   [DNLM: 1. Health Promotion—handbooks.
2. Patient Education—handbooks.   WY 39 P298]
RT90.P376   1987   610.73′06′99   87-6426
ISBN 0-87434-032-2   (v.1)
ISBN 0-87434-066-7   (v.2)

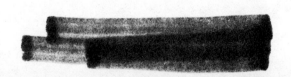

Contents

Contributors

CLINICAL CONTRIBUTORS

Gloria S. Cheeseman, RN, BA, MA
Director, Educational Resources Department
St. Francis Medical Center
Trenton, N.J.
Foreword

Janice Selekman, DNSc, RN
Associate Professor
Thomas Jefferson University
Philadelphia
Chapter 1—"Principles of Patient Teaching"

Basia Belza Tack, RN, MSN
Nursing Consultant
El Camino Hospital
Mountain View, Calif.
Formerly: Clinical Nurse Educator
Allergy and Infectious Disease
    Nursing Service
Clinical Center
National Institutes of Health
Bethesda, Md.
Chapter 9—"AIDS and Its Complications"

Jeannee Parker Martin, RN, MPH
Director
AIDS Home Care and Hospice Center
San Francisco
Chapter 9—"AIDS and Its Complications"

CLINICAL CONSULTANTS

Jo Eland, RN, MA, PhD
Assistant Professor of Nursing
The University of Iowa
Iowa City, Iowa

Christine A. Miaskowski, RN, MS, CCRN
Clinical Nurse Specialist
Jack D. Weiler Hospital of the Albert Einstein
    College of Medicine
New York

Deborah Stephens Mills, RN, MN
Nursing Consultant
Halston Valley Hospital and Medical Center
Kingsport, Tenn.
Formerly: Assistant Professor
Medical-Surgical Nursing
Yale University School of Nursing
New Haven, Conn.

Janice H. Overdorff, RN, BSN
Administrative Nurse III (Head Nurse)
University of Illinois Eye and Ear Infirmary
Chicago

Foreword

Patient teaching has not always been a top priority for the health care professions. In the past, such questions as "What is my blood pressure?", "Why am I taking this pill?", or "Why must I have this test?" often met with the response, "Sorry, but you'll have to ask your doctor for that information." Patients were expected to accept much, if not all, of their diagnostic workups and therapeutic regimens on blind faith. Our traditional view of patient education did not require the dissemination of valuable and sometimes vital information to our patients. Gradually, under the impetus of professional and legal demands for nursing accountability, our philosophy regarding "the patient's right to know" has changed. The nursing process now stipulates patient and family education concerning health problems and health maintenance as a major responsibility of the professional nurse.

Today especially—with the "sicker and quicker" phenomenon clearly reflected in hospital discharge policies—patient care frequently devolves upon the patient or the family. Our goal must be to arm the caregivers with the best and most accurate information available to help them achieve an optimal level of health for the patient.

The Springhouse *Patient Teaching Manuals* were created to help nurses and other health care professionals achieve this goal. These manuals are unique, easy-to-use teaching/learning tools. They permit the nurse to choose from a wide variety of topics and to select from the comprehensive content of each teaching plan the exact level and depth of information needed by her patient. Topics dealt with in the text and patient-teaching aids were selected because they are common, difficult, or otherwise significant teaching problems.

Chapter 1, "Principles of Patient Teaching," provides the nurse with a mini-course in patient teaching. It discusses teaching methods, development and implementation of the teaching plan—even instruction of patients with special needs.

The format of subsequent chapters is consistent. There are five sections in each chapter: Patient-Learner Data Base, Explaining Diagnostic Tests, Explaining Disorders, Explaining Treatments, and Patient-Teaching Aids.

The first section, Patient-Learner Data Base, lists significant areas in which a patient may experience a potential knowledge deficit. Not all data (every risk factor, for example) will apply to each patient. But this comprehensive list tells the nurse those areas which should be questioned so that she can identify those which should be pursued further.

The next three sections, Explaining Diagnostic Tests, Explaining Disorders, and Explaining Treatments, present specific teaching plans that address specific patient problems. For example, in Chapter 5, "Oncologic Disorders," mammography, breast cancer, and chemotherapy are dealt with in the diagnostic tests, disorders, and treatments sections, respectively.

To maximize the quality and effectiveness of the patient education process, the teaching plan content is directly related to the patient objective. The behavioral objectives from which the nurse and patient should select, and upon which they should agree, appear in the left column on each page. The teaching plan content for each patient objective appears in the right column, directly across from the objective.

To individualize her nursing care plan and to promote patient compliance, the nurse must decide which objectives are relevant to that patient's needs, always bearing in mind that prior knowledge is also an important resource for patient learning. Furthermore, she must select information from the teaching plan content based on her knowledge of the patient's ability and desire to learn.

The final section of each chapter comprises selected patient-teaching aids. These aids were chosen either to supplement or complement the textual material, as judged necessary by professional nurses. While they are numerous, they are not intended to be all-inclusive. Several excellent appendices, a list of selected references, and an extensive index appear at the back of each volume.

The Springhouse *Patient Teaching Manuals* provide health care professionals with the tools needed to fulfill their obligation to educate the patient and the family. These tools—basic educational principles telling *how* to teach and specific patient-teaching plans showing *what* to teach—utilized with consistency and continuity, surely will enhance the credibility of the teacher and the receptivity of the learner.

As a nurse and an educator, I am proud and most pleased that these manuals are available to assist health care professionals with their patient education efforts. They engender an awareness of the importance of patient teaching and challenge health care professionals to provide our patients and their families with the knowledge, attitudes, and skills to be true and valuable partners in the promotion, protection, and enhancement of their own health.

GLORIA S. CHEESEMAN, RN, BA, MA

Principles of Patient Teaching

Teaching is an integral component of nursing. To tend only to the physical needs of patients without teaching them to obtain, retain, or regain health is a job half done. While registered nurses and student nurses are expected, and often required, to direct patient teaching, the skill of how to teach patient teaching is often limited in nursing programs. The purpose of this chapter is not only to suggest to the nurse *what* to teach the patient, but also *how* to teach it. We will address such issues as what data the nurse needs before working with a patient, the techniques she can use to aid her teaching, and the variables that interfere with teaching. This chapter will focus on the process of patient teaching.

THE NURSE AS EDUCATOR

Since the turn of the century, nurses have incorporated patient teaching into their professional role. Starting with public health and maternal-child health nurses, the instruction of child care and sanitation measures became the responsibility of the nurse. Lavinia Dock (1858-1956), a pioneer in nursing, emphasized nursing's important role in preventive health care via teaching.

Today, nurses have many opportunities to share their knowledge. This role extends far beyond the treating of acute illness in the hospital setting. While the primary responsibility of nurses is to teach patients the care they need to maintain or regain their health, nurses also inform and support their patients' significant others, especially family members. In addition, nurses promote good public health by working with different groups within society to improve the environment.

While this book focuses on patient teaching, it should be noted that nurses also teach each other by exchanging information, whether during change-of-shift reports or in patient care conferences. This exchange of information promotes continuity of care and, therefore, improves the art of nursing.

Teaching versus learning	Teaching is a collaborative process that involves communication between the nurse and the patient. Its goal is to add to the patient's knowledge base so he can improve or maintain his health and comfort. Teaching can be planned or spontaneous, verbal or nonverbal, individualized or for large groups, affective or cognitive. Learning is a relatively permanent change in behavior that is inferred from a change in performance or cognitive beliefs occurring as a result of experience. Learning helps the patient to increase his understanding, decrease his anxieties, and alter his health care habits.
Patient teaching and the nursing process	The principles of patient teaching correlate directly with the nursing process. Before any interventions can be planned, assessment must occur and goals must be set. The nursing process involves obtaining a data base, assessing this data base (including identifying a list of needs), writing goals, planning and implementing nursing interventions, and making an evaluation. This same process is true in patient teaching. Before teaching can occur, the nurse must assess the patient and his environment, identify his needs, write educational objectives, plan and implement a teaching plan, and evaluate the results.

METHODS OF KNOWING/SOURCES OF KNOWLEDGE

	Every patient has his own values about health and illness and experiences with the health care system. Before assessing the components of the art of teaching, the nurse must understand the different methods of knowing, because from these sources of knowledge spring the roots of both the nurse's and the patient's belief systems and many of their health care practices.
Magic and the supernatural	*Belief in magic and the supernatural* as the cause of events is the first method of knowing. This includes carrying good-luck charms, crossing one's fingers for luck, avoiding the number 13, saying "God bless you" after someone sneezes, or knocking on wood. All are attempts to enhance one's safety and health. Since such practices usually cause no harm to a patient who believes in them, they can readily be acknowledged as important in a teaching plan.
Tradition and culture	Knowledge based on *tradition and cultural norms*, including rituals and beliefs without scientific justification, is the second method of knowing. Using herbal teas to

treat respiratory or gastrointestinal problems, the hot-cold theory followed by some Hispanic groups, using chicken soup or chest rubs for whatever ails you, or the belief that getting one's feet wet in puddles or sitting in a draft will cause illness are examples of this method. The patient at this stage will often say, "I know it is true just because I know it."

When planning to teach someone whose belief system is founded in tradition and culture, it is important for the nurse to assess whether the beliefs interfere with the proposed treatments or are harmful to the patient. If they are not harmful, an attempt can be made to incorporate these beliefs into the treatment regimen. This provides the patient with a familiar, secure base from which to start learning. Why not include herbal teas as part of the patient's required fluid intake or suggest that the patient's "higher power" would want him to comply with proposed treatments? Building on a base of health beliefs familiar to the patient can decrease his anxieties and increase compliance.

Intuition and personal experience

Intuition or personal experience based on trial and error is involved in the third method of developing a knowledge base. The patient's significant others may say, "I know it will work for you; I can just feel it. It worked for me. Try it." Often, personal success with a specific treatment or pressure from a loved one to try a treatment forms the basis of this knowledge (for example, certain positions or exercises for menstrual cramps, concoctions or practices to bring on sleep, or child-rearing directions from a mother based on what worked for her 25 years earlier). Nurses may also have experiences with health measures unrelated to anything taught in nursing school and untested by the scientific community.

Nurses and patients who believe that unproven health measures can prevent or cure ailments need to assess the validity of these measures. If they pose no danger to the patient, the nurse should enhance the patient's knowledge about such measures (based on scientific fact) by discussing rationales for their use; otherwise, the patient's misperceptions should be corrected. The nurse should give the patient credit for his trial-and-error methods and should help him obtain the most accurate and safest knowledge base.

Authority

A fourth method of knowing is based on trust of those in *authority* or those recognized by society as being influential. It refers, in part, to believing what authorities write or say and personalizing the content. The content may or may not be accurate and empirically supported, but this makes no difference to the believer. Accepting health practices without question is common during childhood. Such comments as "My parents said..." or "My teacher said..." can be expanded to include the teachings of physicians, religious leaders, and Nobel prizewinners. Patients like this are not advocates for themselves; rather, they generalize the teachings of these authority figures and relate them to their own condition and health practices.

Since the nurse is often in a role of authority, the patient will follow her say-so if it is logical, sensitive, and presented in an understandable manner. But how should the nurse respond when another authority figure's advice contradicts the patient's medical needs? Some suggestions include presenting equally authoritative information (preferably in writing) that supports the treatment plan; beginning with a simple, but related, example of cause and effect and then building a solid knowledge base from this situation; and avoiding confronting or insulting the patient's belief model while at the same time reinforcing beliefs that are more focused on health promotion. When the patient states, "The Bible says...," an appropriate nursing response would be, "Yes, but the Bible also states...."

Logical reasoning

Logical reasoning, the fifth source of knowledge, includes inductive and deductive processes. Inductive reasoning is a method of obtaining related facts and then making a generalization about these facts; for example, if taking 500 mg of vitamin C is good, then taking 1,000 mg of vitamin C is even better. While this method of thinking may be fine for vitamin C, it could be fatal for cardiac drugs. The nurse must anticipate the patient's thought processes and address his misconceptions in the teaching plan.

In deductive logic, a specific prediction is derived from a generalized statement; for example, multiple studies have documented that decreasing one's intake of carbohydrates and meat improves cardiovascular status. Anorexics may incorrectly believe this is also true for them. It is important for the nurse to impress each patient with the idea that he is special and unique, and then to explain why certain treatments would or would not be helpful. The teaching plan—like the rest of the nursing care plan—must be individualized to meet the specific needs of each patient. Nurses have always believed in providing an individualized plan of care based on the specific needs of each patient.

Scientific method	The highest level of knowing is obtained via the *scientific method,* which requires observation and testing with a reliable and valid instrument while controlling as many variables as possible. It is logical and objective, with controls that prevent error. This method should be the primary source of knowledge for nurses and should provide the basis of material for the teaching plan.

ASSESSMENT OF THE LEARNER

Factors to assess	A patient's belief system is only one area the nurse must assess before preparing a teaching plan. A second, but related, area requiring assessment is the patient's *knowledge base.* How much does he know about his condition or treatment? How accurate is that knowledge base?

A third area is the patient's *ability to learn:* does he understand easily; does he ask questions; or does his body language indicate confusion of the concepts, content, or sequence of events? Can he follow directions, pay attention, and recall information? Can he hear, see, and communicate? Is he easily distracted, or does he demonstrate other signs of learning problems? Does he understand abstract ideas?

Once the nurse has assessed that a patient *can* learn, she needs to assess if he is *ready to learn.* He might say, "I don't want to know; I can't change at this point in my life." If physical or emotional factors interfere with his readiness to learn, the nurse can attempt to clarify the issues by asking open-ended questions. The nurse must also ask herself, "Does the patient really need to know this material or is it *my* need, as nurse, to teach it to him?"

The nurse must also assess the patient's past *history of compliance.* Simply learning to feed back material verbally will not help him maintain or regain his health; he must put the knowledge into practice.

Assessing the following factors will help the nurse complete her patient data base in preparation for developing a comprehensive teaching plan:
—What is the patient's outlook on life?
—What is his past history with health-related material?
—What is his culture's response to pain and illness?
—What is his educational background?
—What are his fears about his illness or the proposed changes in his life-style?

Factors that interfere with learning

Many factors can alter one's readiness or ability to learn. The first is *anxiety.* It has been well documented that, while mild anxiety enhances learning, severe anxiety can be incapacitating. Patients may verbalize their uneasiness, or the nurse may detect it in their body language. Some causes of anxiety include feeling pressure to perform, feeling a loss of control because of the learning situation or because of the health need that requires this new knowledge base, not wanting to expend the energy necessary to learn, lacking trust in the teacher, and dealing with the financial implications of the new knowledge or health practices on one's life-style.

A second factor interfering with learning is *motivation.* In internal motivation, the stimulus and perceived need for change come from the individual himself; in external motivation, the impetus for change comes from significant others. Internally motivated people are more self-directed, and their stimulation for success lasts longer than it does for those who are externally motivated and need repeated reinforcement and praise from others (Redman, 1984).

Motivation is related to *locus of control.* A patient with an internal locus believes that he *can,* if he so desires, change his health by measures he controls. A patient with an external locus believes that his health is controlled by a higher power (God, luck, and/or significant others) and that compliance with treatment would be ineffective. Individuals with such "learned helplessness" feel that they cannot control the outcome of events. Teaching such a patient can be very frustrating for the nurse, for, in addition to presenting needed material, she must also develop and reinforce the idea that the patient can have some control over his condition.

A *lack of trust and honesty* between patient and nurse impedes learning. Providing continuity of care by having a consistent caretaker responsible for the teaching plan can prevent this. In addition, the nurse needs to be prepared, positive, and confident.

The nurse must evaluate the patient's *current physical and emotional status* before attempting teaching. Basic needs must be tended to first. Is the patient hungry or in pain? Is he tired or on drugs that alter his cognitive functioning? Is his mobility limited (this might affect the learning of skills)? Is he lonely or anticipating visitors? Is teaching planned during a time he would rather be with significant others? How much are others pressuring him to perform? What stage of illness is he in? Any of these factors can interfere with learning.

In addition to assessing the patient, the nurse must also evaluate three other factors: the environment, the time factor, and the available resources. *Where* is the teaching/learning to be done? What distractions, such as noise or people, are hindering the patient's ability to concentrate? Is there sufficient privacy? Is there sufficient lighting? Is the room too hot or too cold?

The nurse cannot always control *when* the teaching is to be performed and how much time will be involved. Is one session enough or are many sessions needed? Sessions should be short enough so that patients will have time to absorb the material, both cognitively and psychologically. In some situations, the content to be taught can be presented little by little every time the nurse walks in the room; for example, she can discuss the principles of breathing exercises while setting the patient up for his morning care. Then every time the nurse enters the room that day, she can teach him one new breathing exercise and evaluate his ability to do those already taught. If the nurse does not have enough time to teach the patient adequately or if she does not have a chance to reinforce the material, she should discuss the most important information and provide the remainder of the information in writing.

The final assessment involves exploring the health facility and national organizations for available *educational resources*. A great deal of patient-education material has been developed, and obtaining this material will ease the nurse's teaching role. Clinical specialists are resources for their areas of expertise. The hospital library is often a ready source of ideas and materials. The hospital's continuing education staff may also be able to provide teaching strategies. If a nurse works at a facility affiliated with a nursing school, she can seek help from nursing instructors, who may have access to teaching aids. Also drug and formula companies are often excellent sources of teaching aids, as are national organizations, such as the Cystic Fibrosis Foundation, the American Association of Diabetes Educators, and the American Cancer Society. This material should always be individualized for each patient.

THE TEACHING PLAN

Formulating behavioral objectives

Once the nurse has obtained and interpreted all possible data about the patient and his environment and has identified the problems, needs, or scope of the teaching required, her next step is to identify the patient's long-term and short-term goals by writing behavioral objectives. These objectives will guide the teaching plan and evaluation process.

Behavioral objectives state the change in the patient's behavior expected when "learning" has occurred. Remember that they are *patient* goals, not nursing goals. An effective objective often includes the words, "The patient will...." It is stated in terms of the patient and not the nurse.

To ensure that these objectives are truly patient-oriented, they should be established jointly by the patient and the nurse. Learning is more effective when a patient is motivated to learn, and establishing his own objectives is a reflection of motivation. Defining goals together also decreases the patient's anxiety about learning, since he will have a better idea of what to expect of the nurse and of himself and can have some control over the learning process. This, then, becomes a reflection of the definition of teaching—that of being a collaborative process.

The nurse should ask herself, "What behavioral change do I want to see in this patient? If he only learns one thing from my presentation, what should it be?" Objectives help the nurse focus on the task at hand; they define the expected outcome of the teaching, thereby decreasing the possibility that the patient will be overwhelmed by all available information about the topic.

Behavioral objectives include three major components: the observable behavior and to what degree it will occur; the conditions under which the behavior will be performed; and the criteria to be used to evaluate whether the behavior has been successfully learned. For example: "At the end of the final teaching session about diabetes, the patient will be able to correctly draw up and administer his insulin injection without assistance." In this example, "the end of the final teaching session" indicates *when* the behavior should be learned; the "patient" is *who* will be learning; "drawing up and administering insulin" is *what* will be learned; "correctly" indicates *how* or to what degree the task will be evaluated; and "without assistance" indicates the conditions under which the behavior will be performed.

Behavioral objectives are described in terms of *doing*. In reviewing behavioral objectives, the nurse must ensure that the goal is realistic for the patient and specific to his needs. Can he attain it? Can it be accomplished in the time period specified? What level of cognitive functioning is being addressed, and is it appropriate for the task at hand?

Bloom (1956) developed a system to classify educational objectives for cognitive learning. The stages include knowledge (recalling facts), comprehension (simple understanding), application (applying rules and generalizations to specific situations), analysis (dividing a concept into its parts), synthesis (rearranging the parts into a whole), and evaluation (assessing the value of information).

These stages form a hierarchy, from the easiest cognitive process (rote knowledge) to the most complicated (evaluation). In most situations, patient teaching only involves the first three stages (knowledge, comprehension, and application). However, teaching at any given level can proceed from simple to complex and from concrete to abstract. The nurse should center the objective around an action verb that describes what the patient is expected to accomplish. These verbs are listed in the table on pages 10-11.

While the guidance offered by well-written behavioral objectives usually facilitates learning, a nurse must remain flexible in a teaching situation. She may have to change objectives if the patient's needs change. For example, a patient may verbalize a misconception of something basic to the lesson plan, or the nurse may discover that one part of the teaching plan caused the patient a great deal of confusion and concern.

Writing some behavioral objectives is difficult. First, all learning cannot be anticipated. Also, objectives change as the learning process progresses. The verbs in the table reflect only the cognitive domain (intellectual and problem solving). The descriptors of the psychomotor and affective domains are not as well defined even though the needs of many patients clearly fall into these categories. Nurses should also incorporate these special needs into their teaching plan.

Developing a teaching plan

Once she has written behavioral objectives, the nurse can plan nursing interventions via a teaching plan, which includes the content to be taught and the methods by which it will be presented. Several variables strongly influence the development of a plan: whether teaching will be done one-on-one or in a group; whether material will be presented formally or informally; whether teaching will be performed throughout the shift or at a specific "teaching time"; and how much time is available for teaching. (This is often determined by the institution; for example, how many sessions are available for childbirth education, how many days until a patient is discharged, or how many minutes is a patient willing to stay after a clinic visit?)

An organized and logical teaching plan enhances learning. It is helpful to begin a lesson with content the patient knows and then to progress to new material. *Going from the known to the unknown* decreases

VERBS USED TO DESCRIBE BEHAVIORS OF THE COGNITIVE DOMAIN

Knowledge
(Recalling facts and information)

Accept	Know	Notice	Recognize	Test
Count	Label	Point	Record	Trace
Draw	List	Quote	Reiterate	Underline
Enumerate	Listen	Read	Repeat	Write
Identify	Memorize	Recall	Reproduce	
Indicate	Name	Recite	State	

Comprehension
(Simple understanding of information and ability to draw simple conclusions)

Answer	Contrast	Express	Report
Associate	Define	Inquire	Restate
Classify	Differentiate	Interpret	Review
Compare	Discuss	Locate	Select
Compile	Distinguish	Participate	Tell
Compute	Estimate	Predict	Translate
Consult	Explain	Recognize	

Application
(Applying rules and generalizations to specific problems)

Adopt	Complete	Examine	Schedule	Write
Apply	Decide	Illustrate	Sketch	
Calculate	Demonstrate	Operate	Solve	
Choose	Dramatize	Practice	Use	
Classify	Employ	Present	Utilize	

Analysis
(Breaking down concepts into separate elements and identifying the relationships among them)

Analyze	Construct	Devise	Explain	Realize
Appraise	Contrast	Diagnose	Generalize	Reason
Arrange	Create	Diagram	Infer	Relate
Calculate	Criticize	Discover	Inspect	Solve
Categorize	Debate	Distinguish	Interpret	Summarize
Combine	Detect	Examine	Organize	Support
Compare	Develop	Experiment	Question	Test

Synthesis
(Reassembling elements to create a new idea)

Arrange	Create	Integrate	Plan	Relate
Assemble	Design	Manage	Practice	Set up
Challenge	Determine	Order	Prepare	Transform
Collect	Formulate	Organize	Prescribe	Weigh
Construct	Group	Originate	Propose	

Evaluation
(Assessing the value of materials/ideas)

Appraise	Critique	Evaluate	Rank	Revise
Assess	Determine	Grade	Rate	Score
Assimilate	Establish	Judge	Recommend	Select
Choose	Estimate	Measure	Resolve	Value
Conclude				

anxiety, because the teaching begins on familiar territory. In addition, it helps patients apply information from one setting (past experiences) to their present situation. Starting on comfortable ground reinforces and supports the patient's feelings of having a solid knowledge base. The nurse must ensure that the material is neither too easy nor too hard, so she does not lose the patient's attention or interest.

A second approach involves teaching from *the simple to the complex*. Anatomy, physiology, and pathophysiology involve a language foreign to most patients. Before the nurse can teach them about their myocardial infarction or their beta blockers, she should define the words and approach the concepts simply. Pictures and analogies (if the patient can comprehend these) may help explain normal and abnormal organ functioning. From this simple but solid knowledge base, more complex material can be presented.

The third approach to teaching is to progress from *concrete to abstract* material. Most individuals find it easier to learn new material when they can see, feel, count, hear, or taste it. Since concepts are abstract by nature, they are often difficult to comprehend. Defining the concept of respiratory distress by pointing out the changes it effects, such as increased respiratory rate, wheezing, dusky skin, and retractions, renders it concrete and, therefore, more meaningful.

The final educational concept is that of *multisensory learning*. Perception is necessary for learning. Studies have indicated that a multisensory approach is more effective in learning than a single sensory approach. Some individuals learn better by one approach than another; for example, the pregnant woman listening to a childbirth-preparation lecture experiences only auditory stimulation. This woman may need to *see* a replica of a baby coming through the vaginal canal and *do* the breathing exercises to really understand what will happen during delivery. The nurse needs to plan her teaching so that it involves as many senses as possible.

Additional factors to consider when planning the teaching material include determining what content is most relevant to the patient's condition and needs, prioritizing when performing the teaching role, and avoiding conflict with the patient's culture and past experiences by incorporating his health beliefs into the teaching plan.

Since effective learning requires active participation, the nurse should encourage the patient to participate in each component of the teaching process and should encourage active give-and-take between the teacher and learner. Especially when teaching psychomotor skills, the nurse needs to consider the patient's strength, coordination, and mobility. She must remember that a strong knowledge base enhances the patient's performance of technical skills.

When developing a teaching plan, the nurse can anticipate the patient's fears and concerns and can include questions that decrease the threat of the material with such comments as, "Most new mothers wonder..." or "Many cardiac patients are concerned about...." This type of question reduces the patient's anxiety about the unfamiliar. Being sensitive to psychosocial needs enhances the rapport between the teacher and the learner.

The nurse can use multiple teaching modalities to present material to the patient, including the following:

—*Lecture.* Perhaps the most frequent type of teaching, especially for groups, it is cost effective, uses staff time efficiently, and ensures consistency of material through a structured presentation. However, lectures limit individuality and interpersonal interaction. The nurse should be willing to alter her teaching plan based on the patient's questions and responses. Patients should be involved in the lecture by questions or by challenges to their imagination.

—*Demonstration.* This multisensory presentation involves vision, hearing, and touch, but is limited to very small groups. This method builds skills and is especially effective when a return demonstration is performed by the patient. It is essential for teaching such skills as bathing a baby, walking with crutches, caring for a tracheostomy, and giving insulin injections.

—*Programmed instruction.* This teaching method uses prepared material that is divided into sections or units. The patient must be self-motivated and literate. Working at his own pace, he actively participates in the learning and gets immediate feedback from the source. The nurse does not need to be present, but learning is enhanced if she is involved.

—*Sociodrama.* This group problem-solving technique re-creates a real-life situation by having participants act out roles and feelings of the people involved. It helps patients explore feelings and does require planning. It is effective for attitudinal problems.

—*Role-playing.* This teaching technique allows one person to explore alternative behaviors by putting himself in the shoes of another. This is quite effective for siblings or classmates of handicapped patients or of those with chronic disorders.

—*Simulation.* In this teaching method, the nurse and the patient act out a real situation in a mock environment and behavioral processes are replicated. Learning laboratories in nursing programs and cardiopulmonary resuscitation certification programs are multisensory approaches in a nonthreatening environment that make use of simulation. This approach can be effective in teaching techniques that benefit from demonstration; for example, to prepare a patient to give himself an injection by first giving one to an orange.

—*Behavior modification.* This method is very popular with children, smokers, and those with weight problems. It involves operant conditioning with reinforcement. This means that the nurse gives the patient positive reinforcement for a specific behavior, which causes the desired response to occur more frequently and more intensely. Conditioning is a process of learning. A disadvantage of this method is that, when reinforcement slows or stops, so does behavioral change.

—*Contracting.* In this technique, the nurse and the patient agree on behavior(s) needed to achieve a determined goal. This is often effective with adolescents who may wish to have privileges in return for behavioral changes.

—*Audiovisual materials* (pamphlets, films, printed materials, diagrams, models). Patients must be literate in order to use most of the material involved in this teaching method, since most provide only visual information. In order for this method to be effective, the nurse must offer some verbal intervention and must individualize the material.

—*Play.* This teaching technique is commonly used with children in order that they learn about their world.

Medical play is most effective in preparing children for procedures and in helping them deal with their misconceptions and anger after the procedures.

Additional teaching methods include self-monitoring (keeping records, logs, or diaries of an activity), panels or debates, discussion groups, and using a patient's significant other to teach and monitor the patient.

To determine whether to teach patients individually or in groups, the nurse should consider the following factors. Teaching one-on-one is usually more effective, since the nurse can get to know her patient and can alter the teaching plan to meet his needs. The group process, on the other hand, can handle many individuals at once and, therefore, is less costly to run and takes less time than teaching each person separately. While a group can provide peer support in many situations, it can also make sharing feelings about sexuality or other embarrassing material difficult. The privacy and confidentiality of the one-on-one relationship is lost in the group. (This should not be confused with the principles of group therapy.)

While all of these are structured models in which the nurse can initiate the teaching plan, there is one method of patient teaching that the nurse does every minute she is practicing her profession. The nurse is a *role model* to patients, visitors, and other health professionals without ever saying a word or writing a teaching plan. The way she holds and wraps a baby, lifts an object from the floor, washes her hands, and even what she eats influence those around her. Learning often occurs through imitation. The more the patient respects her, the more he will observe and try to emulate her behavior. This teaching can be planned; if the nurse is aware she is being observed by the family, she should be careful about her performance. She can also verbalize *what* she is doing and *why.*

In conclusion, there are multiple teaching modalities. The same material may be taught effectively in many different ways. Or several modalities can often be used together to provide the best learning plan for the patient.

Implementing the teaching plan

When the nurse has the behavioral objectives and teaching plan before her, the process of implementing it is no more difficult than for any other skill in nursing. It requires the nurse to have a *knowledge base* about the material to be taught and the learning process. Since teaching is a form of communication, she must also have *effective communication skills*. Also teaching is easier and more rewarding when the nurse has *self-con-*

fidence about her ability to teach. The first step in self-confidence is taking responsibility for the teaching role.

The ability to engage in quality interaction and to establish a meaningful rapport with patients enhances the teaching/learning situation. In order to make nurse-patient interaction enjoyable, try the following suggestions:

—*Use your voice* to express enthusiasm and concern. If you are bored or scared, your teaching will reflect it. Be enthusiastic!

—*Use short words and sentences.* This makes it easier for the patient to retain your comments.

—*Repeat yourself* in different ways. Repetition enhances learning.

—*Tell the patient what you expect of him* during the session. This promotes a dialogue between the nurse and the patient and allows the patient to feel more comfortable asking questions or expressing concerns.

—*Let the patient teach you.* Allow him to share what he knows about the subject. This builds his self-confidence and makes him feel a part of the learning process. It also gives you an excellent opportunity to identify where to begin the lesson.

—*Provide reinforcement* for learning. Praise him for the knowledge he retains and/or comprehends.

—Allow time and provide routes for the patient to give *continual feedback.* This provides you with the opportunity to identify additional areas of weakness and confusion.

—*Be flexible.* Adjust your objectives, if necessary, based on the feedback you receive from the patient.

—*Take your time,* if possible. Do not rush through the material. Do not make the patient feel you are pushed for time. Everyone learns at a different speed and this cannot always be accounted for in the teaching plan.

—This is a *team effort* between the nurse and the patient. Work *with* the patient; do not just talk *to* him.

—*Make learning pleasant.* Let your personality shine through, and exude optimism.

If teaching is a new experience for the nurse and she feels overwhelmed by all the objectives and planned interventions, she should ask herself, "What one thing do I want this patient to learn today, and what can I do to help him meet this objective?" In addition, she should ask a peer to observe her during her first teaching session so that she can receive feedback. Seeking assistance while practicing the skill of teaching is akin to seeking support when first passing a nasogastric tube or a urinary catheter.

Evaluating the teaching plan

Just as teaching is a part of the nursing role, so too is evaluation an integral component of teaching. Teaching has little worth until its effectiveness is measured. To begin the evaluation process, the nurse should return to the behavioral objectives. What was the main idea/ concept to be covered? What behavior did she want to change? The next question she should ask herself is, "How do I evaluate whether the material was learned?"

In nursing school, learning was measured by tests and essays. In a patient-teaching situation, evaluation can be accomplished in a variety of ways: continual feedback from the patient during the teaching session by the patient expressing questions and concerns or by the nurse actually seeking patient responses about the content; patient compliance with the treatment plan, or the extent to which a patient carries out a prescribed treatment plan, indicating a change to the desired behavior; and success in attaining the desired goal.

Both the nurse and the patient should evaluate the teaching/learning. Just because the patient says he understands and does not ask any questions, the nurse cannot assume learning has occurred. The objectives spell out how to evaluate the patient. They tell the nurse what to measure, under what conditions, and to what degree the behavior was to be accomplished. If the teaching program was not successful, the nurse should be willing to admit a lack of success and make a new plan.

Evaluation is the most abused component of the teaching process. The nurse may teach a group of patients and feel that she did a good job. She asks if there are any questions, and no one responds. How does she know she has been successful? How does she know learning has occurred? A checklist of content remembered, a verbal quiz, an ungraded posttest, or a return-demonstration are all methods of inferring whether or not learning has occurred.

Remember: Teaching is never complete until you have evaluated the success of your intervention.

Documenting the teaching process

Before a patient undergoes a surgical procedure, it is the physician's responsibility to inform him of the risks and to have him sign a consent form indicating that he has so been informed. The nurse can also be held liable for not recording that a patient has been taught about health care procedures, especially when that teaching is necessary to maintain or regain health: "The nurse...may be liable for failing to instruct the patient in particulars of care; for example, that a certain medication must be taken with food" (Cushing, 1984, p.

721). Legally, it is best to teach verbally and then to reinforce that teaching with written materials. The nurse should document what she taught, how the patient responded to the teaching, the results of the evaluation of the teaching plan, and the materials that were distributed to the patient.

Documenting patient teaching is important not only in legal issues, but is also an integral factor in the concept of continuity of care. Not all teaching can be done in one session or one shift. By noting in the chart how much of the teaching plan was accomplished and what problems the patient had with the materials, nurses and other health professionals will have an idea of how much the patient knows about his disease and treatments. These health professionals can reinforce the learning already accomplished and clarify any misconceptions. Has the patient indicated to the next shift any confusion about what he was told, or is he already practicing his new skills? Documenting these can assist the nurse responsible for the teaching plan. For patients being taught in a clinic setting, documentation helps the nurse remember what content she taught from week to week for each individual patient.

It is not sufficient to just indicate that the patient was taught about a particular concept. This would indicate that the teaching was not a shared process. Learning occurs in the patient. Only to chart what the nurse did and not to document the patient's response is incomplete.

USING CREATIVITY AND HUMOR IN TEACHING

Creativity is both an art and a science, an active way of thinking and behaving that involves a combination of feelings (subjective input) and knowledge (objective input). The goal of creativity is to improve existing conditions by problem solving. There is no perfect way to teach any particular subject or skill. Since each patient's situation, setting, and time constraints are different, creativity by the nurse becomes essential. How does a nurse teach kidney function in 5 minutes or less? Perhaps comparing the filtration process to that of a tea bag may help the patient associate an unknown mechanism with one he deals with daily.

Creativity and humor are closely linked. In the early days of nursing, humor and any form of self-expression by the nurse was considered inappropriate and unprofessional. However, since humor has been identified as an effective tool in promoting healing and health, it is very appropriate for nurses to express their enjoyment of their professional role via humor. Using analogies or rhymes to remember signs of a disorder may prove very helpful to patients. However, humor and clichés can only be used if the nurse has assessed the patient and is confident that the patient can understand and appreciate this method of presentation. Sarcasm has no place in patient teaching.

TEACHING PATIENTS WITH SPECIAL NEEDS

Those with an altered ability to learn, because of aging, congenital disorders, or pathology and disability require the nurse's special attention when she is developing a teaching plan. She must acknowledge their special needs and alter the proposed teaching mechanisms and content accordingly. Most of these patients have significant others who are interested in obtaining the necessary knowledge base to assist in their loved one's care and in promoting his health. Before planning teaching measures, the nurse must assess the needs and concerns of these significant others. They can be a part of the teaching/learning process, either separately or along with the patient.

Teaching the elderly patient

As the aging process progresses, many individuals find that their central nervous system deteriorates. Visual and auditory capabilities decrease, necessitating the use of prostheses (corrective lenses and hearing aids). Cerebral changes cause a decrease in the speed of processing new stimuli and a decrease in short-term memory. Because of the elderly patient's increased incidence of failing health, he may take multiple medications that may further affect his cognitive abilities. In addition, joints lose their flexibility and his mobility may be limited.

Elderly patients have a wealth of past experience on which to build their new knowledge base. Because they have established patterns of living entrenched in habits, they are often more resistant to change. Many elderly patients are on fixed incomes, and the fear of financial burden as a result of the new treatment or proposed change in their life-style threatens their financial security and increases their anxiety. Depression resulting from the health-related problem may make successful learning even more difficult.

As a nurse, some suggestions you must consider before teaching the elderly patient include the following:
—Check that printed materials have print large enough for the patient to see, especially when directions are involved.
—Speak face-to-face with the patient, and check frequently to make sure he can hear you and understands

the words you are using.
—Discover your patient's daily habits. Avoid making
radical changes in his life-style, if possible, and incorporate his daily habits into the teaching plan.
—Give only small amounts of specific information at a
time.
—Plan multiple teaching sessions to reinforce material.
—Because of a decrease in short-term memory, repeat
information often and show the relationships among the
parts of the teaching plan.
—If a skill is involved, multiple return demonstrations
will help the patient learn the material.
—Provide verbal reinforcement and rewards to build
self-esteem.
—In some situations, group work has been found to improve an elderly patient's problem-solving ability.
—Use reminder aids, such as marking pill containers
by the day or hour or making a checklist for exercises
when teaching skills.

Teaching children

Teaching plans for children must be extremely flexible
and creative. The nurse should consider the child's cognitive level of development, his psychomotor skill level,
the amount of trust he has developed with those in his
environment, his fears, and his health needs. A great
deal of health promotion is taught during the childhood
years to assist these young people in developing and
obtaining their highest level of wellness.

The nurse needs to assess the child as she would an
adult; however, in addition to the factors mentioned earlier in this chapter, she must also assess his development. What is his chronologic age? Are his height,
weight, and developmental tasks (fine motor and gross
motor skills) appropriate for his age? Is he psychologically and socially (language skills, accountability) age-
appropriate? What is the relationship/interaction (trust)
between the child and the mother, father, or primary
caretaker? What cognitive concepts (time, cause/effect)
can the child understand?

Pediatric nurses learn never to assess the child
without also evaluating the needs of the parents. What
are their anxieties, fears, and needs? Thus, a teaching
plan for a child is really two teaching plans: one for the
child and one for the parents. For infants, the nurse
must teach the parents instead of the child. But for all
other age-groups, the child must be involved.

Teaching children involves a completely different perspective than that required to teach adults. Children
learn continuously and take in stimuli from all of their
senses. Play is the work of children and the method by

which they learn about their world. Effective teaching plans incorporate these multiple modalities.

Toddlers (12 months to 3 years)	The toddler's greatest fear is separation from his mother. Therefore, teaching should be done in the presence of the mother, even with the child sitting on her lap. This child's favorite word is "no" and he uses it constantly. However, it is not always related to his intent. If the nurse tells him she is going to change a bandage, he may say "no." The nurse can respond, "I know you don't like this, but we have to keep the area clean." The nurse should be honest about when it will hurt and when it will not. Although the patient may not be able to understand the principles of a dressing change, he will begin to trust her.

The toddler has no concept of time. Because of this, the nurse must teach the toddler while she does the procedure. She can explain the blood pressure cuff as she is about to put it on the child. A toddler cannot delay gratification; therefore, he will not understand N.P.O. status prior to a procedure. Teaching for a toddler is continuous, because everything, such as blood pressure cuffs, stethoscopes, and hospital personnel, is new to him. |
| **Preschoolers (3 to 5 years)** | The preschooler fears altered body integrity; for example, he is afraid that he will lose all his blood from a needle stick, thus necessitating the wearing of the magic Band-Aid that uses its sticky ends to hold the skin together and prevent blood loss. He fears any invasion of or treatment to his body.

The preschooler does not understand cause and effect and often has wild fantasies about how his anger or "bad" behavior caused his accident or illness. While the child cannot express these fantasies easily, the nurse must anticipate and respond to them in her teaching plan. Such comments as "You know it's not your fault you got sick" are important in teaching the preschooler.

A preschooler is just beginning to develop a sense of time. He tells time by meals or naps. His attention span is very short, and he learns best when multiple senses are involved. These limitations are important to the teaching plan. A preschooler can be taught immediately before a stressful procedure, but can tolerate preparation for physician's visits and admissions to the hospital at least a week in advance. To tell a child he will be getting an injection in 3 hours will cause him to scream for the next 3 hours. Therefore, wait until 5 minutes before an injection to do the teaching. It is es- |

sential, however, to inform the child about the injection and the reasons for it, to tell him when it will hurt and when it will not, and to allow him to assist in choosing a site and putting on the bandage. All of this promotes trust in the health care system.

Prehospitalization visits, in which the child can tour the pediatric unit, play with the toys, see the beds and the way people dress, and then go home, can be very beneficial. Medical play is an effective means of patient teaching with this age-group. Letting a child play physician and nurse, dress up in surgical gowns, gloves, and masks, give injections to dolls, and bandage the nurse's arm can be more educational than a verbal presentation. Teaching these children is often done with the assistance of their dolls; for example, a cast may be put on a child's doll the day before the child is scheduled for orthopedic surgery. (The nurse should make sure she puts on the same type of cast that the child is expected to have.) This not only helps a child prepare for a procedure, but it is also equally effective after a procedure to allow the child to express his anger and any misconceptions.

School-age children (6 to 12 years)

School-age children are concrete thinkers. This is a period of active cognitive growth and the development of multiple concepts. However, they still may have misconceptions about body functions and some cause/effect thinking. These children are curious about their bodies and may ask the nurse questions completely unrelated to their hospital admission or clinic visit. Their fears need to be addressed in the teaching plan, as they still have some "thinking" reminiscent of their preschool days.

School-age children need preparation and explanations for what is happening to them. The nurse must use language appropriate to their cognitive level. Concrete facts should be used to describe a procedure; this is best done with pictures or models of the procedure. The nurse must be careful of the medical terms she uses. She should not refer to the dye injected during a cardiac catheterization, but rather to the medicine injected. She should not tell a child he is going to have his appendix taken out, but rather to have it fixed. Children's imagination may lead to misperceptions about treatments.

These children like to participate in their teaching. The effectiveness of written materials and audiovisual equipment depends on each child's abilities. They respond better with individual teaching, a great deal of positive reinforcement and praise, and affection. As children enter prepuberty, they begin to separate physically from their parents. They usually want their parents present during teaching. This can be helpful to the nurse, as the parents can provide emotional support during the teaching session and later can reinforce the material being taught.

Adolescents (13 to 18 years)	Cognitively, adolescents are in the process of developing abstract thinking and, therefore, can be taught much of the same material as that presented to adults. While many adolescents may like to appear as if they know all about their body, in fact, their knowledge is minimal. A comment by the nurse should ease the teenager's anxiety about admitting ignorance. Ideally, the teenager can view the nurse as someone from whom he can get reliable information about his body so that he is more knowledgeable than his peers.

In addition, adolescents are aware of their changing bodies, and hospitalization may threaten their self-image. For example, an adolescent female was depressed after an appendectomy, and a nursing assessment determined that she was upset because she thought that now she could never have children. Appropriate nursing intervention resolved the misunderstanding and involved explanations about the anatomy and physiology of the appendix and the uterus.

As they become more conscious of their adult bodies, adolescents desire privacy—for their physical self and for their emotional component. Diaries are a great way of helping adolescents express their concerns. Parents may be present during teaching; however, this should be up to the adolescent. Parents can be taught separately, but the confidences shared by the adolescent should be kept confidential.

Adolescents are social beings. Acting like everyone else is important to them, and, therefore, they are hesitant to ask questions and demonstrate their ignorance in front of peers. The decision of whether to teach individually or in a group depends on the individuals involved and on the ability of the nurse to identify the needs of the group members.

Teenagers want to believe that they are not children anymore, and, therefore, it is important to give them an active role in developing the objectives and the teaching plan. Contracts can be effective with adolescents.

As a nurse working with children of all ages, here are some general guidelines you should use in planning and implementing your teaching plans that are different from the guidelines utilized when working with adults:
—Do not ask "yes/no" questions unless you are willing

to accept a "no" answer.
—Give children choices in their treatment.
—Make sure the language you use fits their cognitive development. Do not use a cliché or a medical term without first explaining it.
—Get on an eye level with the child when teaching him. Sit if he is seated. This decreases the anxiety caused by a large, looming figure standing above him telling him what is wrong with his body.
—Be pleasant. Smile. Children of all ages are quick to pick up on adult body language. They can tell when you care and when you do not.
—Many children regress developmentally while hospitalized. You should address teaching measures first to the level to which the patient has regressed and then to his appropriate developmental level.
—Be honest. All people, especially children, need to feel trust in those responsible for their health care.

Teaching the disabled

Disabilities can be developmental or developed, physical or psychological; they can involve cognitive processes or physical ones. The need to learn among the disabled is just as great as among members of the rest of society; however, their ability to learn may be compromised.

When teaching a blind patient, the nurse must use other senses, especially touch and hearing. A tape recording of the directions for a procedure can be very helpful. On the other hand, the deaf patient needs materials in writing (if he can read) and needs to see demonstrations of what is required of him. Visual models can help him learn.

The patient with arthritis needs a variety of teaching aids to assist him in carrying out physical procedures. A portable percussor will make chest percussion easier to manage. The individual with cerebral palsy needs more verbal teaching because of his deficit in motor function.

The illiterate or non-English-speaking patient is a challenge. If the patient can read, a translator can write the directions in his native language. Demonstration and return demonstration will also be helpful. Try to find a significant other who speaks and understands English; then teach them together.

Children and adults with learning disabilities need special assessments of their areas of confusion and the methods by which they can learn most readily. Some cannot read directions, some confuse numbers, and others cannot remember a sequence of events. The teaching plan needs to present alternative approaches to reaching the desired goal.

Should terminally ill patients be taught? The answer is "yes." As long as there are choices to be made, then there is teaching to be done to assist the patient in making an informed decision.

CONCLUSION

"Teachers are eternal learners" (Clark, 1978, p. 9). The more a nurse teaches others, the more she learns herself. The more comfortable the nurse is with herself and the material she presents, the more sensitive she can be to the patient's needs and the more flexible and creative she can be in her teaching plan.

One of the aims of nursing is to encourage patients to be their own advocates and to assume responsibility for their own health care. In order to make healthy choices for themselves, they need information. Nurses must provide much of this.

Not all teaching can be planned. Often nurses' teaching serves to clarify the teaching of others. Nurses may teach indirectly by allowing a patient to express his feelings and to feel more comfortable with his psychological concerns. Nurses teach about the medications they give a patient or the procedures they are doing, such as taking the pulse, every time they have contact with the patient. And, of course, nurses are always a role model to others.

There is no best way to teach. The best technique is one that works best for each individual nurse and for the patient. The art of teaching takes time to develop.

Organizing and evaluating patient teaching

Before your patient can manage his condition, he has a lot to learn. This patient-teaching checklist will help you to organize your teaching sessions. Because the content to be covered is presented as patient objectives, you can also use the checklist as an *evaluation tool* to determine the effectiveness of your teaching, thus saving valuable time.

PATIENT-TEACHING CHECKLIST FOR _Sally Smith — Endometriosis #1_

PATIENT OBJECTIVES	PRE-TEST RESULTS	SESSION I CONTENT	SESSION II CONTENT	POST-TEST RESULTS
Define endometriosis.	Date: 7/7. Patient unaware of definition of endometriosis. She stated her doctor had explained it was "uterine tissue sitting outside the uterus, but still acting like it was in the uterus."	Date: 7/7. Instructed patient on definition of endometriosis. Also, using a chart, instructed the patient on the menstrual cycle.	Date: 7/8. Reviewed the phases of the menstrual cycle with the patient, making sure she understood the mechanics of how endometrial tissue can leave the uterus and attach to other organs.	Date: 7/8. Patient understands the concept of the disease process. Using charts and illustrations of the female anatomy, she went through the menstrual cycle and answered the nurse's questions with intelligent feedback.
Name three possible causes of endometriosis.	Date: 7/7. Patient knew of only one cause: "at time of menstrual period, the pieces of tissue that flow from the womb can attach to other areas of body."	Date: 7/7. Patient was instructed on the three possible causes of endometriosis, using an illustration of the female anatomy.	Date: 7/8. Started the session by answering relevant questions raised by the patient. Reviewed the material from the last session, making sure she understands the concepts.	Date: 7/8. Using role reversal, patient explained to the nurse the three possible causes of endometriosis. The patient accomplished this smoothly, with very little prompting from the nurse.
Explain the two types or forms of endometriosis.	Date: 7/7. Patient totally unaware of the fact that there are two forms.	Date: 7/7. The forms of endometriosis were explained to the patient.	Date: 7/8. Reviewed the concept of two forms of endometriosis.	Date: 7/8. Patient had no trouble answering nurse's questions about this concept. Demonstrates total understanding of concept.

PATIENT-TEACHING CHECKLIST FOR _Sally Smith — Endometriosis #2_

PATIENT OBJECTIVES	PRE-TEST RESULTS	SESSION I CONTENT	SESSION II CONTENT	POST-TEST RESULTS
Describe the five stages of endometriosis.	Date: 7/7. Patient does not know the five stages of disease process. However, she remembered her doctor telling her she was at Stage II of disease.	Date: 7/8. Using illustrated charts, the five stages of disease were explained to her. She's interested in her stage, and inquired as to whether it could progress to Stages III, IV, V.	Date: 7/9. Once again, went over the five stages of endometriosis. The patient seems very motivated to learn about her disease process.	Date: 7/9. When asked to repeat info back to nurse, the patient did well. She explained the five stages, using medical terminology, and answered the nurse's questions.
Discuss the signs and symptoms of endometriosis.	Date: 7/7. Patient described her symptoms: painful periods and pain a week before her period, which needed very strong medication to give relief; also, some rectal bleeding.	Date: 7/8. Instructed patient on signs and symptoms of endometriosis. Also discussed with her why this pain is different from menstrual cramps.	Date: 7/9. Answered the patient's questions she had from last session. Did not need a review of Session I content.	Date: 7/9. Patient understands signs and symptoms of endometriosis, as illustrated by feedback and her ability to name them for the nurse.
Discuss the differences in signs and symptoms, depending on where her endometrial tissue has implanted.	Date: 7/7. Patient unaware of the fact that symptoms could differ, depending on where her endometrial tissue has implanted.	Date: 7/8. Using illustrations of female anatomy, instructed patient on this concept. Patient had a good number of questions about this.	Date: 7/9. Reviewed material from Session I. Patient appears to understand why different sites of tissue implantation produce the signs and symptoms they do.	Date: 7/9. Patient asked nurse to write down sites with signs and symptoms for her; this was done. Patient understands this concept, but needed prompting from written info to answer the nurse's questions.

PATIENT-TEACHING CHECKLIST FOR _Sally Smith — Endometriosis #3_

PATIENT OBJECTIVES	PRE-TEST RESULTS	SESSION I CONTENT	SESSION II CONTENT	POST-TEST RESULTS
Discuss differential diagnosis.	Date: 7/7 Patient knew that a laparoscopy was going to be done to identify the disease process; was unaware of other tests.	Date: 7/8 After conversing with doctor, teaching of this content has been deferred until it is deemed necessary by laparoscopy results.	Date: 7/10 Reinforced info given to patient by her doctor. Discussed the barium enema procedure with the patient.	Date: 7/10 Patient understands that laparoscopy only tells whether she has endometriosis. Patient also understands that barium enema will provide info to doctor about progression of disease.
Discuss treatments for endometriosis.	Date: 7/7 Patient aware of the fact that "certain hormone pills" may be taken to decrease lesion size.	Date: 7/9 Discussed with patient different treatments used for endometriosis, which depend on stage of disease, lesion site, and her desire for future pregnancies. Reinforced info given by doctor.	Date: 7/10 Reviewed Session I material and zeroed in on her specific stage, site of implantation, and treatment.	Date: 7/10 Patient repeated doctor's info for the nurse. Demonstrates a basic understanding of Session I material and understands her particular treatment regimen.
Describe her medication regimen.	Date: 7/10 Patient could not remember name or dosage of her medication.	Date: 7/10 Patient instructed on medication regimen (name, dosage, side effects, and precautions).	Date: 7/11 Reviewed medication regimen. The patient appears to have a grasp of situation.	Date: 7/11 Patient demonstrated her knowledge of medication regimen by explaining it to the nurse.

PATIENT-TEACHING CHECKLIST FOR _Sally Smith — Endometriosis #4_

PATIENT OBJECTIVES	PRE-TEST RESULTS	SESSION I CONTENT	SESSION II CONTENT	POST-TEST RESULTS
Explain the importance of routine medical follow-ups.	Date: 7/11 Patient told nurse "a yearly exam is important for good health."	Date: 7/11 Discussed with patient importance of an annual pelvic exam and Pap smear for early diagnosis and treatment.	Date: _____	Date: 7/11 Patient understands this concept. Discharged today with a good understanding of her disease process and treatment.
	Date: _____	Date: _____	Date: _____	Date: _____
	Date: _____	Date: _____	Date: _____	Date: _____

A blank sample chart similar to the one above can be found in Appendix C of this manual. You may reproduce the sample chart to use as a tool in organizing and evaluating teaching for your individual patients.

Pain Management

Patient-learner data base*

Areas of potential knowledge deficit
Risk factors for pain:
—Illness or trauma
—Low pain tolerance
—Fear of pain
—Fatigue, boredom, or anxiety
—Personal history of pain
—Treatment delay
—Nonparticipation in a pain management program
—Misconceptions about pain
Personal beliefs about pain and pain management
Definition of pain
Causes of pain
Symptoms associated with pain
Treatment of pain
—Pharmacologic therapy
—Nonpharmacologic therapy
Complications of pain management

Explaining self-management

DISTRACTION

Patient objectives	*Teaching plan content*
1 Define distraction.	Distraction is concentration on something other than pain. Reading a book, watching TV, and simply engaging in conversation are some of the most common examples of distraction.

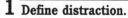

* A general assessment should be done for all patients. For general assessment guidelines, see Chapter 1, Principles of Patient Teaching.

2 Identify the types of pain relieved by distraction.	Distraction is most effective for relieving acute pain; it can also be effective against chronic pain.
3 Explain how distraction relieves pain.	Concentrating on an activity makes it the focus of awareness. Although the exact mechanism is unknown, the result is that the patient feels less pain.
4 Identify four distraction techniques.	Sophisticated techniques of distraction include the following: —Music therapy —Singing —Rhythmic breathing —Description.
5 Describe the use of music therapy for distraction.	This technique may appeal to the patient who likes music. He will need a tape player with a headset and cassettes of his favorite music. —He can sit or lie down in a comfortable position, with his legs and arms uncrossed and relaxed, while he listens to the music through the headset. Depending on his preference, he can either close his eyes and concentrate on the music or stare at a nearby object. —To combine music therapy with guided imagery, he can imagine himself floating or drifting with the music. He can also focus on images suggested by the music, or on a pleasant scene of his own choosing. (See the "Guided Imagery" teaching plan in this chapter.) —Because rhythmic movement can also serve as distraction, the patient may want to keep time with the music by tapping a finger or foot, slapping his thigh, or nodding his head. —He may want to keep his finger on the player's volume-control dial. If his pain increases, he can increase the volume; when the pain subsides, he can decrease it. —This distraction technique has several advantages: It provides a demanding auditory stimulus for the patient without disturbing others, and it works effectively for a tired, sedated, or passive patient. It also allows the patient to respond to varying pain intensities by adjusting the volume.
6 Describe the use of singing for distraction.	This technique also makes use of rhythm as a distractor. —The patient should select a song he likes and then do the following: • Mouth the words, exaggerating the lip movements, while singing them silently. (Children and some

adults may want to sing out loud.)
- Concentrate full attention on the words and rhythm of the song. (Closing the eyes may help.)
- Sing faster or louder when the pain intensifies, slower when the pain subsides.

—Others may sing with him, if they wish.

—If the patient does not like music, he can substitute recordings of comedy routines, stories, or sports events.

7 Describe the use of rhythmic breathing for distraction.	This technique may appeal to a patient who prefers a more structured distraction technique. —To perform rhythmic breathing, the patient follows this procedure: • Stare at a person or an object and inhale slowly and deeply. • Exhale slowly. • Continue breathing slowly and comfortably (but not too deeply) while counting silently: "In, two, three. Out, two, three, four." • Concentrate on the feel of breathing, perhaps closing the eyes and imagining the air moving slowly in and out of the lungs. • Count silently after establishing a comfortable, rhythmic pattern. —If he begins to feel breathless, he can breathe more slowly or take a deep breath. —If rhythmic breathing alone is not sufficient distraction to relieve the pain, the technique can be made more complex. The patient can massage the painful area (or the contralateral area) with a stroking or circular motion as he breathes. Or he can raise his arm as he inhales and lower it as he exhales. Also he may inhale through his nose and exhale through his mouth.
8 Describe the use of description for distraction.	To use this technique, the patient looks at a photo and describes every detail or makes up a story about it. Others present should close their eyes or look away from the photo to avoid influencing his comments. When he finishes, they ask him questions based on his description.
9 Discuss patient guidelines for using distraction techniques.	Distraction is a *short-term* pain-relief measure. The following guidelines explain what to expect and how to benefit from using distraction techniques. —They are simple but effective techniques that can be used whenever pain returns or intensifies; however, pain will probably return when a distraction exercise stops. —Distraction can be tiring, and the resulting fatigue

may intensify the pain after the exercise. Most patients cannot use it for long periods without becoming bored or tired. Rhythmic breathing, for example, can be especially tiring.

—Other pain-relief measures, such as medication, are available for use along with distraction.

—The patient should choose a distraction stimulus (distractor). He will be distracted most effectively by something that interests him (for example, a hobby). If he has used distraction before or if he has developed his own distraction technique for his current pain, he can build on that.

—If the patient is in acute pain and cannot choose a distractor, he can use another distraction technique, such as rhythmic breathing, description, or singing.

—The patient should use distractors that involve more than one sense, if possible. The most effective distractors are those that engage hearing, sight, or touch.

—Distractors that require more concentration should be used when the pain intensifies. A simple distraction, such as listening to music, may help the patient cope with mild pain. But if the pain worsens, a more complex distractor that requires complete attention (such as a chess game) may be more effective.

—If possible, rhythm and repetition should be part of the distraction technique. Many patients have great success with rhythmic breathing patterns: taking shallow or deep breaths; breathing from the chest or abdomen; breathing slowly and deeply; or controlling the length of time for inhalation and exhalation. When rhythmic breathing is impractical (as for obese patients and those with pulmonary disorders), background music, finger tapping, or a repeated word or phrase should be incorporated in the distraction strategy.

—Pain-related distractors should be avoided. Distraction may be ineffective if the patient looks at the painful body part, watches a painful procedure, or even envisions such scenes. If he is using a distraction technique while undergoing a painful procedure, he should stare at a spot on the wall.

PROGRESSIVE MUSCLE RELAXATION

Patient objectives	*Teaching plan content*
1 Define progressive muscle relaxation.	Progressive muscle relaxation is the process of obtaining a state of deep relaxation by systematically tensing and relaxing muscle groups.

2 Identify the types of pain relieved by progressive muscle relaxation.	Progressive muscle relaxation is one of the most widely used nonpharmacologic therapies for acute as well as chronic pain.
3 Explain how progressive muscle relaxation relieves pain.	Progressive muscle relaxation alters the physiologic response to stress by affecting autonomic nervous system (ANS) activity. —Normally, when a stressful condition such as pain occurs, ANS activity causes muscle tension and increases heart rate, blood pressure, and respiratory rate. All of these responses intensify pain. —Relaxation can diminish pain by minimizing ANS activity. It may also reduce muscle tension and contractions that can cause pain. Among other desirable effects, it may enhance comfort measures and other pain-relief interventions and may reduce anxiety.
4 Describe the use of progressive muscle relaxation.	Progressive muscle relaxation requires a systematic approach for best results, and commercially prepared tapes are available to guide the patient. —General instructions are as follows: • Focus on a muscle group, such as the muscles in the hands. Tense the forearm muscles and make a fist. When the muscles are tense, note the sensation. • After 5 to 7 seconds, release the fist and relax the muscles. Concentrate on the difference between the relaxed and tensed states. • Then concentrate on another group of muscles. Continue the procedure until the major muscle groups throughout the body have been tensed and relaxed. —Deep breathing should be incorporated with relaxation of the chest and abdominal muscles. The simplest way to end the exercise is to slowly open the eyes; then to stretch, as if awakening from a deep sleep; and finally, walk around until alertness returns.
5 Describe an alternative method for use with sudden pain.	For pain that occurs suddenly, shorter relaxation exercises can produce quick results. For example, a patient undergoing a lumbar puncture might benefit from one of these 10-second exercises: —Relax the lower jaw as if starting to yawn, and rest the tongue on the floor of the mouth. Then breathe slowly and rhythmically through the mouth: inhaling, exhaling, then resting. Do not even think of words. —Or, close the eyes and imagine a small star about 1″ from the tip of the nose. Breathe deeply and slowly four times through the mouth while focusing on the star.

6 Discuss patient guidelines for using progressive muscle relaxation.	Patient guidelines include the following: —Although relaxation is noninvasive and virtually risk-free, the physician may need to be consulted before it can be used. 　• If the patient has a heart condition, he may respond so well to relaxation that the physician will need to adjust his medication schedule. 　• If the patient has a lung condition, he will have to minimize or eliminate the deep-breathing exercises used in progressive muscle relaxation. These exercises could exacerbate his preexisting condition. —Relaxation is especially useful when waiting for pain medication to work and when facing a painful procedure. However, immediate results are unlikely. —Because relaxation is a learned behavior, it must be practiced regularly—daily, if possible—for best results, in a quiet environment. (See *Progressive Muscle Relaxation*, p. 50.) —If the patient wears contact lenses, he should remove them before beginning a relaxation exercise. Because he will keep his eyes closed during the exercise, his contact lenses would not be lubricated adequately. He would risk corneal abrasion or the adherence of the lenses to his corneas.

GUIDED IMAGERY

Patient objectives	*Teaching plan content*
1 Define guided imagery.	Guided imagery is the use of imagination to create images that decrease pain intensity by focusing the attention elsewhere, relaxing the patient, and reducing his anxiety.
2 Identify the types of pain relieved by guided imagery.	Guided imagery may be used to relieve both acute and chronic pain.
3 Explain how guided imagery relieves pain.	Guided imagery makes use of the mind's ability to affect physiologic response as well as pain perception. And, like other pain-relief strategies, it promotes muscle relaxation and decreases anxiety. Imagery is effective because it can produce physiologic changes. For example, recalling a frightening movie scene long after viewing it can cause the same autonomic nervous system responses experienced at the time, such as rapid respirations and a rapid heart rate.

4 **Describe the use of guided imagery.**

Guided imagery is performed as follows:
—First, the patient should choose a suitable image, one that relaxes and pleases him. For best results, it should be an image based on his experiences, since it will be most meaningful and vivid for him. He can select a particular experience or choose aspects of several experiences and develop a composite image.
—To make the image more vivid, he should engage most or all of his senses. For instance, if he chooses a mountain scene, he should imagine feeling a cool breeze, hearing the wind rustling the leaves, tasting fresh spring water, and seeing brightly colored autumn foliage. Most important, he should imagine how relaxed and peaceful he would feel in such surroundings. Once an appropriate sensory image has been chosen, the exercise begins. The patient finds a comfortable position, takes a deep breath, and tries to relax.
—Next, he closes his eyes and concentrates intensely on the predetermined image. He describes all the sensations suggested by the image. If he is hesitant about describing sensations, he should be asked specific questions; for example, if he chose a mountain scene, he should be asked: "What do you see from the cabin? What color is the sky? Is the ground firm or soft? Can you hear animals or running water?"
—If he still has trouble responding, the image should be introduced gradually. For example, he should be asked what items he packed for his mountain vacation, how long the drive was, what the cabin looked like when he arrived, and how he felt at the time. This helps the patient relax and draws him gradually into the image.
—After a predetermined time (usually 15 to 20 minutes), the patient arouses himself from his deeply relaxed and pain-free state. The session can be ended in several ways, but usually the patient counts silently from one to three. On the last count, he takes a deep breath, opens his eyes, and says, "I feel alert and relaxed."

5 **Discuss patient guidelines for using guided imagery.**

Guidelines for using guided imagery include the following:
—A relaxation exercise should be used just before beginning guided imagery. (See the "Progressive Muscle Relaxation" teaching plan in this chapter.)
—Interruptions should be eliminated and a soothing environment created by dimming the lights, minimizing noise, and drawing the blinds (if a sunny scene has been chosen, the image can be enhanced by opening the blinds).

—Guided imagery can be used for as long as necessary. In most cases, 15 to 20 minutes is long enough.
—A tape of a previous session or a commercial recording can be used to practice guided imagery without assistance.
—Some people feel drowsy after using guided imagery.

 # Explaining treatments

HEAT THERAPY

Patient objectives	*Teaching plan content*
1 Define heat therapy.	Heat therapy is the use of heat to relieve pain.
2 Identify the types of pain relieved by heat therapy.	Heat therapy is effective for chronic pain. Pain from bruises, muscle spasms, and arthritis typically responds well to heat treatment. —Heat therapy is not appropriate in some circumstances. • Because heat dilates blood vessels and increases local blood flow, it is contraindicated after traumatic injuries when swelling and inflammation are present. • It is also contraindicated for patients with clotting defects or with certain cancers, because heat can stimulate cancer cell growth. • Heat should be used cautiously if the patient is severely depressed, because it may intensify his depression.
3 Identify the two types of heat therapy.	Types of heat therapy include superficial heat therapy and deep-heat therapy. Deep-heat therapy requires special training and equipment and is performed only by a person skilled in the technique.
4 Explain how heat therapy relieves pain.	Heat has long been recognized as a simple but effective pain-relief measure. No one knows how it works, but the following factors probably play a part: —Because heat increases blood flow to injured tissues, it may relieve pain by removing the products of inflammation that produce pain locally. —Heat may help reduce pain by stimulating nerve fibers to prevent pain signals from traveling up the spinal cord to the brain.

—By promoting muscle relaxation, heat treatments can promote sleep and diminish tension and anxiety—all of which reduce pain.

---

5 Describe the use of superficial heat therapy.

There are several techniques for applying superficial heat.
—By using covered electric heating pads or heat lamps, dry heat can be applied directly to the skin over painful areas.
—Moist heat is applied by using a hot pack, hot water bottle, or hot bath (such as a sitz bath, for perineal pain).
—A heating pad can be used to apply continuous moist heat by laying a moist towel over the painful area, covering it with a layer of insulation (for example, plastic wrap), and laying the heating pad on top.
—With the exception of hot compresses and hot soaks, heat therapy should be continued for 20 to 30 minutes, or as ordered. Hot compresses should be applied for 15 to 20 minutes; hot soaks, for 20 minutes. CAUTION: Electric heating pads should be checked for frayed cords or other electrical hazards.

---

6 Discuss patient guidelines for using heat therapy.

Guidelines for superficial heat therapy include the following:
—In applying heat directly to the skin, the following temperatures are recommended to prevent burns:
• Hot water bottle or electric heating pad: For infants (to age 2) and geriatric patients: 105° to 115° F. (40.5° to 46.1° C.). For other patients: 115° to 125° F. (46.1° to 51.6° C.)
• Aquamatic K pad: 105° F. (40.5° C.)
• Hot compress: 131° F. (55° C.)
• Hot soak: 105° to 110° F. (40.5° to 43.3° C.).
—Lights or lamps should be set at these distances to prevent burns:
• Infrared or ultraviolet light: 18″ to 24″ (45 to 60 cm) from the affected area (depending on equipment wattage)
• Gooseneck lamp: At 25 watts: 14″ (35 cm) from the affected area. At 40 watts: 18″ (45 cm) from the affected area. At 60 watts: 24″ to 30″ (60 to 76 cm) from the affected area.
—Heat therapy is not appropriate in some circumstances:
• Because heat dilates blood vessels after traumatic injuries when swelling and inflammation are present.
• It is also contraindicated for patients with clotting defects or with certain cancers, because heat can

stimulate cancer cell growth.
• Heat should be used cautiously if the patient is severely depressed, because it may intensify his depression.

COLD THERAPY

Patient objectives	Teaching plan content
1 Define cold therapy.	Cold therapy is the use of cold (in the form of compresses, for example) to alleviate pain.
2 Identify the types of pain relieved by cold therapy.	In contrast to heat therapy, which is effective for chronic pain, cold therapy is more effective for acute pain; for example, pain following soft-tissue injury from trauma, burns, cuts, or sprains. Other painful conditions that respond well to cold therapy include headaches and muscle spasms. Applied before a painful procedure such as an injection, cold can even deaden subsequent pain.
3 Identify four methods of cold therapy.	Methods of cold therapy include the following: —cold towel —ice massage —cold bath —ice pack.
4 Explain how cold therapy relieves pain.	Cold therapy works for several possible reasons: —Cold slows the conduction velocity of nerve impulses, reducing the number of pain impulses that reach the brain. —Perceptual dominance of the cold sensation deadens the pain sensation. —Cold may reduce inflammation (and minimize the local release of pain-producing substances) by constricting peripheral blood vessels.
5 Describe the use of cold therapy.	Cold therapy is used as follows: —A cold towel allows treatment of a large area, such as the lower back. A towel is soaked in ice water (about 40° F. [4.4° C.]), wrung out, and placed directly on the painful area. The towel is covered with plastic wrap as insulation. When the towel becomes warm, it is resoaked. —An ice massage, also used to treat large areas, is given by wrapping a large chunk of ice in a washcloth and rubbing it on the painful area. The ice is removed after about 20 minutes. The skin may no longer feel numb from the cold but may feel warm and tingling.

The ice should not be left on too long: it can cause frostbite.

—A cold bath is used to treat painful knees, ankles, elbows, and hands. The injured part is soaked in 40° F. ice water for about 5 minutes, or held under cold running water.

—An ice pack is used to relieve pain and reduce swelling and bleeding.

• An ice pack is made by filling an ice bag, plastic bag, or disposable glove with ice.

• Ice bags have disadvantages: in addition to being uncomfortably heavy, they may leak or slip out of place. Plastic bags and gloves are lighter and easier to prevent from leaking; they may also conform better to the area being treated. (Other alternatives to ice bags are frozen gel packs or ice placed between towels.)

• The ice pack is wrapped in a towel, pillowcase, or washcloth to protect the skin from a burn. The intensity of cold is adjusted by increasing or decreasing the number of cloth layers surrounding the ice pack, as needed.

• The ice pack and the skin should be checked frequently during treatment. As a rule, the ice should be removed within 20 minutes.

---

6 Discuss patient guidelines for using cold therapy.

Guidelines for cold therapy include the following:

—Cold itself can cause an aching or burning pain and ice can cause burns. Oil may be applied to the skin to reduce the risk of ice burns.

—During cold therapy, the patient or a family member should watch closely for signs of discomfort.

—Time and temperature guidelines for using cold therapy are as follows:

• Ice bag: 50° to 80° F. (10° to 26.6° C.) for 30 minutes

• Cold compress or pack: 59° F. (15° C.) for 15 to 20 minutes

• Chemical cold pack: 50° to 80° F. (10° to 26.6° C.) for 30 minutes

• Cold soak: 59° F. (15° C.) for 20 minutes

• Aquamatic K pad: 59° F. (15° C.) for 20 to 30 minutes.

—Cold-induced numbness can be deceptive. Injured areas should be moved carefully and any strenuous activity avoided until healing is complete.

—Heat therapy alternated with cold therapy can be used as a pain-control measure.

—Cold therapy is contraindicated if the patient has the following problems:

- A history of allergic reaction (hives or joint pain) to cold therapy
- Diabetes
- Rheumatic disease (including arthritis)
- Raynaud's disease (cold may cause arterial spasm in the fingers and toes, reducing blood supply and possibly causing gangrene).

TRANSCUTANEOUS ELECTRICAL NERVE STIMULATION (T.E.N.S.)

Patient objectives	Teaching plan content
1 Define TENS.	TENS is the use of a battery-powered generator to send a mild electrical current through electrodes placed on the skin at or near the pain site. The current produces a pleasant tingling or massaging sensation or stimulates muscle twitching.
2 Identify the types of pain relieved by TENS.	TENS is effective for relief of both acute and chronic pain, but it is most commonly used for chronic pain. TENS is particularly effective for treating acute, well-localized pain and pain following cholecystectomy (gallbladder surgery) and thoracotomy (chest surgery).
3 Explain how TENS relieves pain.	The exact mechanism of pain relief is unknown. According to one theory, TENS stimulates release of endorphins (pain-relieving substances) within the body. Another possible explanation is that electrical stimulation prevents the nervous system from transmitting pain impulses.
4 Describe the use of TENS.	Before therapy begins, the patient should understand how the TENS unit works. —Electrode placement varies with each patient. Initially, the physician, nurse, or TENS specialist may place the electrodes over an area where the nerve is relatively close to the skin's surface and thus more easily stimulated. • If the patient has pain in his arm, shoulder, or chest, the physician may place the electrodes over the ulnar nerve at the elbow. • For radiating pain, he may position the electrodes over the nerve roots along the spine. • To bombard a painful area such as the knee or lower back, he may place them in a crisscross pattern over that area. • For postoperative pain, he will probably place an electrode on either side of the incision. —Placement of electrodes is crucial because a differ-

ence of $\frac{1}{16}''$ (0.16 cm) can mean the difference between pain relief and increased pain. If the initial placement is not effective, the physician may choose sites closer to the painful area (for instance, along an involved nerve or near a painful scar) or along its dermatome. If this placement does not relieve the pain, he may try a location along the corresponding acupuncture meridian or muscle-trigger point. (Once the sites are determined, the patient is taught how to apply the TENS electrodes.) Controls on the TENS unit are adjusted to regulate stimulation. All units have dials or keys that control amplitude (intensity of stimulation), rate (the number of pulses per second), and pulse width (duration of each stimulation pulse). Some units have two channels, permitting the use of two electrode pairs simultaneously, either at the same pain site or at different sites. Each channel can be regulated separately.

• The amplitude dial may be labeled A or AMP (for amplitude), O (for output, on, or off), intensity, or energy. (Some models have increase/decrease buttons and digital display screens.) Although the dial may be calibrated from 1 to 5, 1 to 10, or 10 to 100, the patient should rely on feeling rather than on numbers. The sensation should be mildly or moderately pleasant. A stimulation level that is too high may increase pain and may cause muscle spasms or itching.

• The rate dial regulates the number of electrical impulses per second, ranging from 2 to 200 pulses. Although a high rate may relieve pain more quickly, the rate setting should be increased cautiously. If an unpleasant sensation is felt when turning up the rate, the amplitude or pulse-width dial should be turned down.

• The pulse-width dial determines the duration of each impulse, usually between 50 and 250 microseconds. (On some TENS units, pulse width is incorporated in the rate or amplitude dial.) In most cases, it is best to start with a lower pulse width when stimulating such small muscles as those in the back of the neck. For chronic pain, a mid-range pulse-width setting may deliver stimulation deep enough to relieve the pain without causing muscle spasms or itching.

5 Discuss patient guidelines for applying TENS electrodes.

Patient guidelines for applying TENS electrodes are as follows:

—Apply conductive jelly to each electrode. Use just enough to cover the electrode surface. (Self-adhering electrodes do not require conductive jelly.)

—Position the electrodes so that the distance between them is at least the width of an electrode—otherwise, the skin may be burned. Each electrode should lie flat against the skin.
—Never place electrodes over laryngeal or pharyngeal muscles or over carotid sinus nerves. Also never place electrodes transcerebrally or on the eyes.
—Secure the electrodes. Use strips of tape just long enough to anchor the electrodes securely.

---

6 Discuss patient guidelines for using TENS.

Guidelines for using a TENS unit include the following:
—Because pain relief may not be immediate, the patient should plan to use the TENS unit for at least a week before deciding if it helps. It may take a few days to find the most effective electrode placements and control settings.
—Lock or tape the controls after setting them.
—Remove the electrodes at least once a day (or as recommended), and clean them and the skin. If the TENS unit is worn continuously, the electrodes can then be reapplied.
—Remove the electrodes when swimming or taking a bath or shower. (Removing TENS at bedtime is also recommended; however, if TENS is needed in order to sleep, tape the electrodes and controls securely.)
—Experiment with different control settings to learn which combination best relieves the pain. Record the combinations that work best. NOTE: Do not use excessive voltage. Higher voltage will not necessarily provide better pain relief.
—Clean the unit regularly, using a damp cloth or sponge. To remove stains or adhesive on the stimulator case, use alcohol or a mild cleaning solution. Do not immerse the unit in liquid.
—If skin irritation develops at the electrode sites, substitute hand cream or hydrocortisone cream for the conductive jelly. Other possible solutions include using another brand of conductive jelly, changing the type of adhesive tape or electrode, and varying the electrode positions.

BIOFEEDBACK

Patient objectives

Teaching plan content

---

1 Define biofeedback.

Biofeedback is a technique that uses special electrical equipment to provide information about specific physiologic changes, such as changes in blood pressure or body temperature, that reflect relaxation.

2 **Identify the types of pain relieved by biofeedback.**

Biofeedback can be especially helpful for learning to control the pain of muscle tension and stress, including lower back pain and headaches. For patients with headaches, biofeedback works best for those who experience such prodromes as the bright, flashing lights that sometimes precede migraine headaches. This physiologic warning gives the patient a chance to ward off his headache before it becomes a reality.

3 **Explain how biofeedback relieves pain.**

Biofeedback as a pain therapy teaches the patient to recognize body stress and tension that can precipitate pain. The patient is then taught relaxation techniques to lower body stress and tension and thus to diminish nerve stimulation and decrease pain.

4 **Discuss advantages and disadvantages of biofeedback.**

The advantages and disadvantages of biofeedback are as follows:
—The major advantage is that it is an effective technique that enables the patient to participate in his treatment and gives him a sense of control and accomplishment. In contrast, a more traditional treatment, such as drug therapy, encourages the patient to play a passive role and diminishes his sense of control over his condition.
• If the patient is taking analgesics, biofeedback can have an additional benefit: it may allow the physician to reduce the dosage as the patient learns to effectively manage his pain.
• Biofeedback is also noninvasive and virtually risk-free.
—The major disadvantage is that it is a time-consuming technique that requires a specially trained therapist and special equipment.
• Training is time-consuming because treatment must be individualized and the patient must practice regularly to achieve results. For example, he may need to practice with the special equipment for 20 minutes, one to three times weekly. In addition, he must practice without the equipment several times every day.
• Biofeedback also requires the patient's special interest and enthusiasm. He must be highly motivated to learn the techniques and willing to wait several months or more for results.

5 **Describe the procedure used in biofeedback training.**

A typical biofeedback training session proceeds as follows:
—The therapist takes the patient into a quiet room and seats him in a comfortable chair. He then places elec-

trodes on the patient's forehead. The electrodes will measure forehead muscle tension, since it reflects tension in the rest of the body. The higher the tone emitted from the biofeedback machine, the higher the level of registered tension. To measure skin temperature, the therapist also places electrodes on the patient's hand.
—The therapist then leads the patient through a progressive muscle relaxation session. His goal is to have the patient lower the machine's warning tone by relaxing.
—At the end of the session, the therapist evaluates how the therapy proceeded and teaches the patient how to use the technique at home.

6 Discuss patient guidelines for using biofeedback.

For biofeedback to be effective, it must be practiced every day. A time and location should be chosen that will provide privacy and a quiet environment.

ACUPUNCTURE

Patient objectives	*Teaching plan content*
1 Define acupuncture.	Acupuncture is a Chinese method of producing pain relief by inserting wire-thin needles into the skin at specific sites on the body.
2 Identify the types of pain relieved by acupuncture.	Acupuncture can be used to relieve both acute and chronic pain. It may be effective for headache; musculoskeletal pain; premenstrual or menstrual pain; pain caused by stress, tension, and nervousness; some neuralgias; surgical pain; lower back pain; and dental and facial pain.
3 Explain how acupuncture relieves pain.	The Chinese explain the effectiveness of acupuncture in terms of yin and yang, the two universal life forces represented in the body by spirit and blood, respectively. According to this theory, each force moves along a series of channels called meridians. Pain and illness develop when yin and yang are out of harmony. Inserting acupuncture needles at specific points allows yin and yang to reestablish harmony. Searching for a more scientific explanation, Western researchers have developed several alternative theories. —One explanation is that acupuncture stimulates nerve fibers that carry nonpain impulses and these impulses inhibit pain conduction to the spinal cord from smaller fibers. —Another possible explanation is that acupuncture triggers the release of substances in the body that nat-

urally produce analgesia. This theory is supported by evidence that administration of a morphine antagonist reverses acupuncture's analgesic effects.

4 Describe the procedure used in acupuncture.	Acupuncture is performed in the following manner: —The practitioner inserts long, extremely thin needles into specific acupuncture points (or hoku) located along the meridians. Each meridian runs along a major body part and ends at the fingertips or toes. —Practitioners have identified (by name and number) about 1,000 acupuncture points, each about ⅛″ (0.32 cm) in diameter. Most points belong to one of 14 groups associated with internal organs. —To select appropriate acupuncture points, the practitioner first takes a detailed patient history. He may then use traditional Chinese diagnostic techniques to obtain more information. —To treat the patient's disease or injury, the practitioner may need to stimulate several acupuncture points. For a typical treatment, he will insert 10 to 15 needles at varying angles and depths. (Unlike hypodermic needles, acupuncture needles have rounded tips that push tissue aside without cutting it.) —After insertion, the practitioner may twist or vibrate the needles (either manually or electrically) to maximize stimulation. Or he may heat the needles with burning herbs (moxa). The length of time for each treatment varies according to the intended result.
5 Discuss patient guidelines for acupuncture.	Patient guidelines include the following: —During treatment, the patient may feel sensations ranging from pinpricks, warmth, light-headedness, or heaviness to stinging or a dull, aching throb. The practitioner will then increase stimulation at certain acupuncture points. As treatment progresses, the patient will be able to tolerate more stimulation, although he may feel some discomfort. —The patient may get relief from his pain immediately after the first treatment. Or he may require as many as 20 treatments before feeling significant relief. —Some patients never respond to treatment.

THERAPEUTIC TOUCH

Patient objectives	*Teaching plan content*
1 Define therapeutic touch.	Therapeutic touch is a modern adaptation of the ancient practice of "laying on of hands," used primarily to alleviate chronic pain.

2 **Explain how therapeutic touch relieves pain.**	Although a scientific basis for the effectiveness of therapeutic touch in some cases has not been established, possible reasons include the following: —The laying on of hands may stimulate nerve receptors in the skin at traditional acupuncture points. —It may trigger a placebo response. —It may stimulate the patient's emotional sense of well-being through physical contact with the practitioner.
3 **Describe the procedure used in therapeutic touch.**	The procedure consists of two steps. First, the practitioner meditates to quiet his mental, emotional, and physical energies and to focus on transmitting energy to the patient. Then he uses both hands to locate the painful area and to transmit his healing energy.

NERVE BLOCK

Patient objectives	*Teaching plan content*
1 **Define nerve block.**	A nonsurgical nerve block is a procedure used to stop the transmission of the pain impulse along the nerve, usually through injection of anesthetic or neurolytic agents.
2 **Identify the types of pain relieved by nerve blocks.**	Although especially effective for treating acute pain, nerve blocks also have therapeutic value for treating chronic pain. They may provide immediate pain relief, but a single therapeutic block seldom relieves pain for more than 8 hours. However, for some patients (for example, those with musculoskeletal pain), repeated nerve blocks can produce progressively longer periods of pain relief. In some cases, pain relief lasts for months or even years.
3 **Explain how nerve blocks relieve pain.**	Nonsurgical nerve blocks stop transmission of pain sensations along sensory pathways in the nervous system.
4 **Describe the procedure used in nerve blocks.**	Most nerve blocks are achieved by injecting a local anesthetic into or around a peripheral nerve, into the spine, or into a major nerve plexus. Doing so inhibits pain-impulse conduction and provides local pain relief for 4 to 8 hours in most cases. Neurolytic nerve blocks can provide long-term relief by permanently damaging nerve pathways.

SURGERY

Patient objectives	Teaching plan content
1 **Define surgery as a pain therapy.**	Neurosurgery surgically blocks pain-impulse conduction along sensory nervous system tracts.
2 **Identify the types of pain relieved by surgery.**	Because of its radical nature (sensory impulses other than pain may be blocked), surgery for pain relief is usually reserved for chronic pain relief in the terminally ill.
3 **Explain how surgery relieves pain.**	Surgery interrupts pain pathways by preventing pain impulses from traveling to their destination, thus inhibiting pain perception.
4 **Describe the surgical procedures used to block pain.**	Several surgical procedures are used to block pain transmission. The type of procedure chosen will depend on the location of the pain. The most common procedures are chordotomy, hypophysectomy, and sympathectomy. —Chordotomy is used for one-sided, below-the-waist pain caused by cancer. To perform this procedure, the physician will cut a pain sensory tract called the spinothalamic tract, contralateral to the pain site, using a surgical instrument or electric needle. —Hypophysectomy is done to relieve bone pain from metastatic cancer. To perform it, the physician will surgically remove or chemically destroy the pituitary gland. The pituitary gland produces hormones that influence cancer growth in the body. —Sympathectomy is used to treat pain associated with circulatory disorders, renal and urethral disorders, and biliary and pancreatic disease. To perform it, the physician will cut the sympathetic nerve pathway.
5 **Discuss what to expect before a neurosurgical procedure.**	Before the procedure, the patient and his family should fully understand the risks involved in the particular surgical procedure chosen for him. —The physician will explain the following: • The risks of chordotomy include temporary sleep apnea (after high cervical bilateral percutaneous chordotomy); bowel and bladder dysfunctions (usually transient); sexual impotence; paralysis; and weakness in the arm and leg ipsilateral to the chordotomy (usually transient). NOTE: Bilateral procedures are more likely to cause complications than unilateral procedures. • The risks of hypophysectomy include altered sex

drive; impotence or infertility; hair loss; emotional lability.

• The risks of sympathectomy include ptosis; facial paralysis; masking of subsequent abdominal conditions; failure to relieve pain.

—The patient should feel that all of his questions have been answered before surgery. If they cannot be answered by the nurse, the physician will speak with him again.

—The patient should know about any unusual conditions that will result from the procedure. For example, if he is scheduled for a sympathectomy, he should know that the affected extremity will not perspire.

—The patient should know what type of skin preparation will be ordered for him to prevent contamination of the surgical incision.

---

6 Describe what to expect after surgery.

The patient can expect the following:

—He will be checked frequently during the first 24 to 48 hours, as standard procedure.

—His dressing will be changed every 24 hours or more frequently if it becomes soiled or if the site is exposed to air.

—He will receive antibiotics for up to 7 days after the procedure, as a preventive measure.

—Pain from the incision will be minimized using pain medication, if necessary. He should inform the nurse if he has pain or any other distressing symptoms.

—He will perform active range-of-motion exercises using his unaffected extremities. He will be helped to perform passive range-of-motion exercises using his affected extremities.

—If the patient has had a hypophysectomy, he should keep the head of his bed angled at about 30° (as ordered) to promote venous drainage from his head and to reduce cerebral edema. To prevent cerebrospinal fluid drainage through nasal passages, he should not blow his nose.

—If the patient has had a sympathectomy, he may experience temporary signs and symptoms of neuritis resulting from nerve manipulation during surgery. This condition usually resolves itself spontaneously.

—Discharge teaching will be provided, as appropriate for the surgical procedure performed, to meet his particular needs.

Patient-Teaching Aid

TIPS ON USING YOUR T.E.N.S.

Dear Patient:

Your physician has ordered for you a pain management device called a transcutaneous electrical nerve stimulator (TENS). Before you begin to use your TENS unit, consider these tips:

—Lock or tape the controls after setting them.

—Remove the electrodes at least once a day (or as recommended) and clean the electrodes and your skin. If you are wearing your TENS continuously, you can then reapply the electrodes.

—Remove the electrodes when you swim or take a bath or shower. (Removing TENS at bedtime is also recommended; however, if you need TENS to sleep, tape the electrodes and controls securely.)

—Experiment with different control settings to learn which combination best relieves your pain. Record the combinations that work best. NOTE: Higher voltage will not necessarily provide better pain relief.

—Clean the unit regularly, using a damp cloth or sponge. To remove stains or adhesive on the stimulator case, use alcohol or a mild cleaning solution. Do not immerse the unit in liquid.

—If skin irritation develops at the electrode sites, substitute hand cream or hydrocortisone cream for the conductive jelly. Other possible solutions include using another brand of conductive jelly, changing the type of adhesive tape or electrode, and varying the electrode positions.

Patient-Teaching Aid

HOW TO USE AND APPLY T.E.N.S.

Dear Patient:

Your physician has ordered for you a pain management device called a transcutaneous electrical nerve stimulator (TENS). The TENS unit consists of a battery-powered generator that sends a mild electrical current through electrodes placed on the skin at or near the pain site. TENS also increases blood flow near the electrodes, indirectly relaxing muscles and speeding the healing process. You can use your TENS at home or on the job. Plan to use your TENS unit for at least a week before deciding if it helps.

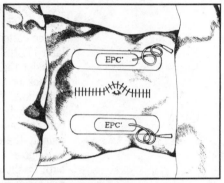

Postoperative placement

Placing the electrodes

Initially, your physician, nurse, or TENS specialist may place the electrodes over an area where the nerve is relatively close to the skin's surface and more easily stimulated. For postoperative pain, the electrodes may be placed on either side of the incision.

If the electrodes do not relieve your pain, inquire as to a more suitable placement site for you.

—Apply conductive jelly to each electrode. Use just enough to cover the electrode surface. (Self-adhering electrodes do not require conductive jelly.)

—Position the electrodes so the distance between them is at least the width of an electrode—otherwise, you will be burned. Make sure each electrode is flat against the skin. CAUTION: Never place electrodes over laryngeal or pharyngeal muscles or over carotid sinus nerves. Also never place electrodes transcerebrally or on the eyes.

—Secure the electrodes. Use strips of tape just long enough to anchor the electrodes securely.

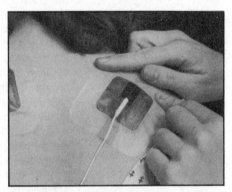

Securing electrodes

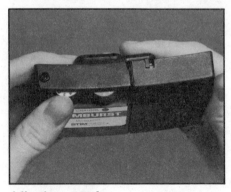

Adjusting controls

HOW TO USE AND APPLY T.E.N.S.—*continued*

Adjusting the controls

All TENS units have dials or keys that control *amplitude* (intensity of stimulation), *rate* (the number of electrical impulses per second), and *pulse width* (duration of each stimulation pulse). Two-channel units will permit you to use two electrode pairs simultaneously—either at the same pain site or at different sites. The amplitude dial may be labeled *A* or *AMP* (for amplitude), *O* (for output, on, or off), *intensity,* or *energy.* (Some models have increase/decrease buttons and digital display screens.) Although the dial may be calibrated from 1 to 5, 1 to 10, or 1 to 100, you should rely on feeling rather than on numbers. When using your TENS, you should feel a mild or moderately pleasant sensation. A stimulation level that is too high may increase your pain and cause muscle spasms or itching.

The *rate* dial regulates the number of electrical impulses per second, ranging from 2 to 200. Although a high rate may relieve pain more quickly, increase the rate setting cautiously. If you feel an unpleasant sensation when turning up the rate, turn down the amplitude or pulse-width dial.

The *pulse-width* dial determines the duration of each impulse, usually between 50 and 250 microseconds. (On some TENS units, pulse width is incorporated in the rate or amplitude dial.) In most cases, you should start with a lower pulse width when stimulating such small muscles as those in the back of the neck.

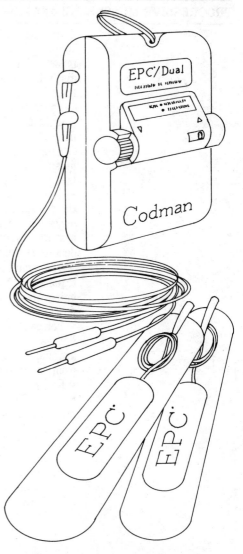

EPC/Dual Electronic Pain Control Unit
This TENS unit, which includes sterile self-adhering electrodes, is designed to control postoperative pain.

Patient-Teaching Aid

PROGRESSIVE MUSCLE RELAXATION

Dear Patient:

Your physician has suggested that you use progressive muscle relaxation, performed by systematically tensing and relaxing muscle groups. Use the following guidelines:

—Focus on a muscle group, such as the muscles in your hands. Tense your forearm muscles and make a fist. When your muscles are tense, note the sensation.

—After 5 to 7 seconds, release your fist and relax your muscles. Concentrate on the difference between the relaxed and tensed states.

—Concentrate on another group of muscles. Continue the procedure until you have tensed and relaxed the major muscle groups throughout your body. NOTE: For best results, choose a systematic approach. Incorporate deep breathing with chest relaxation.

—The simplest way to end the exercise includes these three steps: Slowly open your eyes; stretch, as if awakening from a deep sleep; and finally, walk around until you feel alert.

—For pain that occurs suddenly, shorter relaxation exercises can produce quick results. For example, if you are undergoing a medical procedure, you might benefit from one of the following 10-second exercises:

• Relax your lower jaw as if you were starting to yawn, and rest your tongue on the bottom of your mouth. Breathe slowly and rhythmically through your mouth: inhaling, exhaling, then resting. Do not even think of words.

• Close your eyes and imagine a small star about 1" from the tip of your nose. Then breathe deeply and slowly four times through your mouth while focusing on the star.

Psychiatric Disorders

Patient-learner data base*

Areas of potential knowledge deficit
Psychiatric risk factors
—Stress
—Alcohol and/or narcotic use
—Poor self-esteem
—Sleep deprivation
—Emotional or physical trauma
—Chemical, drug, or toxin exposure
—Family/personal history of psychiatric disorder
Definition of the psychiatric disorder
Causes of the psychiatric disorder
Symptoms associated with the psychiatric disorder
Treatment of the psychiatric disorder
—Diet
—Medications
—Counseling/stress management
—Psychotherapy
—Electroconvulsive therapy
—Other treatments used
Complications of the psychiatric disorder

Explaining diagnostic tests

DEXAMETHASONE SUPPRESSION TEST (D.S.T.)

Patient objectives	*Teaching plan content*
1 Define dexamethasone suppression test (DST).	The DST is a series of blood tests that provides information about neuroendocrine function.

* A general assessment should be done for all patients. For general assessment guidelines, see Chapter 1, Principles of Patient Teaching.

2 State the purpose of the DST.	The purpose of the DST is to assist in diagnosing a depression that will probably respond to somatic intervention.
3 Describe the procedure used in the DST.	The DST involves the following steps: —A baseline blood sample will be drawn. —Dexamethasone (Decadron) 1 mg P.O. at bedtime (11:30 p.m.) will be administered. —The next day, three to five samples of blood will be drawn, depending on how many points the physician wants to assess and track (three points, 8 a.m.-4 p.m.-11 p.m.; five points, midnight-8 a.m.-noon-4 p.m.-midnight). —The samples will then be analyzed and the report returned in a few days.
4 Explain patient guidelines for the DST.	The patient need not restrict foods or fluids before the test. He should know who will perform the test, how many venipunctures he will have, where he needs to go for the test (unit or laboratory), and how to get there, if necessary.

THYROTROPIN-RELEASING HORMONE (T.R.H.) INFUSION TEST

Patient objectives	*Teaching plan content*
1 Define thyrotropin-releasing hormone (TRH) infusion test.	The TRH infusion test is a series of blood tests that provides information about the functioning of the hypothalamic-pituitary-thyroid axis.
2 State the purpose of the TRH infusion test.	The purpose of the TRH infusion test is to assist in differentiating endogenous depression from disorders of the hypothalamic-pituitary-thyroid axis.
3 Describe the procedure used in TRH infusion testing.	The procedure for TRH infusion testing is as follows: —The patient should not eat, drink, or take medications after midnight. He should have a late snack, if possible, since the procedure takes approximately 2½ hours. —The patient should know who will be doing the procedure and where it will be performed, if not on the unit or if he is an outpatient. —An I.V. line will be started in his arm with normal saline at a very slow drip rate. —A stopcock will be placed between the I.V. catheter and tubing line so that blood can be obtained directly from the I.V. line. Once the I.V. has been started, he will not have to undergo any more venipunctures.

—He must rest for about 30 minutes before the hormone injection; therefore, he will lie on a bed, litter, or recliner, in a quiet environment.
—A baseline blood sample will be drawn (probably by the laboratory technician or nurse) before the hormone injection.
—The physician will then administer 500 mcg of synthetic TRH I.V. over 30 seconds.
—Blood samples will then be drawn at 15-, 30-, 60-, and 90-minute intervals.
—The I.V. line will be monitored closely throughout the procedure.
—After the last sample has been drawn, the I.V. line will be discontinued, and the patient will return to his unit.
—The samples will be sent to the laboratory for analysis, and the results will be available in approximately 7 days.

4 **Discuss patient guidelines for TRH infusion testing.**	Patient guidelines include the following: —Fast after midnight the morning before the test. —Remain as calm, quiet, and relaxed as possible during the test. —Hold the arm as still as possible and do not bend it at the elbow during the test. —Urinate before the test. —Inform the nurse of any adverse effects of TRH, such as transient nausea, a feeling of urinary urgency for about 20 seconds after the drug is given, or a bitter taste. —Inform the nurse of any discomfort at the I.V. site.

URINE M.H.P.G. TEST

Patient objectives	*Teaching plan content*
1 **Define urine MHPG test.**	A urine MHPG test measures the level of 3-methoxy-4-hydroxyphenylglycol in a 24-hour urine specimen. MHPG has been found to be relatively low in both major subtypes of affective illness (depression).
2 **State the purpose of a urine MHPG test.**	The purpose of a urine MHPG test is to predict response to drug treatment.
3 **Describe the procedure used in a urine MHPG test.**	A urine MHPG test involves the following: —The patient will be on a specific diet for 3 to 5 days before urine collection begins. —The patient should stop taking all antidepressants, monoamine oxidase inhibitors, and antihistamines 1

week before beginning the urine collection.
—He should obtain a collection container from the laboratory.
—He should begin the 24-hour collection process in the morning after his first void and keep the collection at room temperature.
—When he has completed the collection process, the nurse will send the collection container to the laboratory.

4 Discuss patient guidelines for a urine MHPG test.	Patient guidelines include the following: —All urine voided during the 24-hour test period must be collected. —If one voided specimen is discarded, the staff must report it to the laboratory so it can be taken into consideration. —The patient must rest and relax before and during the test because stress could alter the results.

PSYCHOLOGICAL TESTING

Patient objectives	Teaching plan content
1 Define psychological testing.	Psychological testing is a broad term used to describe the series of tests performed to assess personality and psychological functioning. The two main categories of psychological testing are personality testing and neuropsychological testing.
2 Describe three of the most commonly used personality tests.	Following are descriptions of three of the most commonly used personality tests: —The MMPI is a self-reporting scale consisting of 566 statements. The patient marks each one true or false, meaning that he does or does not view the statement as descriptive of his behavior. —The TAT is used to obtain an idea of the actual thought contents, attitudes, and feelings of the patient. The TAT asks the respondent to look at a picture of people and then tell a story about the picture. —The Rorschach test may be chosen to obtain an understanding of personality structure. The patient looks at a set of random inkblots and then reports what he sees in them to the evaluator.
3 State the purpose of neuropsychological testing.	Neuropsychological testing assists in distinguishing between an organic and a functional disorder.

4 Describe the Halstead-Reitan neuropsychological test battery.

A major component of the Halstead-Reitan neuropsychological test battery is the category test, a series of 208 visual stimuli shown to the patient by a slide projector. The category test assesses complex concept formation and the ability to abstract. These capacities are frequently compromised in the early stages of organic brain syndrome.

—Additional components of the Halstead-Reitan test include the following:
  • the tactile performance test, in which objects are placed in a form board on the basis of touch alone
  • the rhythm test, which calls for differentiation among a variety of rhythms
  • the speech-sounds perception test
  • the finger oscillation (tapping) test.

—Auxiliary tests may also be ordered to assess memory function.

BRAIN SCAN

Patient objectives	*Teaching plan content*
1 Define a brain scan.	A brain scan is a test performed by using a gamma scintillation camera to provide a series of images of the brain after an I.V. injection of a radionuclide (radioactive contrast agent). The scintillation camera detects rays emitted by the radionuclide and converts them into images that are then displayed on an oscilloscope screen (a type of television screen).
2 State the relevant purpose of a brain scan.	A brain scan is performed to assist in differentiating between a functional and an organic disorder.
3 Describe the procedure used in a brain scan.	The following procedure is observed for a brain scan: —The patient should know who will perform the test and where and that each series requires 1 to 1½ hours. —An I.V. line will be inserted after he assumes a comfortable supine position on the X-ray table. —A bolus of technetium 99m pertechnetate (^{99m}Tc) will be injected into the I.V. line. —Rapid-sequence images will be taken immediately after the ^{99m}Tc injection to track the passage of the radionuclide through the carotid arteries and cerebral hemispheres. —When the scanning has been completed, the I.V. line will be discontinued and manual pressure applied until any bleeding has subsided.

—The patient will then be returned to his unit, or, if the scan was done on an outpatient basis, he will be able to leave.

4 Discuss patient guidelines for a brain scan.

Patient guidelines include the following:
—The patient does not have to restrict foods or fluids.
—He may experience slight burning at the injection site and should tell the nurse if there is any significant pain.
—He should keep his arm still and try to relax; therefore, he should know that the scanner will move back and forth and make some noise.
—He should remove all metal objects or jewelry.
—He should know that the procedure is painless, and that the radiation poses no danger to him or his visitors and will clear his body within 6 hours.

INTRACRANIAL COMPUTERIZED TOMOGRAPHY (C.T.) SCAN

Patient objectives	*Teaching plan content*
1 Define an intracranial computerized tomography (CT) scan.	An intracranial CT scan is a series of X-ray images of various layers of the head (tomograms), which are processed by a computer and displayed on an oscilloscope screen as cross-sectional views of the skull (cranium) and the tissues within it.
2 State the relevant purpose of an intracranial CT scan.	The purpose of an intracranial CT scan is to assist in differentiating functional from organic disorders.
3 Describe the procedure used in an intracranial CT scan.	An intracranial CT scan involves the following steps: —The patient will be placed supine on an X-ray table. —His head will be immobilized by straps; then it will be moved into the scanner, which will rotate around it and take radiographs at 1-degree intervals in a 180-degree arc. —On completion of this series, contrast enhancement (the injection of a contrast medium to further outline the area being scanned) will be done, if ordered. —Approximately 50 to 100 ml of contrast medium will be injected I.V. or by I.V. piggyback drip method over 1 to 2 minutes. —The patient will be observed closely for any hypersensitivity. —Another series of scans will be completed. —Information from the scans will be stored on magnetic tapes, fed into a computer, and converted into images on an oscilloscope screen (a type of television screen).

4 **Discuss patient guidelines for an intracranial CT scan.**	Patient guidelines include the following: —If contrast medium has *not* been ordered, the patient will *not* have to restrict foods or fluids. —If contrast medium *has* been ordered, he *will* have to restrict foods and fluids for 4 hours. —The test will cause no discomfort and will take 15 to 30 minutes. The patient should know who will perform the test and where. —He will need to wear a hospital gown and remove all metal objects and jewelry. —He should inform the nurse of any urticaria (hives), rash, or difficulty breathing after the injection of the contrast medium. —He should remain calm, relaxed, and still during the procedure.

ELECTROENCEPHALOGRAPHY

Patient objectives	*Teaching plan content*
1 **Define electroencephalography.**	Electroencephalography is a test in which electrodes attached to areas of the scalp record a portion of the brain's electrical activity. These electrical impulses are transmitted to an electroencephalograph, which magnifies them and records them as lines on moving strips of paper (an electroencephalogram, or EEG).
2 **State the relevant purpose of electroencephalography.**	The purpose of obtaining an EEG is to evaluate the brain's electrical activity in psychiatic disorders.
3 **Describe the procedure used in electroencephalography.**	Obtaining an EEG involves the following steps: —The patient will be positioned comfortably on a bed or reclining chair. —Electrodes will be attached to his scalp. —Before the recording procedure begins, he will be instructed to close his eyes, relax, and remain still. —During the recording, the patient will be carefully observed through a window in an adjoining room, and blinking, swallowing, talking, or other movements that may cause artifacts (unusual marks) on the tracing will be noted. —The recording may be stopped periodically to allow the patient to reposition himself and get comfortable. This is important, since restlessness and fatigue can alter brain wave patterns. —After an initial baseline recording, the patient may be tested in various situations to elicit patterns not obvious in the resting state.

—Photic stimulation, a technique that tests central cerebral activity in response to bright light, may be used to evaluate a patient with suspected hysterical blindness. A strobe light will be placed in front of the patient and flashed 1 to 20 times/second. Recordings will be made with his eyes opened and closed.

—The electrical activity of the brain will also be recorded after a sensory stimulus, such as experiencing a minor electrical shock, observing a black-and-white checkerboard pattern, or listening to sounds through earphones. Since these evoked electrical potentials have low amplitudes, they will be amplified and then separated by a computer from the ongoing brain activity on the recording.

4 Discuss patient guidelines for electroencephalography.	Patient guidelines include the following: —The patient will not have to restrict foods or fluids. —He should know who will perform the test and where it will be performed. —He should be reassured that the procedure is safe and painless, and that the electrodes will not shock him. —He should remove metal objects and jewelry from his head and neck. —He should try to remain quiet and calm throughout the procedure. —He should not take anticonvulsants, barbiturates, tranquilizers, or sedatives for 24 to 48 hours before the test.

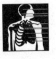 **Explaining disorders**

ALCOHOLISM (Alcohol addiction)

Patient objectives	Teaching plan content
1 Define alcoholism (alcohol addiction).	Alcohol addiction is a chronic illness characterized by physiologic and psychological dependence on alcohol and a pattern of pathologic use that impairs social, emotional, physiologic, and occupational function.
2 Explain the causes of alcohol addiction.	Alcohol addiction may be the result of several factors. —The biological factors include strong evidence that alcoholism is inherited, either as a physical trait or as a predisposition. —The psychological factors include excessive depen-

dency needs that cannot be met in reality. When they are not met, the patient feels rejected. This rejection leads to anxiety. Initially, alcohol reduces the anxiety and induces feelings of power and competence. But as the patient's addiction progresses, the addictive behavior causes further anxiety, guilt, shame, remorse, and self-hatred as the self-enhancing effects of alcohol diminish.

—The sociological factors include widespread approval of the use of alcohol to feel better. In societies where this exists, alcohol addiction is more prevalent and has been tied to stress-related problems, anxiety, and depression.

---

3 Identify the relevant behavioral characteristics of alcohol addiction.

The behavioral characteristics of alcohol addiction include the following:
—Secret drinking
—Morning drinking
—Blackouts
—Binge drinking
—Arguments about drinking
—Denial of the illness
—Rationalization of problems
—Absenteeism from work
—Alcohol-related police record
—High incidence of suicide attempts
—Consumption of alcohol not intended for drinking (mouthwash, ethyl alcohol, cough syrup)
—High incidence of accidental injuries
—Violence during intoxication.

---

4 Identify the relevant physical problems associated with alcohol addiction.

The following physical problems are associated with alcohol addiction:
—Respiratory problems include the following: decreased respiratory rate, decreased cough reflex, pooling of secretions, increased susceptibility to infection, decreased lung capacity because of abnormal accumulation of fluid in the abdominal cavity, and increased incidence of tuberculosis.
—Central nervous system problems include the following: peripheral neuropathy (disturbance in nervous system function or change in sensation); myopathies (disorders of muscle function and sensation), with severe pain and tenderness; changes in gait caused by peripheral nerve damage; muscle weakness; numbness; and prickly sensations.
—Cardiovascular problems include the following: hypertension (high blood pressure), increased heart rate, decreased cardiac output (amount of blood ejected from

the left ventricle), congestive heart failure, shortness of breath, and enlarged heart.

—Gastrointestinal problems include the following:
- acute gastritis (inflammation of the lining of the stomach), which may be accompanied by pain, nausea, vomiting, bleeding, abdominal distention, and belching
- esophagitis (inflammation of the tissue lining of the esophagus), which may be accompanied by pain on swallowing, vomiting, and heartburn—midchest or epigastric pain
- acute/chronic pancreatitis (inflammation of the pancreas), which may be accompanied by nausea, vomiting, and severe upper abdominal pain that radiates to the back
- liver dysfunction, which may be indicated by a swollen, enlarged, "fatty" liver; fever; jaundice (yellowish tinge to skin and whites of eyes); abdominal swelling; foot edema; dilated veins (hemorrhoids); ascites (accumulation of fluid in the peritoneal cavity); and testicular atrophy, menstrual irregularities, gynecomastia (development of breasts in the male), or loss of chest and axillary hair.

—Hematologic problems include the following: anemia, increased infection, destroyed platelets, increased bruising, and decreased clotting time.

—Nutritional problems include the following: malnutrition, decreased vitamin B levels, and decreased niacin levels.

5 Discuss the goals of the treatment regimen for alcohol addiction.

The treatment regimen for alcohol addiction should help the patient do the following:

—Maintain physiologic stability by meeting his safety needs, providing for protection, and assessing his degree of intoxication

—Recognize the signs and symptoms of delirium tremens (DTs) and alcohol withdrawal syndrome, while he is sober

—Acknowledge and accept alcoholism as a disease

—Understand that he will have to make a commitment to himself and to treatment

—Know that counseling may be necessary to help him form positive relationships and confront frustration and anxiety in a healthy manner

—Know that counseling may also help alleviate depression and prevent suicidal thoughts.

6 Identify the components of the treatment regimen for alcohol addiction.	The treatment regimen for alcohol addiction includes these components: —Medications —Vitamin replacement/supplementation —Fluid replacement (if necessary) —A well-balanced, nutritious, high-protein diet (if liver function is adequate) —Reality orientation —Supportive counseling —Aversion or deterrence therapy —Alcoholics Anonymous (AA) meetings —Stress management —Routine medical examinations.
7 Describe the medication regimen.	Some drugs commonly used for this disorder may include amitriptyline, chlordiazepoxide, clorazepate, desipramine, diazepam, doxepin, haloperidol, imipramine, isocarboxazid, maprotiline, nortriptyline, oxazepam, phenelzine, protriptyline, and tranylcypromine. Disulfiram may also be used, but the use of this drug is controversial. For specific medication instructions, see Chapter 10, Drug Therapy.
8 Identify the relevant signs and symptoms associated with alcohol addiction.	The following signs and symptoms are associated with alcohol addiction: —Increased heart rate —Increased blood pressure —Increased temperature —Increased tremors —Excitement —Anxiety —Increased disorientation —Hallucinations —Rigidity —Seizures —Mild alcohol withdrawal (jitters, irritability, profuse sweating, nausea, and vomiting) —Delirium tremens (DTs)—coarse tremors, depression, disorientation, decreased attention span, anorexia, insomnia, tachycardia, fever, profuse sweating, tachypnea, and visual or tactile hallucinations.
9 Identify and describe deep-muscle relaxation techniques.	Deep-muscle relaxation techniques include taped relaxation exercises, relaxation by cue, deep breathing, imagery, and progressive muscle relaxation. —With taped relaxation exercises, the patient listens to a tape recording of a programmed relaxation exercise twice a day, preferably not at bedtime. (If he associates

the exercise with sleep, he may fall asleep during daytime practice sessions.) He should follow all the instructions on the tape and should concentrate on relaxing. With practice, he may be able to relax without the tape.

—Relaxation by cue does not require any special equipment. As a result, the patient can use it anywhere, anytime. The patient selects a cue, which can be anything easily noticed—his watchband, for instance, or a sign on a door near his workplace. He concentrates on the cue as he relaxes. In time, simply looking at the cue may help him relax within minutes.

—In deep breathing, the patient breathes rhythmically while staring at a cue object. As he breathes, he establishes a rhythm by counting: for example, "In, two, three, four; out, two, three, four." The pace should be kept slow. When he has established a comfortable, relaxing rhythm, he concentrates on feeling a little more relaxed with each exhalation. He focuses on how he feels as he relaxes: weightless, pulsating, tingling, warm, or heavy.

—In using imagery, the patient thinks of a place where he usually feels relaxed and carefree—the beach or some other vacation spot, for example. He mentally transports himself to that place and concentrates on the details of every sight, sound, smell, and touch he associates with that location.

—Progressive muscle relaxation depends on the patient's ability to systematically tense and relax muscle groups throughout his body. To perform this technique:
- The patient focuses on a particular muscle group (he might start with the muscles in his hands).
- He tenses these muscles.
- After 5 to 7 seconds, he relaxes the muscles and concentrates on the difference he feels between the relaxed and tensed states.
- Then he concentrates on another group of muscles, tensing and then relaxing them. He continues the procedure until he has tensed and relaxed the muscle groups throughout his body.

—In a similar technique (sometimes called the Benson technique), the patient progressively relaxes his muscles from his feet to his head, without tensing them first. When he is relaxed, he performs deep breathing for about 20 minutes.

---

10 Explain the importance of follow-up care.

Routine medical follow-up during recovery is important, even after initial control and sobriety are attained, because it ensures that treatment maintains optimal physical functioning. Ongoing psychiatric or supportive counseling improves the patient's ability to cope with stress, anxiety, and frustration. In Alcoholics Anonymous (AA), a self-help group, the patient can find emotional support from others with similar problems.

DRUG ADDICTION

Patient objectives	Teaching plan content
1 Define drug addiction.	Drug addiction is a chronic illness characterized by physiologic and psychological dependence on a chemical substance (a drug other than alcohol) that produces an altered physiologic and psychological state. It is evidenced by a pattern of pathologic use and impairment of social or occupational functioning.
2 Explain the causes of drug addiction.	Drug addiction may be the result of several factors. —The biological factors include strong evidence that drug addiction is inherited, either as a physical trait or as a predisposition. —The psychological factors include excessive dependency needs that cannot be met in reality. When they are not met, the patient feels rejected. This rejection leads to anxiety. Initially, drugs reduce the anxiety and induce feelings of power and competence. But as the addiction progresses, the addictive behavior causes further anxiety, guilt, shame, remorse, and self-hatred as the self-enhancing effects of drugs diminish. —The sociological factors include widespread approval of the use of drugs to feel better. In societies where this exists, drug addiction is more prevalent and has been tied to stress-related problems, anxiety, and depression.
3 Identify the relevant behavioral characteristics of drug addiction.	The behavioral characteristics of drug addiction include the following: —Reluctance to talk about self or personal problems —View of self as "different" from others —Minimization of use of chemical substances —Tendency to blame others for problems —Many somatic complaints —Denial of the illness —Anger —Hostility —Self-pity —Use of intellectualization as a defense mechanism (separating the emotion aroused by an event from ideas or

opinions about the event, because the emotion itself is too painful to acknowledge)
—Physical isolation
—Superficial relationships
—Marital/family problems
—Financial problems
—Employment problems.

4 Identify the relevant signs and symptoms of drug intoxication.

The signs and symptoms of drug intoxication are as follows:

—Barbiturates, tranquilizers, and hypnotics are associated with mood lability (emotional instability), decreased inhibition of sexual and aggressive impulses, irritability, slurred speech, ataxia (muscle incoordination), impaired memory, impaired attention, impaired social judgment, and increased verbalization.

—Opioids (heroin, morphine, meperidine, methadone) are associated with pupillary constriction, pupillary dilation due to anoxia (lack of oxygen) from severe overdose, euphoria, dysphoria (a generalized state of feeling unwell or unhappy), apathy, psychomotor retardation (decreased voluntary movements), drowsiness, slurred speech, impaired memory and attention, and impaired social judgment.

—Cocaine, 1 hour after ingestion, is associated with psychomotor agitation (restlessness and purposeless activity), elation, grandiosity (exaggeration, feelings of power and invulnerability), increased verbalization, increased heart rate (over 100 beats/minute), pupillary dilation, increased blood pressure, perspiration/chills, nausea and vomiting, and hypervigilance (increased alertness).

—Cocaine overdose is associated with syncope (lightheadedness, fainting), chest pain, seizures, and cardiopulmonary arrest.

—Amphetamines (speed, diet pills), 1 hour after ingestion, are associated with psychomotor agitation, elation, grandiosity, increased verbalization, hypervigilance, increased heart rate (over 100 beats/minute), increased blood pressure, pupillary dilation, perspiration/chills, and nausea and vomiting.

—Phencyclidine (PCP)/tetrahydrocannabinol (THC), 1 hour after ingestion, is associated with vertical or horizontal nystagmus (involuntary, rhythmic movement of the eyes), increased blood pressure, increased heart rate, numbness or decreased pain response, ataxia, euphoria, psychomotor agitation, marked anxiety, emotional lability, grandiosity, sensation of slowed time, synesthesia (e.g., seeing colors when a loud sound is heard), and possible suicidal thoughts.

—Hallucinogen hallucinosis (LSD, DMT, mescaline) is associated with increased perceptual changes that occur in a state of full wakefulness, pupillary dilation, increased heart rate (over 100 beats/minute), sweating, palpitations (pounding heart), tremors, incoordination, ideas of reference (e.g., subject's belief that the television is speaking to him with a message), fear of "going crazy," and impaired judgment.

—Cannabis, marijuana, and hashish (THC) are associated with increased heart rate (over 100 beats/minute), euphoria, subjective intensification of perceptions, sensation of slowed time, apathy, conjunctival infection, increased appetite, dry mouth, increased anxiety, and impaired judgment.

—Tobacco is associated with no known or reported signs of drug intoxication.

—Caffeine, in amounts greater than 250 mg (1 cup of coffee = 100 to 150 mg), is associated with restlessness, nervousness, excitement, insomnia, flushed face, diuresis (frequent urination), gastrointestinal complaints, muscle twitching, rambling flow of thought and speech, cardiac dysrhythmia, and psychomotor agitation.

5 Identify the relevant signs and symptoms of drug withdrawal.

The signs and symptoms of drug withdrawal are as follows:

—Barbiturates, tranquilizers, and hypnotics are associated with nausea and vomiting; increased heart rate (over 100 beats/minute); increased blood pressure; diaphoresis (sweating); depressed mood; central nervous system irritability; orthostatic hypotension (drop in blood pressure on standing); coarse tremor of hands, tongue, eyelids; seizures; and delirium that occurs within 1 week of cessation.

—Opioids (heroin, morphine, meperidine, methadone) are associated with lacrimation (watery eyes), rhinorrhea (runny nose), piloerection (hair standing up on skin surface), sweating, diarrhea, yawning, mildly increased blood pressure, increased heart rate (over 100 beats/minute), increased temperature, insomnia, pupillary dilation, and persistent back and abdominal pain.

—Cocaine is associated with depression, irritability, disorientation, tremors, and muscle weakness.

—Amphetamines (speed, diet pills), with long-term use at high doses, are associated with a rapidly developing delusional syndrome after cessation, evidenced by persecutory delusions, ideas of reference, aggressiveness, hostility, anxiety, and psychomotor agitation. Within 48 to 96 hours, withdrawal is evidenced by depressed mood, increased dreaming, and overwhelming fatigue.

—Phencyclidine (PCP)/tetrahydrocannabinol (THC) is associated with no known or reported physiologic signs of withdrawal.
—LSD, DMT, and mescaline are associated with no known or reported physiologic signs of withdrawal.
—Cannabis, marijuana, and hashish (THC) are associated with no known or reported physiologic signs of withdrawal.
—Tobacco, with habitual use of more than 10 cigarettes per day (0.5 mg nicotine), is associated with craving for tobacco, irritability, anxiety, decreased ability to concentrate, restlessness, headache, drowsiness, and gastrointestinal disturbances within 24 hours after cessation.
—Caffeine is associated with fatigue, headache, and drowsiness.

---

6 Discuss the goals of the treatment regimen for drug addiction.

The goals of the treatment regimen for drug addiction include the following:
—Preventing and/or treating drug withdrawal syndrome
—Treating physiologic consequences of drug addiction
—Maintaining physiologic stability
—Acknowledging and accepting drug addiction as an illness
—Making a commitment to himself and to treatment
—Understanding that counseling can help him form positive relationships and confront frustration and anxiety in a healthy manner and that it can help alleviate depression and prevent suicidal thoughts.

---

7 Identify the components of the treatment regimen for drug addiction.

The treatment regimen for drug addiction includes these components:
—Medications
—Vitamin replacement/supplementation
—Fluid replacement
—A well-balanced, nutritious, high-protein diet (if liver function is adequate)
—Reality orientation
—Supportive counseling
—Aversion or deterrence therapy
—Narcotics Anonymous (NA) meetings
—Stress management
—Routine medical examinations.

---

8 Describe the relevant medication regimen.

Drug therapy depends on what drug the patient is addicted to. Some drugs used for this disorder are chlordiazepoxide, chlorpromazine, diazepam, haloperidol, methadone, naloxone, pentobarbital, phenobarbital, and secobarbital. For specific medication instructions, see Chapter 10, Drug Therapy.

9 Identify and describe deep-muscle relaxation techniques.	Deep-muscle relaxation techniques include taped relaxation exercises, relaxation by cue, deep breathing, imagery, and progressive muscle relaxation. For a detailed description of these techniques, see the "Alcoholism" teaching plan in this chapter.
10 Explain the importance of follow-up care.	Routine medical follow-up is important, even after initial control and abstinence are attained, because it ensures that treatment maintains optimal physical functioning. Ongoing psychiatric or supportive counseling improves the patient's ability to cope with stress, anxiety, and frustration. In Narcotics Anonymous (NA), a self-help group, the drug-dependent person can find emotional support from others with similar problems.

ANXIETY

Patient objectives	*Teaching plan content*
1 Define anxiety and differentiate it from fear.	Anxiety is a state in which the individual feels uneasy and apprehensive, thereby activating the autonomic nervous system in response to a vague, unidentifiable, nonspecific threat. Anxiety differs from fear because the anxious person is unable to identify the threat. With fear, the threat is easily identified.
2 Explain the causes of anxiety.	Anxiety is usually caused by threats to physical integrity and self-concept that the patient cannot identify. Some current research indicates a possible physiologic link to high serum lactate levels.
3 Identify events that can precipitate anxiety.	The following events can precipitate anxiety: —Threats to physiologic integrity, including interference with the satisfaction of hunger or thirst, of the need for warmth, and of sexual expression. —Real or anticipated threats to self-concept, including disapproval from a significant person, unfulfilled expectations, and unmet needs for respect and self-esteem.
4 Identify the relevant signs and symptoms of anxiety.	Symptoms reported by the patient are likely to include: —anger/hostility —alterations in appetite, either increased or decreased

—apprehensive expectation
—intense apprehension
—chest pain/discomfort/burning/aching
—choking, smothering sensation
—delusions
—diarrhea or constipation
—dry mouth
—dyspnea (shortness of breath)
—faintness/dizziness
—fear of "going crazy"
—fear of dying or "impending doom"
—fear of losing control
—fear/terror
—hot/cold flashes
—hallucinations
—headaches
—increased irritability
—abnormal or absent menstrual cycle
—motor tension and increased psychomotor activity
—numbness/tingling in fingers/toes
—palpitations (pounding heart)
—phobias (fear of objects, things, or situations)
—tinnitus (ringing in ears)
—sweating, especially palms of hands
—trembling/shaking
—"unsteady" feelings
—urinary retention or urgency
—visual disturbances, blurred vision
—increased vigilance (increased alertness).
Signs observed by others (e.g., nurse, physician) are
likely to include:
—altered blood pressure, either higher or lower than
normal
—cold, clammy skin
—dilated pupils
—increased heart rate
—increased respiratory rate and depth of respiration
—release of glucose by liver
—retention of sodium
—shifts in body temperature.

5 Identify the cognitive responses to anxiety.

The following are cognitive responses to anxiety:
—Blocking of thought
—Confusion
—Decreased perceptive ability
—Diminished productivity
—Errors in judgment

—Forgetfulness
—Impaired attention and concentration
—Preoccupation.

6 Discuss the goals of the treatment regimen for anxiety.	The goals of the treatment regimen for anxiety include the following: —Reducing the present level of anxiety —Recognizing anxious behavior and anxiety triggers —Reducing or alleviating maladaptive coping behaviors.
7 Identify the components of the treatment regimen for anxiety.	The treatment regimen for anxiety includes these components: —Medications —Supportive counseling —Psychotherapy (individual/group/family therapy) —Stress reduction and management —Systematic desensitization —Biofeedback.
8 Describe the medication regimen.	Some drugs commonly used for this disorder are chlordiazepoxide, clorazepate, diazepam, and oxazepam. For specific medication instructions, see Chapter 10, Drug Therapy.
9 Identify and describe deep-muscle relaxation techniques.	Deep-muscle relaxation techniques include the following: —Taped relaxation exercises —Relaxation by cue —Deep breathing —Imagery —Progressive muscle relaxation. For a detailed explanation on how to perform these techniques, see the "Alcoholism" teaching plan in this chapter.
10 Explain the importance of follow-up care.	Routine medical follow-up is important, even after initial control of the anxiety is attained, especially if the patient is on medication to decrease anxiety, because it ensures that the patient is functioning well on the treatment prescribed. Ongoing psychiatric or supportive counseling to effectively manage his anxiety is also important. It may improve his ability to cope with stress, anxiety, and frustration. A self-help group may allow the patient to find emotional support from others with similar problems.

DEPRESSION

Patient objectives	Teaching plan content
1 Define depression.	Depression refers to a mood state, a symptom, or a syndrome. As a mood state, depression is the feelings of sadness, disappointment, and frustration occasionally felt by all individuals. The syndrome, or disorder, of depression is distinguished from depression symptoms by the severity and duration of the depressed mood.
2 Differentiate between endogenous and exogenous depression.	The difference between endogenous and exogenous depression can be explained as follows: —Endogenous depression: • A clear-cut, identifiable precipitating factor does not always exist. • The patient has a strong family history of depression. • The patient has experienced a major episode of depression in the past. • The patient responds better to electroconvulsive therapy and antidepressants than to environmental stimuli and psychotherapy. —Exogenous depression (reactive depression): • An identifiable situation or stressful event was a precipitating factor. • The patient usually responds to psychotherapy.
3 Explain the causes of the two categories of depression.	The possible causes of the two categories of depression are as follows: —Endogenous depression is primarily explained by the biogenic amine hypothesis (at present, however, much research is being conducted in this area). This hypothesis proposes that there is an impairment in the activity of biogenic amines, particularly the monoamine neurotransmitters norepinephrine and serotonin. Therefore, there is a correlation between the depletion of norepinephrine and serotonin and depression. —Exogenous depression occurs when a real or perceived loss is experienced, and the patient believes that he will never be the same. An interruption of goals and plans ensues, and a period of grief develops. If the grief turns into hopelessness and despair, the individual believes that he will never achieve any goals or feel good again. Another psychodynamic theory proposes that depression is a result of anger turned inward. The real or perceived loss causes the individual to experience anger, not always on a conscious level. The indi-

vidual who develops depression is most likely unable to acknowledge and accept being angry.

4 Identify the relevant conditions associated with depression.	The following conditions can be associated with depression: —Bereavement, uncomplicated —Bipolar disorder (manifested by agitation and depression) —Cyclothymic disorder (a mild form of bipolar disorder) —Dementia (a progressive, organic mental disorder) —Dysthymic disorder (depressive neurosis) —Major depressive episodes —Organic-affective syndrome with depression —Personality disorders —Depressed reaction to the impairments of physical illness —Schizoaffective disorder (similar to manic-depressive disorder) —Schizophrenia —Separation-anxiety disorder.
5 Identify the relevant signs and symptoms of depression.	The signs and symptoms of depression include the following: —Emotional manifestations of affect or mood, such as depression, sadness, hopelessness, discouragement, emptiness, anhedonia (inability to experience pleasure), low self-esteem (negative feelings about self), feelings of worthlessness, shame and guilt, anxiety or agitation, anger, dependence and demanding behavior, self-doubt, and feelings of powerlessness. —Cognitive manifestations/thoughts, such as worry, preoccupation, self-criticism, self-devaluing thoughts, slow and impoverished thoughts, difficulty thinking, impairment of memory and concentration, short attention span, negative outlook or expectations, indecision, ambivalence, exaggeration of problems, distorted perception, distorted body image, excessive concern with physical health (can progress to somatic delusions), self-devaluing hallucinations/delusions, and thoughts of death or suicide. —Motivational manifestations/behavior, such as psychomotor retardation (slowed speech, lack of energy, fatigue), psychomotor agitation (inability to sit still, pacing, hand wringing, and pulling or rubbing hair, skin, clothing, or other objects), labored speech, sad facial expression, lack of attention to personal hygiene, passivity and dependency, panic attacks/phobias, crying/weeping, avoidance, escapism, and withdrawal. —Physical manifestations/symptoms, such as increased

or decreased appetite, weight loss or gain, insomnia (difficulty falling asleep, interrupted sleep, early morning waking), constipation, dry mouth, general aching, amenorrhea (no menstrual periods), impotence, loss of sexual desire, headaches, and blurred vision.

6 Discuss the goals of the treatment regimen for depression.

The goals of the treatment regimen for depression are as follows:
—Maintaining physiologic stability by treating suicidal tendencies, when apparent, and treating physical symptoms
—Assessing changes or perceived threats/losses in the patient's life and investigating and clarifying possible misperceptions
—Recognizing, accepting, understanding, and ventilating feelings, especially anger
—Building a self-image that is more accurate and healthy.

7 Identify the components of the treatment regimen for depression.

The treatment regimen for depression includes these components:
—Medications
—Suicide precautions/restraints (if the patient is potentially suicidal)
—Electroconvulsive therapy
—Psychotherapy (individual/group/family therapy)
—Supportive counseling
—Stress reduction
—Bereavement counseling.

8 Describe the medication regimen.

Some drugs commonly used for this disorder are amitriptyline, desipramine, doxepin, imipramine, isocarboxazid, nortriptyline, phenelzine, protriptyline, and tranylcypromine. For specific medication instructions, see Chapter 10, Drug Therapy.

9 Explain the importance of follow-up care.

Routine medical follow-up is important, even after initial elimination of the depression, especially if the patient is taking antidepressive medications, because it ensures that the patient is functioning well. Depression can mask parallel physiologic problems or can even produce physical illness. If he is taking antidepressive medication, close monitoring is important. Ongoing psychiatric or supportive counseling to effectively manage the patient's depression is also important. It may improve his ability to cope with loss, perceived threats, and frustration. A self-help group may allow the patient to find emotional support from others with similar problems.

MANIA

Patient objectives	*Teaching plan content*
1 Define mania.	Mania, the manic phase of a bipolar disorder, is characterized by expansiveness, elation, and hyperactivity.
2 Explain the causes of mania.	Hypotheses about the causes of mania are as follows: —There appears to be a strong genetic influence in the development of mania, which may be mediated by an inherited biochemical abnormality. —Biogenic amines appear to play a role. A disturbance in the balance of neurotransmitters (norepinephrine and serotonin) and an increase in their activity may produce mania. —The psychodynamic hypothesis places mania and depression at opposite ends of one spectrum. It proposes that mania is a defense against depression, as the individual tries to deny his feelings of worthlessness, helplessness, and powerlessness. His elated state, agitation, and hyperactivity are overt pleas for attention, love, and protection from depression. —A unified hypothesis that the causes of mania include hereditary, developmental, biochemical, and interpersonal factors is possibly the most accurate.
3 Identify the signs and symptoms of mania.	The signs and symptoms of mania include the following: —Emotional manifestations of mood or affect, such as elation, euphoria, inappropriate humor (laughing at nothing), inflated self-esteem, lack of shame or guilt, and decreased tolerance of criticism or suggestions. —Cognitive manifestations/thoughts, such as unrealistic ambitions, denial of real danger, short attention span, flight of ideas, grandiose thoughts, illusions, lack of judgment, loose associations, racing thoughts, and hallucinations/delusions/delirium (in mania's severe, hyperacute form). —Motivational manifestations/behavior, such as aggression, argumentative behavior, excessive spending of money, grandiose acts, hyperactivity, increased motor activity, flamboyant or bizarre dress or makeup, irresponsibility, irritability, poor personal hygiene/grooming, provocative behavior, sexually inappropriate behavior, overactive social life, and verbosity. —Physical manifestations/symptoms, such as dehydration, increased heart rate and blood pressure, diminished sleep or inability to perceive the need for sleep, and weight loss.

4 Discuss the goals of the treatment regimen for mania.

For the patient, the treatment regimen for mania includes these goals:
—Maintaining physiologic stability through adequate rest and sleep, nutrition, and hydration
—Carrying out his activities of daily living and meeting his basic needs
—Building trusting relationships
—Decreasing hyperactivity, anxiety, and agitation
—Finding outlets for the relief of tension and energy
—Recognizing, accepting, understanding, and ventilating feelings, especially anger
—Knowing that a safe, controlled environment will be provided if he is or becomes suicidal.

5 Identify the components of the treatment regimen for mania.

The treatment regimen for mania includes these components:
—Medication
—Restraints
—Electroconvulsive therapy (ECT)
—Psychotherapy
—Supportive counseling.

6 Describe the medication regimen.

The drug of choice for this disorder is lithium. For specific medication instructions, see Chapter 10, Drug Therapy.

7 Explain the utmost importance of follow-up care.

Frequent medical follow-up is of the utmost importance, even after initial control of the mania is attained, especially if the patient is taking lithium, neuroleptics, or antidepressants (singly or in combination). With lithium, careful monitoring at set intervals is needed to ensure a therapeutic rather than a toxic dosage. Ongoing psychiatric or supportive counseling may improve the patient's ability to cope with loss, perceived threats, and depression. A self-help group may allow the patient to find emotional support from others with similar problems.

PSYCHOTIC BEHAVIOR

Patient objectives | *Teaching plan content*

1 Define psychotic behavior.

Psychotic behavior results from a serious disturbance of the personality that involves an impairment of the ego function: specifically, reality testing. Psychotic behavior can take many forms. The individual may experience disruption in one or all of the following activities: conscious thought, reality orientation, problem solving, judgment, and comprehension.

2 Differentiate between the functional and organic causes of psychotic behavior.	The difference between the functional (psychiatric) and organic (physical) causes of psychotic behavior is as follows: —Functional psychosis results from disturbed mental functioning in the absence of any structural changes that affect brain function. —Organic psychosis involves gross, microscopic, or submicroscopic (chemical) changes that affect brain function.
3 Identify the causes of psychotic behavior.	The causes of psychotic behavior include the following: —Functional causes include paranoid, schizophrenic, or schizophreniform disorders. —Organic causes include chemicals/drugs, toxins, physical damage or trauma, and sleep deprivation.
4 Identify the relevant signs and symptoms of psychotic behavior.	The signs and symptoms of psychotic behavior include the following: —Functional psychosis may result in bizarre behavior; delusions; disturbances of self-initiated, goal-directed activity; appetite disturbances; aggression against self and others; hallucinations; disorganized, illogical thinking; difficulty with verbal communication; increased anxiety/agitation; low self-esteem; alteration in ego boundaries (inability to differentiate the self from the external environment); poor interpersonal relationships; withdrawn behavior; inappropriate/inadequate emotional responses; sexual conflicts; and regressive behavior. —Organic psychosis may result in impaired concentration, delusions, disorientation, aggressiveness/hostility, fear, inattention to personal hygiene and grooming, impaired sleep cycle, disturbances in eating, physical acting out, clouding of consciousness, marked apathy and indifference, incoherent speech, perceptual disturbances, repetitive questioning, and poor impulse control.
5 Discuss the goals of the treatment regimen for psychotic behavior.	For the patient, the treatment regimen for psychotic behavior includes these goals: —Maintaining physiologic stability by following adequate hydration, nutrition, and elimination patterns; receiving therapy for the causative factor (if known) in organic psychosis; and living in a safe environment —Becoming oriented to reality —Increasing his ability to differentiate between himself and the external environment —Increasing his self-esteem and feelings of self-worth —Decreasing his withdrawn, seclusive behavior

—Reestablishing ego boundaries
—Decreasing bizarre behavior, anxiety, and agitation/
aggression.

6 Identify the components of the treatment regimen for psychotic behavior.	The treatment regimen for psychotic behavior includes these components: —Medication —Psychotherapy —Restraints —Supportive counseling.
7 Describe the relevant medication regimen.	Some drugs commonly used for this disorder are chlorpromazine and haloperidol. For specific medication instructions, see Chapter 10, Drug Therapy.
8 Explain the importance of follow-up care.	Routine medical follow-up is important, even after elimination of the psychotic behavior, especially if the patient is taking neuroleptic medication that produces an altered state of consciousness. Ongoing psychiatric or supportive counseling may improve his ego function and his ability to maintain adequate reality testing. A self-help group may allow the patient to find emotional support from others with similar problems.

 Explaining treatments

ELECTROCONVULSIVE THERAPY (E.C.T.)

Patient objectives	*Teaching plan content*
1 Define electroconvulsive therapy (ECT).	ECT is the use of electrical stimulation of the brain to produce a series of major motor seizures.
2 State the purpose of ECT.	The purpose of ECT is to rapidly relieve the following symptoms in major depressive episodes: —Anorexia —Catatonia (a condition characterized by motor disturbances, manifested by immobility and muscle rigidity) —Delusions —Diurnal mood swings (those associated with time of day) —Inability to concentrate —Inhibition of motor activity —Insomnia —Stupor

—Suicidal thoughts and attempts
—Uncontrolled excitement and exhaustion
—Weight loss.

3 Identify the appropriate uses of ECT.	ECT is an appropriate treatment modality for patients with the following diagnoses: —Catatonia —Mania —Depression (geriatric, postpartum, unipolar/bipolar) —Major affective disorder (disturbed personal coping pattern) —Psychotic depression —Psychotic behavior that does not respond to other therapies.

4 Describe the procedure used in ECT.	The procedure used in ECT is as follows:
	—The patient will receive atropine (a drug used to dry up secretions in the mouth and nose) I.M. about 30 to 60 minutes pretreatment.
	—He will be escorted to the treatment area in the morning.
	—His vital signs will be monitored throughout the treatment, which will be performed by a physician.
	—The patient will be placed supine on the bed/stretcher.
	—Any dentures will be removed.
	—His temples will be prepared as follows:
	  • For bilateral ECT, the anterior portion of the patient's temples will be wiped with an alcohol sponge and conductive jelly applied.
	  • For unilateral ECT, the anterior portion of the patient's nondominant temple (if right-handed, the right temple) and the posterior scalp at any location 2″ from the anterior temple will be wiped with an alcohol sponge and conductive jelly applied. Round, flat metal electrodes will be applied to a band around the patient's head and conductive jelly applied to the electrodes.
	—An I.V. injection of a muscle-relaxing drug will be given.
	—Oxygen will be administered pretreatment.
	—The electric shock will be delivered.
	—The patient will experience a seizure.
	—The nurse will gently protect the patient during the seizure.
	—When the seizure is finished, an anesthetist will give him oxygen.
	—The nurse will awaken the patient by calling his name and reassuring him.

—When awake and aware of his surroundings, the patient may get down off the stretcher.
—The patient will be returned to his unit or home (if ECT was done on an outpatient basis).

5 Explain patient guidelines for ECT.	Patient guidelines include the following: —The patient should not drink or eat anything after midnight before the treatment. —He should urinate and defecate before treatment. —He should dress in loose clothes, preferably a hospital gown. —He will probably experience some memory deficit as a result of treatment, and staff members will reorient him afterward.

INDIVIDUAL PSYCHOTHERAPY

Patient objectives	*Teaching plan content*
1 Define individual psychotherapy.	Individual psychotherapy is a method of therapeutic intervention in which a therapist and patient engage in a confidential and primarily verbal series of interactions over an agreed-upon period of time, with mutually agreed-upon goals that focus on behavioral changes for the patient.
2 State the goals of individual psychotherapy.	The goals of individual psychotherapy include the following: —Removing, modifying, or retarding existing symptoms —Alleviating or diminishing disturbed behavior patterns —Promoting positive personality growth and development.
3 Describe the phases of individual psychotherapy.	The phases of individual psychotherapy may be described as follows: —The introductory phase is the period when the patient and therapist become acquainted and assess each other's limits and boundaries. —The working phase develops as the patient comes to the sessions prepared to discuss problems and issues and actively participate in problem solving. —The termination phase occurs when patient and therapist agree to terminate the psychotherapeutic relationship, or the patient or therapist relocates, or the patient decides to end treatment.

GROUP PSYCHOTHERAPY

Patient objectives	Teaching plan content
1 Define group psychotherapy.	Group psychotherapy is a method of therapeutic intervention in which both individual and intrapsychic structures are explored and analyzed within the group process. As members interact in a group over time, they are able to observe their own and one another's desires, conflicts, and motivations.
2 State the purposes of group psychotherapy.	The purposes of group psychotherapy are to examine the behavior of group members and help them adopt more satisfying modes of interaction.
3 Describe group psychotherapy.	Group psychotherapy may be described as follows: —All prospective members are seen at least once on an individual basis before admission to the group. —The patient is not coached or prepared for what will happen in the group or who will be there. —General information is provided, such as "The group is a place to discuss feelings, issues, and problems and to explore reactions and solutions." —Group members sit in a circle with no table between them, and no one sits on the floor. —Generally, weekly sessions last for 1½ hours, and daily sessions last for 1 hour. —Sessions begin and end on time. —There is a standing rule against physical violence.
4 Explain patient guidelines for group psychotherapy.	Patient guidelines for group psychotherapy are as follows: —The patient should attend every session or inform the group leader beforehand of his expected absence or of a crisis. —He should be as open as possible. —He must not become physically violent. —He should not discuss group matters outside the group.

RAPID NEUROLEPTIZATION (Rapid tranquilization)

Patient objectives	Teaching plan content
1 Define rapid neuroleptization.	Rapid neuroleptization is the rapid administration of antipsychotic chemotherapy.
2 State the purpose of rapid neuroleptization.	The purpose of rapid neuroleptization is to rapidly diminish severe symptoms of acute psychosis (severely

aggressive, assaultive, violent behavior; agitation; delusions; hallucinations; and disoriented thinking) and to reduce the patient's psychic pain.

3 Describe the procedure used in rapid neuroleptization.	The procedure for performing rapid neuroleptization is as follows: —The patient's baseline vital signs will be obtained. —He will receive an initial dose of the medication ordered by the physician, either by mouth or by injection. —The nurse will monitor his vital signs and symptom reduction. —A dosing schedule will be determined and the drug repeated within that schedule (every 15 to 60 minutes) until symptom reduction is obtained. —The nurse will help assess the patient's drug tolerance, thereby establishing a maximal daily dose and determining his susceptibility to adverse effects. —The nurse will also monitor the patient closely for any changes in vital signs, especially blood pressure, or adverse effects in the extrapyramidal tract (areas of the brain that control postural, static, supporting, and locomotor mechanisms and cause contractions of muscle groups sequentially and simultaneously). Adverse effects include uncoordinated movement of muscle groups. An antiparkinsonian agent may be ordered by the physician and administered by the nurse to diminish extrapyramidal effects.
4 Explain patient guidelines for rapid neuroleptization.	The following are patient guidelines for rapid neuroleptization: —Report any adverse effects of the neuroleptics, including dizziness or light-headedness. —Call the nurse for help in walking because this treatment can cause orthostatic hypotension (dizziness or light-headedness on arising), which may precipitate a fall.

SUICIDE PRECAUTIONS

Patient objectives	Teaching plan content
1 Define suicide precautions.	Suicide precautions are intense observations of a patient who is suicidal and/or engaging in self-destructive behavior. Varying levels of suicide precautions reflect how intensely self-destructive the patient is at any time.
2 State the purpose of suicide precautions.	The purpose of suicide precautions is to protect patients from their own self-destructive behavior.

3 **Describe suicide precautions.**	Suicide precautions are as follows: —After evaluation and assessment, suicide precautions may be instituted by either the physician or the registered nurse. —The patient will be told why he is on suicide precautions, and the procedure will be explained to him. —The patient's belongings and body will be searched for such dangerous items as razor blades, cords, belts, drugs, and glass objects. —If the patient is on level 1 (constant-awareness precautions), 15-minute checks of his behavior will be made and documented. If he is on level 2 (constant observation), nurses will be assigned to stay with him on a one-to-one basis everywhere he goes, especially the bathroom. —All off-unit privileges will be discontinued, or he will be accompanied off the unit by a staff member. —The administration of medication will be monitored and medication given in liquid form, if necessary. —The order for suicide precautions will be communicated to all members of the staff. The order will be noted on the Kardex and on the front of the chart. —Daily assessment of the continued need for suicide precautions will be made by the physician and the patient's nursing staff.
4 **Explain patient guidelines for suicide precautions.**	The patient's role in observing suicide precautions is as follows: —He is an active member of the team that is trying to see him through this self-destructive period; therefore, he needs to honestly inform staff members of improvements of positive feelings or intensifications of negative feelings. —He enters into a "no-suicide" contract with the staff.

Patient-Teaching Aid

WHAT YOU SHOULD KNOW ABOUT LITHIUM

Dear Patient:

To get the most from your drug therapy, follow these instructions carefully:

• If you experience diarrhea, vomiting, drowsiness, muscle weakness and coordination failure, tremors, restlessness, or confusion, call the physician immediately. But do not abruptly stop taking your drug.

• Expect transient nausea, frequent urination, and thirst during the first few days of therapy.

• Expect a time lag of 1 to 3 weeks before you notice the drug's beneficial effects.

• Avoid activities that require complete mental alertness, such as driving or operating machinery, until your response to the drug is determined.

• Do not switch brands of lithium without asking the physician first.

• Drink a full glass of water when you take your medication. Take your medication after meals to help minimize nausea.

• Carry an identification card that gives instructions and toxicity and emergency information (available from your pharmacy).

Patient-Teaching Aid

FOODS TO AVOID WHEN TAKING M.A.O. INHIBITORS

Dear Patient:

When your physician prescribes an antidepressant, ask if it is an MAO (monoamine oxidase) inhibitor. If it is, avoid foods with a high tyramine content. These include:

- most cheeses, but especially blue, brick, Brie, Camembert, cheddar, Emmentaler, Gruyère, mozzarella, Parmesan, Romano, Roquefort, and Stilton
- caviar
- herring
- sausage meats, especially bologna, pepperoni, salami, and summer sausage
- yeast extracts; that is, those foods containing live yeast, such as compressed yeast cakes (Cooking kills yeast cells, so baked goods will not cause adverse reactions.)
- chocolate
- Chianti wine and imported beers. (Feel free to drink white wines because, unlike red wines, they are made without the grape pulp and seeds, the possible sources of the amino acid tyramine.)

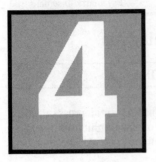

Eating Disorders

Patient-learner data base*

Areas of potential knowledge deficit
Risk factors
—Age (under 30)
—Female sex
—Body image disturbance
—Premorbid personality
—Dominant mother
—Unpleasant and forced eating patterns in childhood
Definition of the eating disorder
Causes of the eating disorder
Symptoms associated with the eating disorder
Treatment of the eating disorder
—Diet
—Behavior modification
—Psychotherapy
—Family therapy
—Other treatments used
Complications of the eating disorder

Explaining diagnostic tests

NUTRITIONAL ASSESSMENT

Patient objectives	Teaching plan content
1 Define nutritional assessment.	Nutritional assessment is the process of gathering information about the patient's food-related behavior and

---

* A general assessment should be done for all patients. For general assessment guidelines, see Chapter 1, Principles of Patient Teaching.

intake of calories and nutrients and evaluating physical and metabolic signs of nutritional status. It involves a dietary survey, anthropometry (body measurement), and clinical and biochemical appraisals.

2 State the purpose of a nutritional assessment.

The purpose of a nutritional assessment is to aid in the diagnosis of an eating disorder and to identify malnutrition.

3 Describe the procedures used in a nutritional assessment.

The procedures used in a nutritional assessment include the following:

—A dietary survey provides information on food or nutrient intake, nutritional practices, food preparation and procurement, and quantity and quality of food consumed by the patient.

Data are collected in the following categories:

- Demographics: age, sex
- Food intake: actual foods consumed and their frequency, food likes and dislikes, dosage of vitamins and other supplements
- Type of feeding: oral, enteral, parenteral
- Appetite: taste and smell perception, loss or gain of appetite, anorexia
- Physical activity: occupation, length and types of exercise, duration of sleep
- Food avoidances: allergies and intolerances, reasons for avoiding foods
- Dental/oral health: teeth and gum health, properly fitted dentures, salivation, swallowing
- Gastrointestinal abnormalities: heartburn, bloating, gas, distention, diarrhea, constipation, GI fistula
- Medications: antacids and laxatives, frequency of usage and dosage of other medications
- Home life-style: who shops, who cooks, type of cooking and storage facilities, number in household
- Economic condition: source of income and food dollars
- Ethnicity: ethnic, cultural, religious background (if immigrants, which generation).

—Clinical appraisal is the physical examination of the body, especially the eyes, hair, mucous membranes, skin, and mouth, to detect symptoms of nutritional deficiency.

—Anthropometry is the measurement of a body part or of the entire body. The most commonly used measurements are height and weight, skin-fold thickness, and arm, chest, and head circumference.

—Biochemical appraisal measures levels of nutrients, their metabolites, and enzymes associated with compounds directly related to the nutrient being investigated in the blood, urine, or body tissues such as liver and bone.

4 Discuss patient guidelines for height and weight measurements.

Patient guidelines for height and weight measurements are as follows:
—She should be weighed or weigh herself on the same scale each time.
—She should weigh herself nude; if that is not possible, she should wear the same amount and weight of clothing for each weighing.
—She should measure her standing height on a standard scale, standing erect, with no shoes on.

5 Describe the procedure used in measurement of skin-fold thickness.

Measuring skin-fold thickness involves the following:
—The evaluator uses calibrated calipers to pinch the patient's skin fold so that the two surfaces are parallel. This is done carefully, so that muscle and bone are not touched.
—He then measures the thickness by using the standard calipers while exerting constant pressure.
—The most common assessment sites are the deltoid triceps, the subscapular region, and the upper abdomen.

BLOOD UREA NITROGEN (B.U.N.)

Patient objectives	*Teaching plan content*
1 Define BUN test.	The BUN test measures the nitrogen fraction of urea, the chief end product of protein metabolism.
2 State the purpose of a BUN test.	The purpose of a BUN test is to aid in an assessment of hydration and nutritional status. It may also be used to evaluate renal function.
3 Describe the procedure for obtaining a BUN test specimen.	To obtain a specimen for the BUN test, a venipuncture will be performed and 10 to 15 ml of blood collected. —The patient should know who will perform the venipuncture and where it will be performed. —Collecting the sample will take only a few minutes. —The patient may experience some discomfort from the needle puncture and the pressure of the tourniquet.
4 Discuss patient guidelines for a BUN test.	Patient guidelines for a BUN test are as follows: —She need not restrict food or fluid before the test.

—She should remain calm, relaxed, and still to aid in the collection of the specimen.
—She should help maintain pressure on the venipuncture site for about 1 minute after the procedure.

TOTAL CHOLESTEROL

Patient objectives	Teaching plan content
1 Define total cholesterol test.	This test, a quantitative analysis of serum cholesterol, measures the circulating levels of free cholesterol and cholesterol salts. Cholesterol is a structural component in cell membranes and plasma and is a precursor of glucocorticoids, sex hormones, and bile acids. It is absorbed from food, metabolized and synthesized in the liver, and secreted in the bile.
2 State the relevant purpose of a total cholesterol test.	The purpose of a total cholesterol test in evaluating eating disorders is to evaluate fat metabolism.
3 Describe the procedure for obtaining a total cholesterol test specimen.	To obtain a specimen for total cholesterol testing, a venipuncture will be performed and approximately 7 to 8 ml of blood collected. —The patient should know who will perform the venipuncture and where it will be performed. —Collecting the sample will take only a few minutes. —The patient may experience some discomfort from the needle puncture and the pressure of the tourniquet.
4 Discuss patient guidelines for total cholesterol testing.	Patient guidelines for total cholesterol testing are as follows: —She will need to restrict food and fluid for 8 hours before the test. —She must abstain from alcohol for 24 hours before the test. —She should help maintain pressure on the venipuncture site for about 1 minute after the procedure.

COMPLETE BLOOD COUNT (C.B.C.)

Patient objectives	Teaching plan content
1 Define CBC.	This test provides a complete picture of all the blood's formed elements. It includes determinations of hemoglobin concentration and hematocrit, red and white blood cell counts, and stained red blood cell examinations.

2 State the purpose of a CBC.	The purpose of a CBC is to detect and determine the severity of anemias and to differentiate specific types of anemias.
3 Describe the procedure for obtaining a CBC specimen.	To obtain a specimen for a CBC, a venipuncture will be performed and approximately 10 to 15 ml of blood collected. —The patient should know who will perform the venipuncture and where it will be performed. —Collecting the sample will take only a few minutes. —The patient may experience some discomfort from the needle puncture and the pressure of the tourniquet.
4 Discuss patient guidelines for a CBC.	Patient guidelines for a CBC are as follows: —She need not restrict food or fluid before the test. —She should remain calm, relaxed, and still to aid in the collection of the specimen. —She should help maintain pressure on the venipuncture site for about 1 minute after the procedure.

SERUM CREATININE

Patient objectives	*Teaching plan content*
1 Define serum creatinine test.	This test measures creatinine, a nonprotein end product of creatine metabolism. As does creatine, creatinine appears in serum in amounts proportional to the body's muscle mass; unlike creatine, it is easily excreted by the kidneys. Since creatinine levels normally remain constant, elevated levels usually indicate diminished renal function.
2 State the purpose of a serum creatinine test.	The purpose of serum creatinine testing is to assess glomerular filtration and to screen for renal damage.
3 Describe the procedure for obtaining a serum creatinine test specimen.	To obtain a specimen for serum creatinine testing, a venipuncture will be performed and approximately 10 to 15 ml of blood collected. —The patient should know who will perform the venipuncture and where it will be performed. —Collecting the sample will take only a few minutes. —The patient may experience some discomfort from the needle puncture and the pressure of the tourniquet.
4 Discuss patient guidelines for serum creatinine testing.	Patient guidelines for serum creatinine testing are as follows: —She will need to restrict food and fluid for 8 hours before the test.

—She should remain calm, relaxed, and still to aid in the collection of the specimen.
—She should help maintain pressure on the venipuncture site for about 1 minute after the procedure.

ELECTROLYTE PANEL

Patient objectives	Teaching plan content
1 Define electrolyte panel.	This series of tests measures serum levels of the important electrolytes, which are substances that dissociate into ions when dissolved in the blood. Serum concentrations of electrolytes influence movement of fluid within and between body compartments. Commonly assessed electrolytes include sodium, potassium, calcium, magnesium, chloride, bicarbonate, and phosphate.
2 State the purpose of an electrolyte panel.	The purpose of an electrolyte panel is to evaluate fluid-electrolyte and acid-base balance and related neuromuscular, renal, and adrenal functions.
3 Describe the procedure for obtaining an electrolyte panel specimen.	To obtain a specimen for an electrolyte panel, a venipuncture will be performed and approximately 15 ml of blood drawn. —The patient should know who will perform the venipuncture and where it will be performed. —Collecting the sample will take only a few minutes. —The patient may experience some discomfort from the needle puncture and the pressure of the tourniquet.
4 Discuss patient guidelines for an electrolyte panel.	Patient guidelines for an electrolyte panel are as follows: —She need not restrict food or fluid before the test. —She should remain calm, relaxed, and still to aid in the collection of the specimen. —She should help maintain pressure on the venipuncture site for about 1 minute after the procedure.

FASTING BLOOD SUGAR (F.B.S.)

Patient objectives	Teaching plan content
1 Define FBS test.	The FBS test (or fasting plasma glucose test [FPG]) is the measurement of plasma glucose levels after a 12- to 14-hour fast.
2 State the relevant purpose of an FBS test.	The purpose of an FBS test in diagnosing an eating disorder is to assess carbohydrate metabolism during changes in nutritional status (weight gain or loss).

3 Describe the procedure for obtaining an FBS test specimen.	To obtain a specimen for an FBS test, a venipuncture will be performed and approximately 5 to 7 ml of blood collected. —The patient should know who will perform the venipuncture and where it will be performed. —Collecting the sample will take only a few minutes. —The patient may experience some discomfort from the needle puncture and the pressure of the tourniquet.
4 Discuss patient guidelines for an FBS test.	Patient guidelines for an FBS test are as follows: —She will need to restrict food and fluid for 12 to 14 hours before the test. —She will need to report the exact time of her last meal. —She should report any signs of hypoglycemia (weakness, restlessness, nervousness, hunger, sweating) immediately to laboratory personnel or the nurse. —She should remain calm, relaxed, and still to aid in collection of the specimen. —She should help maintain pressure on the puncture site for about 1 minute after the procedure.

SERUM PROTEIN ELECTROPHORESIS

Patient objectives	*Teaching plan content*
1 Define serum protein electrophoresis.	This test measures serum albumin and globulins, the major blood proteins, in an electric field by separating the proteins according to their molecular size and shape and their electric charge at pH 8.6. Because each protein fraction moves at a different rate, this movement separates the fractions into recognizable and measurable patterns. This test also provides a numerical value for total protein.
2 State the purpose of serum protein electrophoresis.	Serum protein electrophoresis aids in the diagnosis of protein deficiency.
3 Describe the procedure for obtaining a serum protein electrophoresis specimen.	To obtain a specimen for serum protein electrophoresis, a venipuncture will be performed and approximately 7 to 8 ml of blood collected. —The patient should know who will perform the venipuncture and where it will be performed. —Collecting the sample takes only a few minutes. —The patient may experience some discomfort from the needle puncture and the pressure of the tourniquet.

| **4** Discuss patient guidelines for serum protein electrophoresis. | Patient guidelines for serum protein electrophoresis are as follows:
—She need not restrict food or fluid before the test.
—She should remain calm, relaxed, and still to aid in obtaining the specimen.
—She should help maintain pressure on the venipuncture site for 1 minute after the procedure. |

SERUM URIC ACID

Patient objectives	*Teaching plan content*
1 Define serum uric acid test.	This test measures serum levels of uric acid, the major end metabolite of purine. Serum uric acid levels are usually raised by: —disorders of purine metabolism —rapid destruction of nucleic acids —conditions marked by impaired renal excretion.
2 State the purpose of the serum uric acid test.	The purpose of the serum uric acid test is to help detect kidney dysfunction.
3 Describe the procedure for obtaining a serum uric acid test specimen.	To obtain a specimen for the serum uric acid test, a venipuncture will be performed and approximately 10 to 15 ml of blood collected. —The patient should know who will perform the test and where it will be performed. —Collecting the sample will take only a few minutes. —The patient may experience some discomfort from the needle puncture and the pressure of the tourniquet.
4 Discuss patient guidelines for the serum uric acid test.	Patient guidelines for the serum uric acid test are as follows: —She need not restrict food or fluid before the test. —She should remain calm, relaxed, and still to aid in collection of the specimen. —She should help maintain pressure on the venipuncture site for about 1 minute after the procedure.

THYROID FUNCTION TESTS

Patient objectives	*Teaching plan content*
1 Name the tests that are used as thyroid function tests.	The following tests are used as thyroid function tests: —Serum thyroxine (T_4) —Serum triiodothyronine (T_3) —Serum thyroxine-binding globulin —T_3 resin uptake.

2 State the relevant purpose of thyroid function tests.

The purpose of thyroid function tests is to evaluate thyroid function and to assist in ruling out thyroid dysfunction as a cause of malnutrition or obesity.

3 Describe the procedure for obtaining a blood specimen for thyroid function tests.

To obtain a specimen for thyroid function tests, a venipuncture will be performed and approximately 7 ml of blood per test collected.
—The patient should know who will perform the venipuncture and where it will be performed.
—Collecting the sample will take only a few minutes.
—The patient may experience some discomfort from the needle puncture and the pressure of the tourniquet.

4 Discuss patient guidelines for thyroid function tests.

Patient guidelines for thyroid function tests are as follows:
—She need not restrict food or fluid before the test.
—She should remain calm, relaxed, and still to aid in collection of the specimen.
—She should help maintain pressure on the venipuncture site for about 1 minute after the procedure.

ROUTINE URINALYSIS

Patient objectives | *Teaching plan content*

1 Define routine urinalysis.

Routine urinalysis is an important test used to screen for urinary and systemic pathologies. Normal urine findings suggest the absence of major disease, while abnormal findings suggest its presence and mandate further urine or blood tests to identify a specific disorder. The elements of routine urinalysis include the following:
—Evaluation of physical characteristics (color, odor, and opacity)
—Determination of specific gravity and pH
—Detection and approximate measurement of protein, glucose, and ketone bodies
—Examination of sediment for red and white blood cells, casts, and crystals.

2 State the purpose of a routine urinalysis.

The purpose of a routine urinalysis is to screen for renal or urinary tract disease and to help detect metabolic or systemic disease unrelated to renal disorders.

3 Discuss the criteria for a urinalysis specimen.

The criteria for a urinalysis specimen are as follows:
—A specimen of at least 15 ml of urine should be voided directly into a plastic container.

—The specimen should be a first-voided morning urine, since this contains the greatest concentration of solutes (substances dissolved in urine).

4 **Discuss patient guidelines for a routine urinalysis.**	Patient guidelines for a routine urinalysis are as follows: —She need not restrict food or fluid before the test. —She should avoid strenuous exercise before urine collection, since exercise may cause transient myoglobinuria (presence in the urine of myoglobin, the compound that gives muscle its color and acts as a store of oxygen).

ELECTROCARDIOGRAPHY

Patient objectives	*Teaching plan content*
1 **Define electrocardiography.**	Electrocardiography is a procedure for evaluating cardiac status by recording the electrical current (electrical potential) generated by the heart. These currents are transmitted to the electrocardiograph machine by electrodes placed on the body, amplified, and graphically displayed on a strip chart recorder. The graphic display, or tracing, is called an electrocardiogram (EKG).
2 **State the relevant purpose of an EKG.**	The purpose of an EKG in diagnosing or evaluating an eating disorder is to assist in assessing the effects of electrolyte disturbances by detecting and locating conduction problems and dysrhythmias.
3 **Describe the procedure for an EKG.**	Just before the test, the patient will be placed supine, unless she becomes short of breath; in this case, she will be allowed to sit at a 45-degree angle. —The electrode placement sites will be cleaned with alcohol and shaved, if necessary. Electrode gel will be applied to the inner wrists and ankles. —The limb electrodes will be secured with rubber straps. —After recordings from the limb leads have been completed, electrode placement sites will be marked on the patient's chest. —A suction-cup electrode will be moved across the chest to where each chest lead position has been marked. —After recordings from the chest leads have been completed, the equipment will be disconnected and the gel on the patient's chest and limbs cleaned off.

4 Discuss patient guidelines for an EKG.	Patient guidelines for an EKG are as follows: —She need not restrict food or fluid before the EKG. —She must disrobe to the waist and expose both legs for electrode placement. A hospital gown will be provided for her. —She should try to relax, lie still, and breathe normally. —She should not talk during the procedure because the sound of her voice could distort the EKG tracing. —The procedure takes about 15 minutes. —She should not touch the metal handrail of the bed or allow her feet to touch the footboard; this will distort the EKG tracing.

EATING ATTITUDES TEST (E.A.T.)

Patient objectives	*Teaching plan content*
1 Define EAT.	The EAT is a 40-item, self-reporting questionnaire that provides information about the patient's eating attitudes and behaviors. The EAT measures symptoms commonly found in anorexia nervosa.
2 State the purpose of an EAT.	The purpose of an EAT is to assist in diagnosing anorexia nervosa.
3 Describe the procedure used in an EAT.	The patient will be given a pencil and the test. She is to read and honestly answer each question. The investigator will then score the questionnaire and discuss the results with the patient and the treatment team.

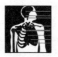 **Explaining disorders**

ANOREXIA NERVOSA

Patient objectives	*Teaching plan content*
1 Define anorexia nervosa.	Anorexia nervosa is a conscious and relentless determination to attain and maintain a very thin stature, despite the presence of an appetite and an interest in food. Anorexia nervosa is most common in preadolescent girls; however, it can surface from late adolescence up to the early thirties.

2 Identify the diagnostic criteria for anorexia nervosa.	The following are the diagnostic criteria for anorexia nervosa: —Disturbance of body image (claiming to be fat when actually emaciated) —Intense fear of becoming obese, which does not lessen as weight loss progresses —Refusal to maintain body weight over a minimal normal weight for age and height —Loss of at least 25 percent of original body weight —No known or documented physical illness that accounts for the weight loss.
3 Identify the relevant signs and symptoms of anorexia nervosa.	The signs and symptoms of anorexia nervosa include the following: —Manifestations in the patient's appearance include dry hair, with possible alopecia (loss of hair); emaciation; hollow face and sunken eyes; lanugo (fine body hair); and yellowish skin. —Behavioral manifestations include bizarre eating habits; calorie counting and preoccupation with recipes and exercise; cooking for others and forcing them to eat; denial of hunger, thinness, or need for treatment; denial of illness; excessive dawdling over food; demanding and bargaining behavior; delusional denial of thinness; hoarding of food; irritability and arrogance; inability to separate from parents; need to be special; phobias about the scale; theft of food and money; lying, teasing, deceitful behavior; pride in self-denial; refusal of food as a threat; suicide attempts after forced weight gain; perfectionism; and use of laxatives, enemas, and diuretics. —Mood manifestations include depersonalization, fear of becoming fat accompanied by a desire for food, depression and suicidal thoughts, guilt after having eaten, inability to recognize feelings, separation anxiety, and a view of life as a constant struggle with weight. —Physiologic manifestations include amenorrhea, decrease in body temperature, constipation, decrease in or loss of appetite in the late stage of the disease, bradycardia, and death caused by starvation or alteration in body chemistry.
4 Explain the causes of anorexia nervosa.	The causes of anorexia nervosa are complex. They include developmental issues, personality traits, mental processes, and family patterns. —Developmental issues include the following: • Early feeding experiences were mechanical, rigid, and usually not enjoyed by the mother. • Feeding schedules were imposed in a regimented

way by a dominant mother, without an assessment of the child's need for feeding, holding, and nurturing.

• As this pattern continued over the years, the dominating control by the mother led to an inability in the child to recognize bodily sensations such as hunger, fatigue, body temperature, tactile pleasure, anxiety, bowel and bladder sensations, and sexual impulses and sensations.

• Over the years, initiative from the child was overwhelmed by the parent and was subjected to correction and criticism. Therefore, a sense of body image was poorly developed.

—The following personality traits are usually demonstrated in childhood:

• compliance
• obedience
• passivity
• perfectionism
• dependence
• obsessive neatness
• high level of intelligence
• high need for achievement in school
• above-average athletic ability
• serious attitude, with little or no sense of humor
• superficial friendships, preference for friendship with one person at a time
• high need to please—especially parents, teachers
• guilt when expressing a want.

—The patient's mental processes may reveal the following:

• The child experiences her developing body as an extension of her dominating, controlling mother.
• Her body begins to represent the bad mother image.
• Feeding the body causes it to further develop and grow and thereby become overpowering, just as the child had previously experienced the mother.
• Therefore, the child must keep her body in control. The intent is not to destroy herself, but to attain and maintain control.
• As adolescence arrives, the child is desperately searching for an independent identity and for control.
• The eating and not-eating behaviors represent a struggle for control.

—Family patterns include the following:

• The parents of anorexics are seldom divorced.
• Anorexics are usually from middle- or upper-class families.
• Mothers have usually had careers and given birth in their mid-thirties.

• The average number of children is two or three, usually girls.
• The anorexic is overvalued by both parents.

---

5 State the goals of the treatment regimen for anorexia nervosa.

The goals of the treatment regimen include the following:
—Restoring the anorexic's nutritional status to normal by increasing caloric and nutritional intake
—Establishing normal eating behaviors
—Promoting weight gain
—Helping the patient develop non-food-related coping mechanisms
—Decreasing the association between food and control
—Establishing a trusting therapeutic relationship
—Assisting in clarifying and resolving family dynamics that contribute to the patient's illness.

---

6 Identify the relevant complications associated with anorexia nervosa.

The complications associated with anorexia nervosa include the following:
—Endocrinologic: amenorrhea (no menstrual flow), growth arrest, and osteopenia (reduced bone mass caused by a decrease in the rate of bone synthesis)
—Fluid- and electrolyte-related: abnormalities in water balance, chronic potassium depletion, decreased chloride, metabolic alkalosis (a decrease in acid or overproduction of alkaline substances in the blood), and increased or decreased sodium
—Biochemical: hypophosphatemia (an abnormally low amount of phosphates in the blood) because of chronic laxative use and zinc deficiency
—Gastrointestinal: increased liver enzymes, increased serum amylase, acute gastric dilation and rupture (stretching of the stomach), delayed gastric emptying, constipation, painless parotid swelling, and altered glucose metabolism
—Cardiovascular: bradycardia, hypotension, decreased maximal heart rate (heart rate on exercise), decreased cardiac output, dysrhythmias, decrease in size of left ventricle, left atrium, and aorta, and decompensation (decreased cardiorespiratory function)
—Hematologic and immunologic: anemias (low blood counts), leukopenia (low white blood cell count), thrombocytopenia (decrease in number of platelets), low erythrocyte sedimentation rates, low fibrinogen levels, and bone marrow alterations
—Neurologic: generalized, reversible cerebral and cerebellar atrophy, seizures caused by profound hyponatremia (low sodium in the body), and peripheral neuropathies (pain, anesthesia, or tingling sensations in the arms, legs, toes, or fingers)

—Dental: extensive decay of teeth, nonreversible peri-myolysis (enamel erosion), and decreased saliva production.

7 Identify the components of the treatment regimen for anorexia nervosa.	The treatment regimen for anorexia nervosa includes these components: —Medications —Individual psychotherapy —Group psychotherapy —Family therapy —Behavior modification —Dietary replacement and realignment: • frequent meals • tube feedings • hyperalimentation.

BULIMIA

Patient objectives	*Teaching plan content*
1 Define bulimia.	Bulimia is a disorder characterized by binge eating, accompanied by an awareness that the eating pattern is abnormal. Eating binges may be planned. A binge is usually terminated by abdominal pain, sleep, or induced vomiting.
2 Identify the diagnostic criteria for bulimia.	The diagnostic criteria for bulimia include the following: —Recurrent episodes of binge eating (rapid consumption of a large amount of food in a discrete amount of time, generally less than 2 hours) —Consumption of high-calorie, easily ingested food during a binge —Inconspicuous eating during a binge —Termination of such eating episodes by abdominal pain, sleep, or self-induced vomiting —Frequent, small weight fluctuations caused by alternating binges and fasts —Awareness that the eating pattern is abnormal and fear of not being able to stop binge eating voluntarily —Depressed mood —Self-deprecating thoughts after eating binges —Bulimic episodes not traceable to anorexia or any known physical disorder.
3 Identify the relevant symptoms of bulimia.	The symptoms of bulimia include the following: —Bloated/full feeling —Abdominal pain —Nausea

—Headache
—Tiredness
—Induced vomiting
—Laxative use
—Diuretic use
—Diarrhea
—Electrolyte disturbances
—Fairly stable body weight
—Menstrual irregularity.

4 Explain the causes of bulimia.	The causes of bulimia are the same as the causes of anorexia nervosa. (See the "Anorexia Nervosa" teaching plan in this chapter.)
5 State the goals of the treatment regimen for bulimia.	The goals of the treatment regimen for bulimia include the following: —Restoring the bulimic's nutritional status to normal —Establishing normal eating behaviors —Helping the patient develop non-food-related coping mechanisms —Decreasing associations between food and control —Establishing a trusting therapeutic relationship —Assessing, clarifying, and resolving family dynamics that contribute to the patient's illness.
6 Identify the relevant complications associated with bulimia.	The complications associated with bulimia include the following: —Endocrinologic: dysmenorrhea (painful menstruation) —Fluid- and electrolyte-related: potassium deficiency, decreased chloride, and increased or decreased sodium —Dental: extensive decay of teeth and nonreversible perimyolysis (enamel erosion).
7 Identify the components of the treatment regimen for bulimia.	The components of the treatment regimen for bulimia include the following: —Individual psychotherapy —Group psychotherapy —Family therapy —Dietary realignment —Behavior modification.

BULIMAREXIA

Patient objectives	*Teaching plan content*
1 Define bulimarexia.	In bulimarexia, the patient consumes huge quantities of food during short intervals, later ridding herself of the calories by self-induced vomiting, laxatives, or extreme

fasting. This definitive binge-and-purge syndrome encompasses behaviors of both anorexia nervosa and bulimia.

2 **Identify the characteristics of a bulimarexic patient.**	The characteristics of a bulimarexic patient include the following: —Binge-and-purge behavior —Insistence on secrecy in treatment —Ability to maintain normal body weight and attractiveness accompanied by dissatisfaction with weight and body proportions —Perfectionism —Desire to please everyone —Isolation from others —Strong need for success —Strong need to achieve.
3 **Explain the causes of bulimarexia.**	The causes of bulimarexia are the same as the causes of anorexia nervosa and bulimia. (See the "Anorexia Nervosa" teaching plan in this chapter.)
4 **State the goals of the treatment regimen for bulimarexia.**	The goals of the treatment regimen for bulimarexia include the following: —Restoring the patient's nutritional status to normal (if necessary) —Establishing normal eating behaviors —Helping the patient develop non-food-related coping mechanisms —Decreasing associations between food and stress reduction —Establishing trusting therapeutic relationships within the group therapy framework.
5 **Identify the components of the treatment regimen for bulimarexia.**	The treatment regimen for bulimarexia includes these components: —Short-term group psychotherapy —Behavioral contracting —Family therapy, if possible —Establishment of a "sponsor," similar to the method used by Alcoholics Anonymous.

OBESITY

Patient objectives	*Teaching plan content*
1 **Define obesity.**	Obesity is characterized by excessive accumulation of fat in the body.

2 Explain the cause of obesity.	Obesity occurs when more calories are eaten than are expended or "burned off." Theories about the reasons why fat accumulates include the following: —Hypothalamic dysfunction of satiety and hunger regulation centers —Genetic predisposition —Abnormal absorption of nutrients —Impaired action of gastrointestinal tract, growth hormones, hormone regulators, and insulin —Environmental and social factors (activity levels and learned patterns of eating) —Psychological/emotional disturbances.
3 Describe the assessment process for diagnosing obesity.	The assessment process for diagnosing obesity is as follows: —Physical observation of appearance —Comparison of patient's weight/height ratio to standardized weight chart (20 percent over standardized table indicates obesity) —Measurement of the skin-fold thickness.
4 Identify the health hazards associated with obesity.	The following health hazards are associated with obesity: —Diabetes (five times more common among the obese) —Gallbladder disease —Osteoarthritis —Shortness of breath —Hypertension —Stroke —Coronary artery disease (more common among obese men less than 40 years old than among the general population) —Menstrual irregularities.
5 Identify the goals of the treatment regimen for obesity.	Weight reduction and maintenance of reduced weight are the goals of the treatment regimen for obesity.
6 Identify the components of the treatment regimen for obesity.	The following are components of the treatment regimen for obesity: —Well-planned, prescribed diet, managed by a dietitian —Pharmacological intervention —Physical activity —Surgical intervention —Group self-help (Overeaters Anonymous, Weight Watchers, Take Off Pounds Sensibly [TOPS]).

| 7 Identify the relevant benefits of weight reduction. | The benefits of weight reduction include the following:
—Reduction in blood pressure
—Improved cardiac function
—Improved pulmonary ventilation
—Reduction in osteoarthritis pain and low-back pain
—Improved peripheral vascular circulation
—Reduction in fatigue; increase in energy
—Improved self-esteem
—Increased sociability
—Improved body image
—Improved relationships, including sexual ones. |

 Explaining treatments

FAMILY THERAPY

Patient objectives	Teaching plan content
1 Define family therapy.	Family therapy is a psychotherapeutic technique in which the entire family is viewed as a system instead of a group of separate individuals.
2 State the purposes of family therapy.	The following are the purposes of family therapy: —To observe and collect data about the family's interactional patterns —To observe and collect data on the "identified" patient or patients in relation to the family as a whole —To formulate a workable hypothesis for use in exploring the family's dysfunction —To help the family understand what interpersonal factors are fostering the dysfunctional behavior by the entire family or by individual members.

INDIVIDUAL PSYCHOTHERAPY

Patient objectives	Teaching plan content
1 Define individual psychotherapy.	Individual psychotherapy is a relationship between a patient and therapist who engage in a confidential and primarily verbal series of interactions over an agreed upon period of time, with mutually agreed-on goals that focus on behavioral changes for the patient.
2 State the purposes of individual psychotherapy.	The purposes of individual psychotherapy are as follows:

—To remove, modify, or retard existing symptoms
—To alleviate or diminish disturbed behavioral patterns
—To promote positive personality growth and development.

3 **Describe the phases of individual psychotherapy.**

The phases of individual psychotherapy are as follows:
—The introductory phase is the period when the patient and therapist become acquainted and assess each other's limits and boundaries.
—The working phase develops as the patient comes to the sessions prepared to discuss problems and issues and to actively participate in problem solving.
—The termination phase occurs when there is a mutual decision to terminate, the therapist or patient relocates, or the patient decides to end treatment.

GROUP PSYCHOTHERAPY

Patient objectives	*Teaching plan content*
1 **Define group psychotherapy.**	Group psychotherapy is a method of therapeutic intervention in which individual and intrapsychic structures are explored and analyzed within the group process. As individuals interact in a group over time, they are able to observe their own and one another's desires, conflicts, and motivations.
2 **State the purposes of group psychotherapy.**	The purposes of group psychotherapy are as follows: —To examine and explore the behavior of group members —To help them adopt more satisfying modes of interaction.
3 **Describe the process of group psychotherapy.**	Group psychotherapy is conducted as follows: —All prospective members are seen at least once on an individual basis before admission to the group. —The patient is not coached or prepared for what will happen in the group or who will be there. —General information is provided, such as "The group is a place to discuss feelings, issues, and problems and to explore reactions and solutions." —Group members sit in a circle with no table between them, and no one sits on the floor. —Generally, weekly sessions last for 1½ hours, and daily sessions last for 1 hour. —Sessions begin and end on time. —There is a standing rule against physical violence.

4 Discuss patient guidelines for group psychotherapy.	Patient guidelines for group psychotherapy are as follows: —She should attend every session or inform the group leader beforehand of her expected absence or of a crisis situation. —She should be as open as possible. —She must not become physically violent. —She should not discuss group matters outside the group.

BEHAVIOR MODIFICATION

Patient objectives	*Teaching plan content*
1 Define behavior modification.	Behavior modification is a therapeutic intervention in which patients are reeducated, based on the principles of Pavlovian conditioning. It is designed to change their behavior in a desired direction (i.e., weight loss or weight gain).
2 State the goals of a behavior modification program.	The following are goals of a behavior modification program: —To strengthen the patient's adaptive behaviors —To weaken the patient's maladaptive behaviors —To teach the patient new behaviors for living with herself, her family, and her environment.
3 Identify the components of a behavior modification program.	The components of a behavior modification program answer the following questions: —What are the target behaviors? —In what settings do the target behaviors occur? —What are reinforcers and punishers for the patient? —Can these reinforcers and punishers be easily controlled? —What schedule of reinforcement or punishment should be used?

NASOGASTRIC TUBE (N.G.T.) FEEDING

Patient objectives	*Teaching plan content*
1 Define NGT feeding.	NGT feeding involves the insertion of a tube through the patient's nose into her stomach to administer medication and supplemental feedings.
2 State the relevant purpose of NGT feeding.	The purpose of NGT feeding in the treatment of eating disorders is to improve nutritional status when the patient is emaciated and to administer medications.

3 Describe the procedure used in NGT feeding.	NGT feeding is performed as follows: —The patient will be seated upright. —The tube will be advanced slowly into her nose and downward. —She will be encouraged to swallow to help the tube pass into the esophagus. —The tube will be advanced as the patient swallows. —When the tube is thought to be in place, it will be tested for placement by injecting air into the tube and listening to the stomach and attempting to aspirate contents from the patient's stomach. —On confirmation of tube placement, feeding will be started. —The tube feeding may be a continuous flow, and the flow rate will be monitored mechanically to ensure accuracy. —The tube feeding may be intermittent, with a flow of 30 to 60 minutes every 4 to 6 hours. The NGT will be removed between feedings to prevent the patient from siphoning out the nutritional supplement.
4 Discuss patient guidelines for NGT feeding.	Patient guidelines for NGT feeding are as follows: —She will have to blow her nose before tube insertion. —She should tell staff members before NGT insertion if she has had nasal surgery. —She will have to swallow and take deep breaths during the insertion phase. —She will have to make a contract to leave the NGT in place and not change the flow rate or siphon out the tube feeding.
5 Identify the potential complications of NGT feeding.	The potential complications of NGT feeding are as follows: —Skin erosion at the nostril —Sinusitis —Esophagitis —Esophagotracheal fistulas —Gastric ulceration —Pulmonary infection —Oral infection.

TOTAL PARENTERAL NUTRITION (T.P.N.)

Patient objectives	*Teaching plan content*
1 Define TPN.	TPN, or intravenous hyperalimentation (IVH), is the I.V. administration of a solution of dextrose, proteins, electrolytes, vitamins, and trace elements in amounts that exceed the patient's energy expenditure to help

her achieve an anabolic (building-up) state and to gain weight. The usual route of administration is by the superior vena cava, through an I.V. line inserted in the subclavian vein.

2 State the purpose of TPN.

The purpose of TPN is to restore the patient's normal nutritional status and promote weight gain.

3 Describe the procedure used in TPN.

TPN is performed as follows:
—The patient will be placed supine, with her head turned away from the catheter insertion site.
—A sterile drape will be placed over her.
—The physician will prepare the insertion site with a cold antiseptic solution.
—The physician will insert the I.V. catheter into the patient's subclavian vein and connect it to an I.V. solution.
—After insertion, anchoring, and dressing of the catheter line, a chest X-ray will be taken to check the position of the catheter.
—The hyperalimentation solution is high in glucose content, so the infusion will start slowly to allow the patient's pancreatic beta cells to adapt to it by increasing insulin output.
—The catheter dressing will be changed every 24 hours or if it becomes wet or soiled.
—The nutrients and the I.V. site will be frequently monitored.
—The hyperalimentation flow rate will be monitored and controlled by an I.V. pump. The patient who is able to walk may be able to wear an ambulatory hyperalimentation vest.

4 Discuss patient guidelines for TPN.

Patient guidelines for TPN are as follows:
—She must not alter the flow rate unless instructed to do so.
—She needs to "bear down" or hold her breath while the I.V. tubing is changed to increase intrathoracic pressure and prevent air embolization.
—She should not touch the I.V. line or dressing.
—She should inform staff members *immediately* if the line becomes disconnected or dislodged.
—She should inform staff members if she experiences any pain, tenderness, or discomfort at the site of insertion.

5 Identify the possible complications of TPN.

The possible complications of TPN include the following:
—Catheter-related sepsis (infection)

—Subclavian/jugular vein thrombosis (blood clot)
—Air embolism (air obstruction, or air bubble)
—Extravasation (pouring out of the catheter's contents into the skin), which can cause necrosis.

SURGICAL INTERVENTION: JEJUNOILEAL BYPASS OR GASTRIC PARTITIONING (PLICATION)

Patient objectives	Teaching plan content
1 Describe the jejuno-ileal bypass as a treatment for obesity.	The jejunoileal bypass creates a shunt between the jejunum and the terminal ileum that leaves only 14″ to 18″ of small intestine; this induces a permanent malabsorption syndrome. (An illustration can be used to demonstrate the location of these structures in the gastrointestinal tract.)
2 Describe gastric partitioning (plication) as a treatment for obesity.	Gastric partitioning creates a small pouch by introducing two rows of staples across the stomach, approximately 1.5 cm distal to the gastroesophageal junction, leaving a small opening through which food passes. Patients are satisfied after eating small amounts of food and do not experience the nutritional problems associated with the bypass.
3 List the potential complications of surgical treatment for obesity.	The potential complications of surgical treatment for obesity are as follows: —Severe diarrhea —Electrolyte disturbances —Urinary calculi (stones) —Liver failure —Polyarthritis.

Patient-Teaching Aid

GIVING T.P.N. THROUGH YOUR HICKMAN CATHETER

Dear Patient:

At home, you will use the Hickman catheter to feed yourself special I.V. fluid. These feedings are called TPN (total parenteral nutrition).

Your nurse has helped you learn how to give yourself TPN. Use this patient-teaching aid as a reminder of what you have learned. Carefully read this aid before you leave the hospital. If you have questions, be sure to ask your nurse. If you have questions or problems after you go home, contact _____.

Follow all the daily-care guidelines your nurse has taught you. By doing so, you will reduce the risk of a complication, such as infection.

Now, here is how to prepare for a TPN feeding:

1

First, gather the infusion pump, pump tubing, filter, needle, tape, and TPN solution. Set up this equipment according to the instructions for your pump. Then, use the tape to secure all tubing junctions, as shown here.

If you have long hair, tie it back. Make sure your catheter's clamp is secure. Then, thoroughly wash and dry your hands.

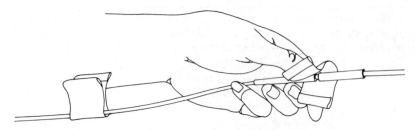

2

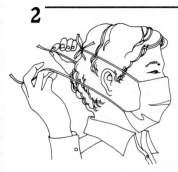

Chances are, the hospital or clinic has provided you with supplies for this procedure. For this patient-teaching aid, we will assume you are using prepackaged supplies. If you are not, gather this equipment: two alcohol swabs, two povidone-iodine swabs, four sterile gauze pads, two pairs of sterile disposable gloves, a face mask, a sterile disposable towel, clean tape, an empty plastic bag, scissors, a bottle of alcohol, and a clean cloth.

Put on the face mask.

GIVING T.P.N. THROUGH YOUR HICKMAN CATHETER—*continued*

3

Using alcohol, wipe the table where you will lay your supplies. Unbutton or take off your shirt, to expose the catheter. While the table dries, again wash and dry your hands.

Put the clean tape and scissors on the table, to one side. Tape the empty plastic bag to the table's edge to collect soiled equipment.

Among your prepackaged equipment, the sterile supplies are contained in a kit wrapped with sterile paper. Place the kit on the clean table and unwrap it. As you do, take care to touch only the *outside* of the paper. Remember, everything *inside* the paper is sterile. You will find that the sterile gloves have been placed on top of your sterile equipment. IMPORTANT: Do not let the sterile equipment touch *anything* that is not sterile: for example, your hands, the tape, or the scissors.

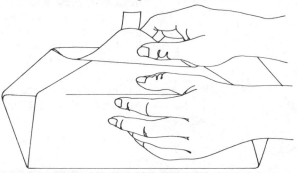

4

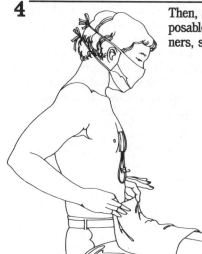

Then, sit down near the table and put the sterile disposable towel on your lap. (Handle it only by the corners, so most of it stays sterile.)

GIVING T.P.N. THROUGH YOUR HICKMAN CATHETER—*continued*

5

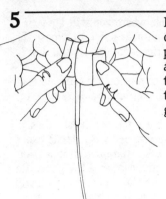

Free your catheter by removing the tape holding the catheter cap to the dressing. Discard the tape in the plastic bag. Also remove and discard the gauze pad and tape around the cap. Then, drop the capped catheter tip onto the sterile towel. NOTE: Once the catheter tip touches the towel, this part of the towel is no longer sterile.

6

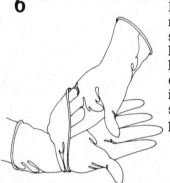

Put on a pair of sterile gloves, using the special technique your nurse has taught you. Then, put another sterile glove on your dominant hand. If you are right-handed, you now have two sterile gloves on your right hand and one sterile glove on your left hand. Now you can handle your sterile equipment without contaminating it. Unwrap the alcohol swabs, povidone-iodine swabs, and gauze pads. Spread them out on the sterile paper, so you can see and grasp everything.

7

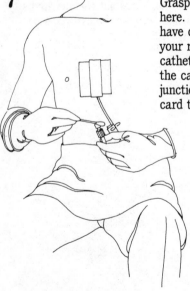

Grasp the catheter tip with your left hand, as shown here. (Your left hand is no longer sterile, because you have contaminated it by touching the catheter.) Using your right hand, pick up an alcohol swab and clean the catheter tip. To do so, first clean the junction between the catheter tip and the catheter cap (catheter-cap junction); then, clean above and below the junction. Discard the alcohol swab in the plastic bag.

GIVING T.P.N. THROUGH YOUR HICKMAN CATHETER—*continued*

8

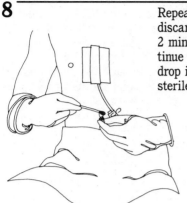

Repeat the procedure with a povidone-iodine swab, and discard the swab. Let the povidone-iodine dry for about 2 minutes, so it has time to work. While you wait, continue to hold the catheter in your left hand; do not drop it on the towel, because the towel is no longer sterile.

9

Then, pick up one dry gauze pad with your right (sterile) hand, and wipe the povidone-iodine from the catheter. Discard the gauze pad.

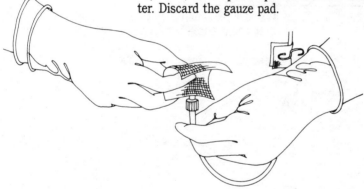

10

With your right hand, pick up a fresh gauze pad by a corner, so it falls open. Lay it on a dry part of the towel. Remember, this pad is sterile, so do not allow anything to contaminate it.

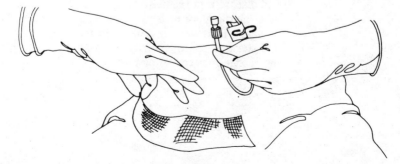

GIVING T.P.N. THROUGH YOUR HICKMAN CATHETER—*continued*

11

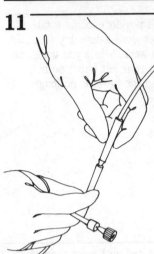

Using your right hand, unscrew the catheter cap and discard it in the plastic bag. (Your right hand is no longer sterile.) Then, still using your right hand, pick up the capped needle on the end of the infusion pump's tubing as shown here. Slip the cap between the second and third fingers of your left hand, and remove the needle from the tubing.

12

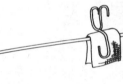

Connect the pump tubing to the catheter. Now, gently drop the junction between the catheter and pump tubing (catheter-tubing junction) into the center of the open sterile gauze pad, as shown.

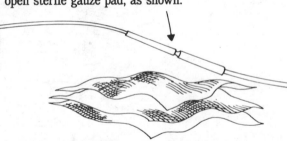

13

Check the pump setting for accuracy. Then, start the pump and immediately remove the clamp on your catheter. Place the clamp away from your sterile supplies.

Now, remove the outer glove from your right hand, and discard it in the plastic bag. Because you have another sterile glove underneath, your right hand is sterile again. Hold your right hand away from the catheter and sterile supplies, and rub your right hand's fingers together to remove any powder.

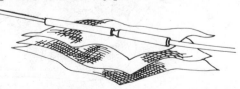

GIVING T.P.N. THROUGH YOUR HICKMAN CATHETER—*continued*

14

With your left hand, lift the catheter. Using your right (sterile) hand, clean the catheter-tubing junction with an alcohol swab. Repeat the procedure with a povidone-iodine swab. Wait at least 2 minutes; then, wipe the junction off with a sterile gauze pad as shown here.

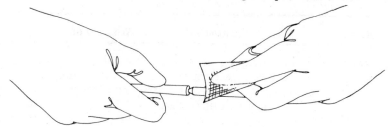

15

With your right hand, pick up another gauze pad by one corner, so it falls open. Drop it on a dry area of the towel. Gently drop the junction onto it as shown here.

Holding your hands away from the catheter-tubing junction and sterile supplies, remove your gloves. Rub your hands to remove any powder.

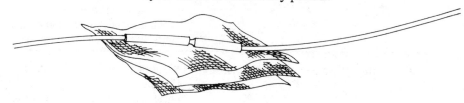

16

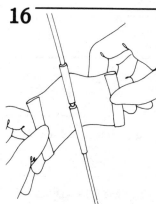

Cover and secure the junction with tape. (Do not touch the adhesive side of the tape or the junction with your hands.) Fold over the edges of the tape to make tabs for easier removal. Tape around the junction, and place another tabbed piece of tape lengthwise along the junction.

Remove your mask. Discard the mask, the towel, and the gauze pads in the plastic bag. Retape the catheter to the exit site dressing. Finally, make sure the tubing is free of kinks and all its connections are secure.

Patient-Teaching Aid

TROUBLESHOOTING HOME TOTAL PARENTERAL NUTRITION

Dear Patient:
Complications, although rare, may develop while you are undergoing home total parenteral nutrition. Here are signs and symptoms to watch for, and what to do about them:

Problem	What to watch for	What to do
Infiltration	Swelling of tissues around catheter insertion site (shoulder, neck, or arm), discomfort, pain in shoulder or arm on catheter side, swollen tissues cooler than rest of body tissues	• Call the physician immediately if you think the catheter has come out of the vein or has ruptured. • Slow the flow rate if you cannot reach the physician immediately.
Cloudy solution or sediment in solution	Solution cloudy or showing undissolved particles	• Do not use. Solution may be contaminated. Return solution container to pharmacy at once for exchange. • If you are mixing your own solution, take extra care with preparation, and do not prepare more than 24 hours' worth of solution at a time.
Too-rapid infusion	Nausea, headache, lassitude	• Check to be sure solution is flowing at the rate ordered by your physician. If you are using an infusion pump, check for mechanical problems. • If the flow rate is correct and symptoms persist, contact your physician.
Catheter dislodgment	Catheter pulled out of vein	• Place a sterile gauze pad on insertion site, and apply pressure. • Notify your physician.
Crack or break in catheter tubing	Fluid leaking out through crack or break in tubing	• Apply padded hemostat above break, to prevent entry of air. • Call your physician at once.
Clotted catheter	Solution flow stops and does not enter the vein	• Notify physician. He may instill streptokinase or heparin into the catheter to try to dissolve clot.

TROUBLESHOOTING HOME TOTAL PARENTERAL NUTRITION—*continued*

Problem	What to watch for	What to do
Hyperglycemia (high blood glucose level)	Fatigue, restlessness, confusion, anxiety, weakness, urine tests positive for sugar, and possibly delirium and/or coma	• Notify physician at once.
Phlebitis	Pain, tenderness, skin redness and warmth	• Rest, and apply gentle heat to the site. Elevate your arm if the catheter is inserted in your arm. • Relief should occur within 24 to 72 hours, and condition should subside within 3 to 5 days. • Notify your physician immediately. He may want to examine you or give you additional care instructions.
Infection	Fever (body temperature above 100° F. [37.8° C.]), redness and/or pus at insertion site	• Notify your physician so he can determine the fever's source. • If infection is present, the physician will remove the catheter to have the tip cultured.
Thrombosis	Redness and swelling around catheter entrance site, swelling of catheterized arm and of neck or face on catheter's side of body, pain at insertion site and along vein, rapid heartbeat, fever	• Notify your physician at once. He will evaluate the catheter for removal. • These symptoms usually indicate blood clot formation around the catheter, a problem that requires prompt medical and nursing treatment.
Air embolism	Apprehension, chest pain, rapid heartbeat, low blood pressure resulting in dizziness and fainting, bluish appearance; problem caused by air entering catheter, usually during bottle changes	• Call your physician immediately. If symptoms are severe, go to hospital emergency department at once. • Lie on your left side, with your head slightly lower than the rest of your body.

NOTE: Complications from home total parenteral nutrition are uncommon if proper technique is maintained. Despite the possibility of these problems, home total parenteral nutrition results in decreased hospitalization and significant cost savings for you. In addition, this therapy lets you maintain a more normal life-style.

Patient-Teaching Aid

HOME CARE FOR TOTAL PARENTERAL NUTRITION (T.P.N.)

Dear Patient:

At home, you will use a Hickman catheter to give yourself total parenteral nutrition (TPN). To prevent problems and detect early signs of rare complications, follow these guidelines:

1   Take your temperature every day, just after getting up in the morning, and write it down. Also, weigh yourself every morning, and write down your weight. (Wear similar clothing and use the same scale for each weighing.)

2   Every morning, test a second-voided urine specimen for ketones and glucose. Keep a record of the results for your physician.

3   For convenience, try keeping your records on a small calendar; also, jot down any problems you are having. These records help the physician determine how you are doing.

4   Do not forget to keep your appointments for regular blood testing (once a week, or as directed by your physician). If you cannot regularly visit the physician or clinic, a visiting nurse can help you at home. A weekly blood test helps the physician decide if any changes need to be made in your TPN solution.

5   Keep your TPN containers in the refrigerator. For your comfort during feeding, let a container warm to room temperature for about 1 hour before using it. NOTE: Do not freeze the solution.

6   Store your TPN solution in a safe part of the refrigerator: for example, the top shelf, where nothing is likely to spill on it.

7   Before using any TPN solution, hold it up to the light and make sure it looks clear. Do not use it if it looks cloudy or has an unusual color. (Some solutions look yellow, depending on the additives; make sure you

HOME CARE FOR TOTAL PARENTERAL NUTRITION (T.P.N.)—*continued*

know your solution's normal color.) Also, do not use it if the container is cracked, torn, or damaged. Finally, check the container's expiration date to make sure the solution is fresh. Your pharmacist will probably mark on the container the date he mixed the solution. Use the solution within a week of this date, unless the pharmacist or physician directs differently.

8

Put all your supplies together in a box or basket, so you can easily find everything you need for each TPN administration. To keep your supplies clean, put them in a place where they will not get dusty or be disturbed. Also, place them out of children's reach.

9

Never reuse any supplies, unless your physician or nurse says it is permitted.

10

Change your Hickman catheter's cap after each TPN administration.

Oncologic Disorders

 Patient-learner data base*

Areas of potential knowledge deficit
Cancer risk factors:
—Tobacco use
—Diet high in fat or salt-cured, smoked, and nitrate-
cured foods
—Personal or family history of cancer
—Overweight
—Alcohol use
—Exposure to sun
—Exposure to industrial agents
—Excessive exposure to X-rays
Anatomy and physiology of the involved body site
Definition of the specific oncologic disorder
Causes of the oncologic disorder
Symptoms associated with the oncologic disorder
Treatment of the oncologic disorder
—Chemotherapy
—Radiation therapy
—Surgery
—Diet
Complications of the specific oncologic disorder

 Explaining diagnostic tests

BONE MARROW BIOPSY/ASPIRATION

Patient objectives	*Teaching plan content*
1 Define bone marrow biopsy.	In bone marrow biopsy, a core of bone marrow cells is removed with a needle, under a local anesthetic.

*A general assessment should be done for all patients. For general assessment guidelines, see Chapter 1, Principles of Patient Teaching.

2 Define bone marrow aspiration.	In bone marrow aspiration, fluid from the bone marrow is removed with a needle, under a local anesthetic.
3 State the purposes of a bone marrow biopsy/aspiration.	The purposes of bone marrow biopsy/aspiration include the following: —To diagnose thrombocytopenia, leukemias, granulomas, and aplastic, hypoplastic, and pernicious anemias —To diagnose primary and metastatic tumors —To determine the cause of infection —To aid in the staging of a disease, such as Hodgkin's disease —To evaluate the effectiveness of chemotherapy and help monitor myelosuppression (bone marrow suppression).
4 Describe the procedure used in a bone marrow biopsy/aspiration.	Just before the procedure, the patient may receive a mild sedative. —He will be positioned to allow easy access to the bone marrow site selected by the physician. —The skin over the biopsy site will be cleansed with an antibacterial agent, and then drapes will be placed around the site. —A local anesthetic will be injected into the skin to numb the area. —After the area is numb, a needle will be inserted into the bone marrow to obtain a specimen. —The patient will feel pressure when the biopsy needle is inserted and a brief, pulling pain when the marrow is removed. —When the specimen has been obtained, the needle will be withdrawn and pressure applied to the site for 5 to 15 minutes. —The site will then be cleansed again and a sterile dressing applied.
5 Explain patient guidelines for a bone marrow biopsy/aspiration.	Patient guidelines include the following: —Food or fluids are not restricted before the procedure, which usually takes 5 to 10 minutes. —A consent form must be signed. —The patient should know which bone—sternum, anterior or posterior iliac crest, vertebral spinous process, rib, or tibia—will be the biopsy site. —The patient should know where the procedure will take place and who will be present. —During the procedure, the patient must remain as still as possible but may talk. —For 4 to 12 hours after the procedure, the biopsy site will be checked for bleeding and inflammation. Temperature, pulse, blood pressure, and breathing patterns will be monitored during this period.

BONE SCAN

Patient objectives	Teaching plan content
1 Define bone scan.	A bone scan is a test in which images of the skeleton are recorded by a camera after I.V. injection of a radioactive substance to identify abnormal bone.
2 State the purpose of a bone scan.	The purposes of a bone scan include the following: —To detect or rule out malignant bone lesions —To detect bone trauma caused by pathologic fracture.
3 Describe the procedure used in a bone scan.	The patient will receive an I.V. injection of a radioactive substance in his room. This substance is harmless and emits less radiation than a standard X-ray machine. —He will be asked to drink several glasses of water or tea in the interval between injection of the radioactive substance and the actual scanning (about 1 to 3 hours). —He will be asked to void and will then be taken to the Nuclear Medicine Department for the scan. —He will be placed on the scanner table and may be asked to assume various positions. —The procedure takes about 1 hour and is painless. —Someone will be available to explain things and reassure him during the procedure.
4 Explain patient guidelines for a bone scan.	Patient guidelines include the following: —The patient will have to sign a consent form. —Fluid intake will be kept to a minimum before the radioactive substance is injected. —The patient should know who will perform the test and when it will be done. —After the procedure, he will be returned to his room and may resume his usual activities. —His injection site will be checked for redness or swelling. Warm soaks can be applied to lessen discomfort at the site.

LIVER-SPLEEN SCAN

Patient objectives	Teaching plan content
1 Define liver-spleen scan.	A liver-spleen scan is a test in which the distribution of radioactivity within the liver and spleen is recorded by a camera after I.V. injection of a radioactive substance. The image recorded can be used to identify abnormal tissue.

2 State the purpose of a liver-spleen scan.	The purposes of a liver-spleen scan include the following: —To screen for liver metastasis (spread of cancer cells to sites other than the primary site) —To detect tumors, cysts, and abscesses in the liver and spleen.
3 Describe the procedure used in a liver-spleen scan.	The patient will receive an I.V. injection of a radioactive substance just before the scan, which takes about 1 hour and is painless. The radioactive substance is harmless and emits less radiation than a standard X-ray machine. —He will be placed on the scanner table and will be asked to assume various positions. —He will be asked to lie still and to breathe quietly as the images are recorded. He may also be asked to hold his breath briefly. —The scanner may touch his abdomen or make a soft clicking noise as it moves across his abdomen. —Someone will be available to explain things and reassure him during the procedure.
4 Explain patient guidelines for a liver-spleen scan.	Patient guidelines include the following: —The patient will have to sign a consent form. —He should know who will perform the test and when and where it will be done. —After the procedure, he will be returned to his room and may resume his usual activities. —He will be observed for signs of fever or reaction to the radioactive substance, such as itching or difficulty breathing. If he feels uncomfortable in any way, he should report this development.

MAMMOGRAPHY

Patient objectives	*Teaching plan content*
1 Define mammography.	Mammography is an X-ray of the breast(s).
2 State the purpose of mammography.	The purposes of mammography include the following: —To screen for breast malignancy —To investigate palpable and unpalpable breast masses, breast pain, or nipple discharge —To help differentiate between benign and malignant breast disease.
3 Describe the procedure used in mammography.	During mammography, the patient can expect the following: —She will be seated on a chair and asked to rest one of her breasts on a table above an X-ray cassette. A

plastic compressor will be placed on her breast, and she will be asked to hold her breath as an X-ray is taken.
—The X-ray machine will be rotated, the breast compressed again, and another X-ray taken.
—The procedure will then be repeated on the other breast.
—Although the test takes only about 15 to 30 minutes to perform, the patient may be asked to wait while the films are checked to make sure they are readable.

4 Explain patient guidelines for mammography.	Patient guidelines include the following: —The patient should know who will perform the test, when and where it will be done, and that it is painless. —Just before the test, she will be asked to remove all jewelry and clothing above her waist and to put on a gown that opens in the front. —After the test has been completed, she may resume her normal activities.

COMPUTED TOMOGRAPHY (C.T.)

Patient objectives	*Teaching plan content*
1 Define CT.	CT is a procedure in which multiple X-ray beams are directed at selected layers of the body and converted by computer into cross-sectional images (tomograms), which are displayed on a screen similar to a TV screen. CT can be used to examine any part of the body and may include injection of a radioactive substance to produce clearer images of certain body structures.
2 State the purpose of CT.	The purposes of CT include the following: —To detect primary tumors or metastases —To identify the specific location and shape of a tumor —To show the progression of a tumor, as well as the effects of therapy.
3 Describe the procedure used in CT.	During CT, the patient can expect the following: —He will be positioned on an X-ray table and moved into a large, ring-shaped X-ray machine, which will rotate around him. The machine may be noisy. —He will have to lie still during the test and may be asked to hold his breath a few times. —A radiopaque substance may be injected into a vein in his arm. The amount of radiation exposure will be minimal, but he may experience a warm feeling, salty taste, or slight nausea. —Someone will be available to explain things and reassure him during the procedure.

4 Explain patient guidelines for CT.	Patient guidelines include the following: —The patient will have to sign a consent form. —He should know who will perform the test, when and where it will be done, and that it usually takes 1½ hours. —He will be asked if he is sensitive to iodine or radiographic dyes. —If a radiopaque contrast medium will be used, food and fluids will be restricted for 4 hours before the test. —He will have to remove all jewelry before the test. —After the procedure, he will be returned to his room and may resume his usual activities. —He will be observed for signs of a reaction to the radiopaque substance, such as itching, low or high blood pressure, or difficulty breathing. If he feels uncomfortable in any way, he should report this development.

MAGNETIC RESONANCE IMAGING (M.R.I.)

Patient objectives	*Teaching plan content*
1 Define MRI.	MRI provides images of body structure by directing radio and magnetic waves at body tissues.
2 State the purpose of MRI.	The purposes of MRI include the following: —To detect structural and biochemical abnormalities —To detect small lesions or tumors that other scans are unable to detect —To detect metastatic bone disease and soft-tissue masses.
3 Describe the procedure used in MRI.	During MRI, the patient can expect the following: —He will be positioned on a table that will then be moved into a long tunnel in the machine. The machine will be quiet. —He will have to lie very still (usually a strap is placed around the patient to prevent mobility) and may occasionally be asked to hold his breath. —The procedure is painless, but he may feel claustrophobic. (Many institutions have mirrors set up so that the patient can see outside the machine.) Someone will be in the room or in voice contact with him at all times. —For examination of the head, a plexiglass helmet containing radio transmitters or a cloth containing surface body wires will be taped to his head. —For examination of the chest or spine, a cloth containing surface body wires will be secured to his body.

4 Explain patient guidelines for MRI.

Patient guidelines include the following:
—He should know who will perform the test, when and where it will be done, and that it may take from 15 minutes to 1 hour.
—All metal objects and jewelry must be removed before the test. Patients with implanted surgical clips and pacemakers should not undergo this test.
—After the procedure, he will be returned to his room and may resume his usual activities.

INCISIONAL BIOPSY

Patient objectives	*Teaching plan content*
1 Define incisional biopsy.	Incisional biopsy is a technique for removing tissue specimens from large, multiple, hidden lesions. It may be done by aspiration (removal of a small quantity of cells), needle (removal of a core of tissue), or punch (removal of tissue from the core of a lesion).
2 State the purpose of an incisional biopsy.	The purpose of an incisional biopsy is to provide tissue for microscopic examination that can distinguish between benign and malignant tissue.
3 Explain patient guidelines for an incisional biopsy.	Patient guidelines include the following: —The patient will be asked to sign a consent form. —He should know who will perform the procedure and where and when it will be done. —During the procedure, he will be asked not to move. —He will be positioned to allow easy access to the biopsy site. —A local anesthetic will be injected into his skin to numb the site after it has been cleansed. —A dressing may be placed over the biopsy site after the procedure. —If a dressing is in place, it should be kept clean and dry. —The site should be observed for tenderness, bleeding, or redness. The physician should be notified if any of these are present. —If the area is painful, an analgesic, such as aspirin, acetaminophen, or codeine, may relieve the discomfort.

EXCISIONAL BIOPSY (OPEN BIOPSY)

Patient objectives	*Teaching plan content*
1 Define open biopsy.	An open biopsy allows surgical removal of suspicious tissue or a mass under a local or general anesthetic, depending on the biopsy site.
2 State the purpose of an open biopsy.	The purposes of an open biopsy include the following: —To provide tissue for microscopic examination that can distinguish between benign and malignant disease —To provide treatment by removing a malignant mass.
3 Describe the procedure used in an open biopsy.	During an open biopsy, the patient can expect the following: —If a local anesthetic is to be used, the biopsy may be performed at the bedside, in a treatment room, or in the physician's office. • The patient will be positioned to allow easy access to the biopsy site. • The site will be cleansed and the local anesthetic injected into the skin to numb the area. —If a general anesthetic is to be used, the biopsy will be performed in the operating room. • The patient will be positioned on the operating table to allow the surgeon easy access to the biopsy site. • The general anesthetic will be given by a physician or nurse trained in the administration of anesthetics.
4 Explain patient guidelines for an open biopsy.	Patient guidelines include the following: —The patient must sign a consent form. —He should know who will perform the procedure and where and when it will be done. —If sutures are in place after the procedure, the area should be kept clean and dry. —If a dressing is in place, it should be kept clean and dry. (Adhesive strips should not be removed without the physician's approval.) —The site should be observed for tenderness, redness, or bleeding. The physician should be notified if any of these are present. —If the area is painful, an analgesic, such as aspirin, acetaminophen, or codeine, may relieve the discomfort. —If a general anesthetic was used, the patient may be groggy for several hours. His vital signs will be checked frequently to make sure they are normal, and an I.V. line may be in place for several hours after surgery.

Explaining disorders

BREAST CANCER

Patient objectives	*Teaching plan content*
1 Define cancer.	Cancer is the uncontrolled growth and reproduction of cells. Cancer cells differ from normal cells in their structure, size, function, and rapid rate of growth. They can spread throughout the body through the bloodstream or through the lymphatic system, or by direct extension from one site to another. The spread of cancer cells from their primary site to secondary sites is called metastasis. At secondary sites, these cells reproduce and form tumors or lesions.
2 Describe breast cancer.	Breast cancer is the most common malignancy affecting women. It is classified by the appearance of the cells and the location of the lesion or tumor. Treatment and prognosis are based on tissue type, location, and size of tumor; involvement of any lymph nodes; and the presence of metastasis. There are two types of breast cancer: —Ductal carcinomas make up over 90% of all breast cancers. In this form, the malignant cells arise from the mammary ducts. —In lobular carcinomas the malignant cells arise from the mammary lobules.
3 Identify the risk factors associated with breast cancer.	Risk factors associated with breast cancer include the following: —History of breast, endometrial, or ovarian cancer —Family history of breast cancer (Daughters and sisters of those with breast cancer have a higher risk of developing the disease.) —Age greater than 50 years —Reproductive history that includes no pregnancies, first child after age 30, early menarche, or late menopause —Long-term hormonal replacement for menopausal symptoms —Exposure to radiation —History of fibrocystic breast disease. In addition, the following potential risk factors are under investigation:

—Obesity
—High-fat diet
—Exposure to viruses
—Oral contraceptive use
—Stress.

---

4 Identify the symptoms of breast cancer.

The symptoms of breast cancer include the following:
—A lump or mass in the breast
—A change in breast symmetry or size
—A change in breast skin (thickening, dimpling, swelling, or ulceration)
—A change in skin temperature (warm, hot, or flushed areas)
—Unusual drainage or discharge
—A change in the nipple (itching, burning, erosion, or retraction).

---

5 Identify the screening methods for detection of breast cancer.

The following are screening methods for breast cancer detection:
—Yearly breast examination by a health care professional
—Monthly breast self-examination
—Yearly mammography after age 40.

---

6 Identify components of the treatment regimen for breast cancer.

Treatment of breast cancer is based on the stage of the disease and the patient's age and menopausal status. The following are possible components of the treatment regimen:
—Surgery
—Chemotherapy
—Radiation therapy
—Hormonal therapy.

---

7 Describe the relevant surgical procedure.

The following surgical procedures may be used alone or in combination with radiation therapy, chemotherapy, and/or hormonal therapy to treat breast cancer:
—In radical mastectomy, the entire breast, major and minor pectoral muscles, axillary lymph nodes, and fat are removed. This procedure is used when the tumor is large or invasive or when there is lymph node involvement.
—In modified radical mastectomy, the entire breast, some fat, and most of the axillary lymph nodes are removed, but the pectoral muscles are not removed. This procedure is often preferred over radical mastectomy because it may be just as effective without causing severe functional and cosmetic losses.
—In total or simple mastectomy, the entire breast and some fat tissue are removed, but muscles and axillary lymph nodes are left in place. This procedure is used for a large tumor without muscle or lymph node involvement.

—In partial or segmental mastectomy, the tumor, overlying skin, and a wedge of breast tissue (2 to 3 cm of tissue surrounding the tumor) are removed. This procedure is used for a small, self-contained tumor near the nipple.

—In local wide excision (lumpectomy), the tumor and a small amount of surrounding breast tissue are removed, but muscles and most of the skin are left intact. This procedure is used for very small, self-contained tumors or fibroid tumors that do not respond to conservative treatment.

8 Discuss postoperative procedures.

Postoperative procedures after a mastectomy are as follows:

—A dressing will be in place, and the patient may have a drain (Hemovac) in the operative area; this drain will be removed when drainage becomes minimal.

—The patient should never allow anyone to take her blood pressure, insert an I.V. line, withdraw blood, or inject medication into the affected arm. (To decrease the likelihood of this, a sign should be hung over the patient's bed and on the door of her room.)

—The affected arm will be elevated above the level of her heart on pillows.

—She may ease pain by lying on the affected side or by placing a hand or pillow on her incision. Pain medication will be available, and she should tell the nurse when she is in pain.

—The patient will need to turn in bed, to cough, and to deep-breathe for several days after surgery.

—She will need to exercise the affected arm to prevent lymphedema. Arm exercises should be planned with the physician, to avoid potential problems with the suture line.

—The following exercises can begin the day of surgery:
  • opening and closing the hand tightly six to eight times every 3 hours while awake
  • using the affected arm to wash the face, comb the hair, and eat.

—The following exercises can begin with the physician's approval: wall climbing, pendulum swing, pulley, and rope turning. (See *Strengthening Exercises: After Your Mastectomy,* pp. 152-153, for specific instructions on how to perform these exercises.)

—With the physician's approval, a volunteer from the American Cancer Society's Reach to Recovery program will visit the patient. Volunteers are former breast cancer patients who provide support and information.

9 Discuss patient guidelines to follow after discharge.

Patient guidelines after discharge include the following:
—Breast self-examination should be performed monthly. (See *Breast Self-Examination*, pp. 154-155, for step-by-step instructions.)
—Hand and arm exercises (if applicable) should be performed several times a day. The patient should stop these exercises when she feels pain. (See *Strengthening Exercises: After Your Mastectomy*, pp. 152-153.)
—The patient should know how to care for the surgical incision.
—The patient should know how to prevent postmastectomy complications (if applicable). (See *Preventing Postmastectomy Complications*, p. 151.)
—Swelling in the affected arm (if applicable) can be prevented by elevating the arm on pillows or by resting it across the back of a chair or sofa.
—All health care appointments should be kept.
—The patient should continue with her usual activities as much as possible.
—Breast surgery does not interfere with sexual function; the patient may resume sexual activity as soon as desired after surgery.

10 Discuss the use of breast prostheses.

Breast prostheses may be worn externally or implanted surgically during breast reconstruction.
—Once the suture line has healed, the patient can wear a prosthesis. Prostheses come in various sizes, so the size of the remaining breast can be closely matched.
—Many women are able to have breast reconstruction either at the time of the initial surgery or at a later date, depending on the invasiveness of the cancer and the need for further local treatment. Breast reconstruction is a surgical procedure in which a prosthesis is placed under the skin. Its size and shape matches the remaining breast as closely as possible. The physician should be asked about this option.

11 State the purpose of chemotherapy in treating breast cancer.

Chemotherapy for breast cancer involves the use of anticancer drugs to destroy cancer cells. Its goals are to eliminate the cancer, to stop its progression, and to relieve pain.

12 Describe the use of chemotherapeutic drugs in treating breast cancer.

Chemotherapeutic drugs used to treat breast cancer are usually most effective in combination. Drugs with different sites of attack on cancer cells and with different adverse effects are used together to destroy the greatest number of cancer cells and allow the patient to recover more quickly from any adverse effects. The drugs are given intermittently for prolonged periods (6 to 24 months) to ensure the elimination of cancer cells. The specific drugs and dosages depend on the stage of the cancer (progressive or regressive), the location of the tumor, and the patient's age and tolerance of the drugs.

13 Explain the medication regimen.	The following drugs may be used in the treatment of breast cancer: cyclophosphamide, methotrexate, 5-fluorouracil, prednisone, vincristine, doxorubicin, vinblastine, and chlorambucil. See Chapter 10, Drug Therapy, for specific medication instructions. For additional information, see the "Chemotherapy" teaching plan in this chapter.
14 State the purpose of radiation therapy in treating breast cancer.	The purpose of radiation therapy for breast cancer is to destroy cancer cells while damaging normal cells as little as possible. (Because cancer cells tend to divide more rapidly than normal cells, they are more vulnerable to radiation. Generally, normal cells recover from radiation faster than cancer cells do.) Radiation therapy has two goals: —The curative goal is to destroy all cancer cells in the primary tumor and surrounding lymph nodes. —The palliative goal is to relieve or prevent symptoms by shrinking tumor size.
15 Describe the use of radiation therapy in treating breast cancer.	Curative therapy is often administered 4 days a week for 5 to 7 weeks. Palliative therapy is usually administered in 3 to 10 treatments. Radiation may be delivered externally or internally. (See the "Radiation Therapy" teaching plan in this chapter for additional information.) —In external therapy, the source of radiation is an X-ray beam. Therapy is administered to the chest and axilla, in divided doses; it is painless. —In internal therapy, radiation is administered through a needle or tube placed beneath the skin (interstitial implants). • This therapy delivers a high radiation dose relatively quickly. • Interstitial implants are used to treat breast cancer in combination with lumpectomy and external beam radiation therapy. The implants direct additional radiation right to the tumor bed with fewer adverse effects than with external beam radiation. • This procedure is relatively quick and painless and can be performed under a local or general anesthetic.
16 State the purpose of hormonal therapy in treating breast cancer.	The purpose of hormonal therapy for breast cancer is to alter the cancer cells' environment, resulting in their death. It can be used only if the individual's body is

receptive. (A test will be done to determine if the patient is estrogen receptor-positive or -negative.)

17 **Discuss concerns about the diagnosis and treatment of breast cancer.**

A patient with breast cancer can discuss her concerns by verbalizing her feelings about having cancer, undergoing treatment, and accepting possible changes in body image. She should share her feelings with loved ones and seek information about services available to people with cancer, such as financial assistance and support groups.

LUNG CANCER

Patient objectives	Teaching plan content

1 **Define cancer.**

Cancer is the uncontrolled growth and reproduction of cells. Cancer cells differ from normal cells in their structure, size, function, and rapid rate of growth. They can spread throughout the body through the bloodstream or through the lymphatic system, or by direct extension from one site to another. The spread of cancer cells from their primary site to secondary sites is called metastasis. At secondary sites, these cells reproduce and form tumors or lesions.

2 **Describe lung cancer.**

Lung cancer refers to several types of cancer. (The physician should tell the patient what type of lung cancer he has.) The specific type is determined by microscopic examination of a tissue specimen and the location of the lesion. Treatment and prognosis depend on type of lung cancer, location of tumor, involvement of any lymph nodes, and presence of metastasis. The four most common types of lung cancer and their locations are as follows:
—Squamous cell (epidermoid) carcinoma, the most common type, tends to be centrally located within the lungs.
—Small-cell (including intermediate cell and lymphocyte or oat cell) carcinoma tends to be centrally located but metastasizes easily. It is the type of lung cancer most responsive to chemotherapy.
—Adenocarcinoma (including bronchioalveolar) is often located in the periphery of the lung.
—Large-cell carcinoma may occur in any part of the lungs.

3 **Identify the risk factors associated with lung cancer.**

The following risk factors are associated with lung cancer:
—Smoking (the most significant cause of all types of lung cancer)

—Family history of lung cancer
—Exposure to industrial carcinogens, such as asbestos, uranium, arsenic, nickel, iron oxides, chromium, radioactive dust, and coal dust.
In addition, the following potential risk factors are under investigation:
—Passive smoking (inhaling cigarette smoke generated by others)
—Stress.

---

4 Identify the symptoms of lung cancer.

The symptoms of lung cancer differ according to the location of the primary tumor and metastases. They may include the following:
—Persistent cough
—Productive cough
—Shortness of breath
—Wheezing
—Bloody sputum
—Hoarseness
—Chest pain (involving the chest, shoulder blades, and back)
—Chest wall pain (tends to be localized and sharp and to increase on inspiration)
—Fever
—Weakness
—Weight loss
—Loss of appetite.

---

5 Identify the screening methods for detection of lung cancer.

Screening methods for lung cancer detection include the following:
—Chest X-ray
—Sputum cytology (study of the cells within the sputum specimen).

---

6 Identify components of the treatment regimen for lung cancer.

The following are possible components of a lung cancer treatment regimen:
—Surgery
—Chemotherapy
—Radiation therapy
—Immunotherapy.

---

7 Describe the relevant surgical procedure.

The following surgical procedures may be used in the treatment of Stage I, Stage II, or Stage III squamous cell carcinoma, adenocarcinoma, and large-cell carcinoma:
—Wedge resection (segmental resection) is the removal of a segment of the involved lobe.
—Lobectomy is the removal of an entire lobe of the lung. This is the most common surgical procedure.
—Pneumonectomy is the removal of an entire lung (right or left).

8 **Discuss postoperative procedures for a lobectomy.**

After a lobectomy, the patient should expect the following:
—A large pressure dressing will be in place.
—One or two chest tubes will be in place on the affected side, to remove air and allow drainage from the affected lung. The tubes are usually removed several days after surgery.
—To prevent secretions from building up, the patient will be helped to cough and deep-breathe at least every 2 hours, using hands and pillows for support. (These procedures should be demonstrated to the patient preoperatively.)
—If the patient cannot cough effectively, he may need to be suctioned to remove secretions.
—The patient will have to change his position, since remaining in one position causes retention of secretions. He may lie supine (with the head of the bed elevated) or turn from side to side. (The surgeon may not want the patient to lie on the operative side or flat on his back.)
—An I.V. line will remain in place for several days. (The patient should know the signs and symptoms of infiltration.)
—The patient will begin exercises to strengthen chest muscles after surgery:
 • Immediate postoperative exercises include washing the face, combing the hair, and eating with the affected arm. The patient should use the affected arm whenever possible.
 • After obtaining the physician's approval, more advanced exercises can begin. (See *How to Strengthen Your Muscles After Lung Surgery*, pp. 156-157, for specific instructions.)
—Pain may be eased by adding support to the incision site or changing position. Pain medication will be available, and the patient should tell the nurse when he is in pain.

9 **Discuss patient guidelines to follow after discharge.**

Patient guidelines after discharge are as follows:
—Muscle-strengthening exercises should be performed several times a day (see *How to Strengthen Your Muscles After Lung Surgery*, pp. 156-157).
—The patient should know how to care for the surgical incision site.
—The patient should continue his usual activities as much as possible and should keep all health care appointments.

10 **State the purpose of chemotherapy in treating lung cancer.**

Chemotherapy for lung cancer involves the use of anticancer drugs to eliminate cancer cells. It is effective in treating small-cell (oat cell) carcinoma. Its goals are to shrink the tumor and to relieve the symptoms of pain and pressure.

11 Describe the use of chemotherapeutic drugs in treating lung cancer.

Chemotherapeutic drugs used to treat lung cancer are usually most effective in combination. Drugs with different sites of attack on cancer cells and with different adverse effects are used together to destroy the greatest number of cancer cells and allow the patient to recover more quickly from any adverse effects. The drugs are given intermittently over a period of time to aid in the elimination of cancer cells. The specific drugs and dosages depend on the stage of the cancer (progressive or regressive), the type of cancer, and the patient's age and tolerance of the drugs.

12 Explain the medication regimen.

The following drugs may be used in the treatment of lung cancer: doxorubicin, lomustine, methotrexate, cisplatin, mitomycin, and vincristine. See Chapter 10, Drug Therapy, for specific medication instructions. For additional information, see the "Chemotherapy" teaching plan in this chapter.

13 State the purpose of radiation therapy in treating lung cancer.

The purpose of radiation therapy in treating lung cancer is to destroy cancer cells while damaging normal cells as little as possible. (Because cancer cells tend to divide more rapidly than normal cells, they are more vulnerable to radiation. Generally, normal cells recover from radiation faster than cancer cells.) Radiation may be used to reduce tumor size before surgery and is often used to treat squamous cell carcinoma and small-cell (oat cell) carcinoma. A painless procedure, it is also often used to relieve the symptoms of coughing, shortness of breath, bloody sputum, and bone, chest, and liver pain. (For additional information, see the "Radiation Therapy" teaching plan in this chapter.)

14 State the purpose of immunotherapy in treating lung cancer.

The purpose of immunotherapy is to assist the body in regaining its defense mechanisms, since normal defense mechanisms act to reject unknown body substances such as tumors and abnormal cells. The immune systems of patients with cancer are not working as they should, so live vaccines, such as bacille Calmette-Guérin (BCG) or *Corynebacterium parvum* (*C. parvum*), are administered in an attempt to stimulate the immune system to destroy residual tumor cells after surgery.

15 **Discuss concerns about the diagnosis and treatment of lung cancer.** The patient with lung cancer can vent his concerns by verbalizing his feelings about having cancer and undergoing treatment. He can share his feelings with loved ones and seek information about services available to people with cancer, such as financial assistance and support groups.

COLORECTAL CANCER

Patient objectives	*Teaching plan content*
1 Define cancer.	Cancer is the uncontrolled growth and reproduction of cells. Cancer cells differ from normal cells in their structure, size, function, and rapid rate of growth. They can spread throughout the body through the bloodstream or through the lymphatic system, or by direct extension from one site to another. The spread of cancer cells from their primary site to secondary sites is called metastasis. At secondary sites, these cells reproduce to form tumors or lesions.
2 Describe colorectal cancer.	Colorectal cancer, the third most common cancer, affects men and women in equal numbers. It tends to progress slowly and remain localized for a long time. Treatment and prognosis are based on the location and size of the tumor and the presence of metastasis. The predominant type of colorectal cancer is adenocarcinoma.
3 Identify the risk factors associated with colorectal cancer.	Risk factors associated with colorectal cancer are as follows: —High-fat/low-fiber diet —Family history of colorectal cancer —Age greater than 40 years —History of ulcerative colitis (average interval before onset of cancer is 11 to 17 years) —Other diseases of the digestive tract, such as diverticulitis or familial polyposis (development within the family of multiple polyps with high malignancy potential).
4 Identify the symptoms of colorectal cancer.	The symptoms of colorectal cancer may include the following: —Lesions of the right side of the colon are associated with pain, weakness, black stools, anemia, nausea, and abdominal mass. Late symptoms include diarrhea, constipation, weight loss, loss of appetite, and shortness of breath.

—Lesions of the left side of the colon are associated with pain (cramps), black stools, constipation, nausea, vomiting, and rectal bleeding. Late symptoms include diarrhea, pencil-shaped stools, and frank blood in the stool.

—Lesions of the rectum are associated with change in bowel habits (morning diarrhea, or constipation alternating with diarrhea) and blood or mucus in the stool. A late symptom is pain, ranging from a feeling of rectal fullness to a dull, constant ache of the rectal or sacral area. (An illustration may be used to show the relevant site of the cancer.)

5 Identify the screening methods for detection of colorectal cancer.	Screening methods for colorectal cancer include the following: —Digital rectal examination —Examination of stool for blood (guaiac test) —Sigmoidoscopy or proctoscopy.
6 Identify components of the treatment regimen for colorectal cancer.	The following are possible components of a colorectal cancer treatment regimen: —Surgery —Chemotherapy —Radiation therapy.
7 Discuss the relevant surgical procedure.	Surgery is the primary method of treating colorectal cancer. The following surgical procedures may be performed, depending on the location of the tumor: —Right hemicolectomy (resection of the right half of the colon) for advanced cancer of the cecum and ascending colon —Right colectomy (excision of a portion of the colon) for cancer of the proximal and middle transverse colon —Resection for cancer of the sigmoid colon and upper rectum —Abdominal resection for cancer of the lower rectum.
8 Discuss postoperative procedures.	After bowel resection, the patient should expect the following: —A dressing will be in place. —An I.V. line will remain in place for a few days. (The patient should know the signs and symptoms of infiltration.) —An indwelling urinary (Foley) catheter will be in place for a short time after surgery. —A nasogastric tube will be in place to keep air and fluid out of the stomach. This tube will remain in place for 1 to 3 days after surgery. —To prevent secretions from building up, the patient

will be helped to turn, cough, and deep-breathe at least every 2 hours, using hands and pillows for support. (These procedures should be demonstrated to the patient preoperatively.)
—Depending on the specific surgical procedure, a colostomy may be present. (See Chapter 6, Gastrointestinal Disorders, in Volume I, for colostomy care.)
—The patient may ease his pain by adding support to the incision or changing position. Pain medication will be available, and the patient should tell the nurse when he is in pain.

9 Discuss patient guidelines to follow after discharge.	Patient guidelines after discharge include the following: —The patient should know how to care for the surgical incision and the colostomy, if applicable. (See Chapter 6, Gastrointestinal Disorders, in Volume I, for colostomy care.) —He should continue with his usual activities as much as possible and should keep all health care appointments. —He should know the importance of following dietary restrictions.
10 State the purpose of chemotherapy in treating colorectal cancer.	Chemotherapy for colorectal cancer involves the use of anticancer drugs to eliminate cancer cells. Its goals include the following: —To stop progression of the cancer if it is too widespread to remove surgically or to stop disease progression following surgery —To treat metastases —To treat recurrent tumors.
11 Describe the use of chemotherapeutic drugs in treating colorectal cancer.	Chemotherapeutic drugs used to treat colorectal cancer are usually most effective in combination. Drugs with different sites of attack on cancer cells and with different adverse effects are used together to destroy the greatest number of cancer cells and allow the patient to recover more quickly from any adverse effects. The drugs are given intermittently over a period of time to aid in the elimination of cancer cells. The specific drugs, dosage, and route of administration depend on residual disease at the primary site, metastases, and the patient's age and tolerance of the drugs.
12 Explain the medication regimen.	The following drugs may be used in the treatment of colorectal cancer: fluorouracil, lomustine, mitomycin, methotrexate, and vincristine. See Chapter 10, Drug Therapy, for specific medication instructions. For additional information, see the "Chemotherapy" teaching plan in this chapter.

13 State the purpose of radiation therapy in treating colorectal cancer.

The purpose of using radiation therapy in colorectal cancer is to destroy cancer cells while damaging normal cells as little as possible. (Cancer cells tend to divide more rapidly than normal cells, which increases their vulnerability to radiation. Generally, normal cells recover from radiation faster than cancer cells.) Radiation is also used to shrink the tumor before surgery and/or to eliminate any remaining cancer cells after surgery. (For additional information, see the "Radiation Therapy" teaching plan in this chapter.)

14 Discuss concerns about the diagnosis and treatment of colorectal cancer.

The patient with colorectal cancer can verbalize his feelings about having cancer, undergoing treatment, and accepting possible changes in body image. He can share his feelings with loved ones and seek information about services available to people with cancer, such as financial assistance and support groups.

SKIN CANCER

Patient objectives	*Teaching plan content*

1 Define cancer.

Cancer is the uncontrolled growth and reproduction of cells. Cancer cells differ from normal cells in their structure, size, function, and rapid rate of growth. They can spread throughout the body through the bloodstream or lymphatic system, or by direct extension from one site to another. The spread of cancer cells from their primary site to secondary sites is called metastasis. At secondary sites, these cells reproduce and form tumors or lesions.

2 Describe skin cancer.

Skin cancer, the most common type of cancer, is classified by the appearance of the cells. The two types of skin cancer are as follows:
—Basal cell carcinoma, a superficial, slow-growing, destructive tumor that usually develops on the face, ears, and neck and occasionally on the trunk
—Squamous cell carcinoma, an invasive tumor with metastatic potential that usually develops on the face, back of the hands, lips, and mucous membranes.

3 Identify the risk factors associated with skin cancer.

Risk factors include the following:
—Lightly pigmented skin
—Prolonged exposure to the sun
—Burns
—Exposure to radiation

—Exposure to carcinogens, such as arsenic, tar, and oil
—Chronic skin irritation and inflammation.

4 Identify the symptoms of skin cancer.	Symptoms include the following: —A basal cell carcinoma appears as a small, waxy, or pearly nodule with a depressed center. The surface of the nodule may be pigmented, ulcerated, crusted, or bleeding, and telangiectatic blood vessels commonly mark the nodule's borders. —A squamous cell carcinoma appears as a hard, opaque, reddish brown, dome-shaped, scaly papule that may resemble a wart. On sun-damaged skin, it appears as a painless, red, hard, scaly plaque that enlarges and ulcerates in a few months; in an advanced state, it resembles a cauliflower-like mass.
5 Discuss components of the treatment regimen for skin cancer.	Treatment depends on the type, stage, location, and responsiveness of the tumor and on the patient's tolerance of the treatment protocol. Several of the following treatment methods may be used: —Chemotherapy (for basal cell carcinoma) consists of topical application of fluorouracil, which causes inflammation, necrosis, and sloughing of malignant tissue. —Surgical excision consists of surgical removal of the tumor as well as a margin of normal tissue. —Radiation therapy is most commonly used in older patients; it requires shielding for ear and nose lesions. —Electrosurgery involves the use of needle, blade, or disk electrodes to cut and coagulate the lesions. —Cryosurgery involves the use of liquid nitrogen to freeze the lesion, resulting in necrosis. —Chemosurgery (for basal cell carcinoma) consists of periodic applications of a fixative paste, such as zinc chloride, and subsequent removal of the fixed pathologic tissue. Treatment continues until the tumor is completely removed.
6 Discuss concerns about the diagnosis and treatment of skin cancer.	The patient with skin cancer can verbalize his feelings about having cancer, undergoing treatment, and accepting possible changes in body image. He can share his feelings with loved ones and seek information about services available to people with cancer (such as financial assistance and support groups).
7 Discuss patient guidelines to follow during and after treatment.	Patient guidelines during and after treatment include the following: —Avoid excessive exposure to sun. —Wear protective clothing, such as hats, long sleeves, and shirts.

—Use maximum-strength sunscreen on exposed areas, including lips.

—If applicable, relieve local inflammation after the topical application of fluorouracil with cool compresses or corticosteroid ointment.

 Explaining treatments

SURGERY

Patient objectives	*Teaching plan content*
1 State the purpose of cancer surgery.	The purposes of cancer surgery include the following: —To establish a diagnosis. Examining a suspicious lesion microscopically or visually confirms or rules out the presence of cancer. —To remove a precancerous lesion. The physician may eliminate benign lesions that have a tendency toward malignant transformation; for example, leukoplakia, colonic and rectal polyps, and certain pigmented moles. —To stage a disease. Staging determines the extent of the cancer's invasion. —To cure. The physician may attempt to remove the cancer completely, which, in radical approaches, may necessitate removal of one of the patient's limbs, breasts, organs, or other body parts. When cancer is diagnosed early, surgery may cure the patient without disfiguring him. —To reconstruct after a radical procedure. Reconstructive surgery after a mastectomy, radical neck dissection, or other disfiguring procedure may relieve a patient's psychological trauma. —To palliate. When cancer is advanced and a cure is not probable, surgery may relieve pain, pressure, infection, and hemorrhage. Palliative procedures for intractable pain include rhizotomy, peripheral neurotomy, cervical or thoracic cordotomy, tractotomy, thalamotomy, sympathectomy, and frontal lobotomy.
2 Briefly describe the relevant surgical procedure.	For information about specific surgical procedures used in treating cancer, see the "Breast Cancer," "Lung Cancer," "Colorectal Cancer," and "Skin Cancer" teaching plans in this chapter. Also see the "Surgery" teaching plan in Chapter 2, Pain Management.

CHEMOTHERAPY

Patient objectives	*Teaching plan content*
1 Explain how chemotherapeutic drugs work.	Chemotherapeutic drugs stop cancer cell production by interrupting the cell cycle, which is divided into distinct resting and replication phases. (Replication is a series of phases in which genetic materials and proteins in the cell produce an exact copy of it.) Because repeated administration of one chemotherapeutic drug tends to produce resistant cancer cells, alternative drugs must be substituted. The success of any chemotherapeutic program depends on the extent to which drugs may be combined. There are two types of chemotherapeutic drugs: —Cell-cycle-specific drugs act at one or more specific cell-cycle phases. —Cell-cycle-nonspecific drugs can act on both replicating and resting cells.

2 Discuss the route of administration of chemotherapeutic drugs.	The routes of administration of chemotherapeutic drugs include oral, intravenous (I.V.), subcutaneous (SQ), intrathecal, intraperitoneal, and intraarterial. The frequency and duration of administration depend on the treatment protocol being used, the patient's tolerance of the drug(s), and the effectiveness of the therapy.
	—In oral administration, the patient may be given drugs in pill form. The frequency and duration of medication depend on the treatment protocol being followed.
	—In I.V. administration, a needle is placed in a vein, usually in an arm or hand.
	  • The drug may be injected directly into the vein or mixed in a solution and infused over a period of time, which depends on the treatment protocol being followed.
	  • The frequency and duration of administration depend on the treatment protocol being followed.
	  • Signs and symptoms of infiltration include burning and tingling, and redness and swelling around the I.V. insertion site.
	  • The I.V. line should be checked frequently and any discomfort from it should be reported.
	—In SQ administration, a needle (attached to a syringe) is inserted into the tissue under the skin and the medication is then injected.
	  • The medication is absorbed from the subcutaneous tissue into the patient's bloodstream.
	—Intrathecal administration involves delivery of drugs within the sheath of tissue surrounding the brain and spinal cord. Because most drugs cannot cross the

blood-brain barrier, this route may be used to attack cancer cells in the central nervous system.
- A lumbar puncture may be performed and the drug injected into the patient's spinal cord.
- An Ommaya reservoir (an implantable pump) may be surgically implanted in the patient's head. This avoids multiple lumbar punctures while allowing chemotherapeutic drugs to enter the brain directly.

—In intraperitoneal administration, a catheter is placed in the abdominal and pelvic cavity to allow direct access of chemotherapeutic drugs to tumor(s) within the cavity. This route of administration permits localized drug absorption and helps to eliminate diffuse toxicities, but some systemic absorption may still occur, causing visible adverse effects of the specific drug.
- The chemotherapeutic drug is instilled by infusion into the cavity.
- The patient may be asked to change position (turn from side to side, sit, lie flat) to allow the drug to reach all areas of the peritoneal cavity.
- After a period of time (usually 2 to 6 hours), the fluid is drained from the peritoneal cavity.

—In intraarterial administration, the drug is infused into a major artery leading directly into a tumor. This route of administration is used in the treatment of head, neck, liver, and lung cancers. It permits localized drug absorption and helps eliminate diffuse toxicities, but some systemic absorption may still occur, causing diarrhea, nausea, and vomiting. Local adverse effects may include edema, hemorrhage, necrosis, and infection.

---

3 Discuss the adverse effects of chemotherapeutic drugs and the interventions used to manage them.

The adverse effects of chemotherapeutic drugs include nausea and vomiting, alopecia (hair loss), stomatitis and mucositis (inflammation of the mouth), diarrhea, constipation, infection, bleeding, and anorexia (loss of appetite).

—Nausea/vomiting may require the following interventions:
- Eat four to six small meals rather than three large meals a day.
- Eat cold foods or drink clear liquids.
- Drink clear liquids if unable to eat solid foods.
- Avoid spicy, fatty, or sweet foods.
- Select foods high in calories and protein.
- Eat in a pleasant environment. Eliminate sights, sounds, or smells that stimulate nausea.
- Alter eating patterns before or after therapy.
- If possible, sleep during periods of nausea.
- Rinse mouth frequently to eliminate any unpleasant taste.

- Use relaxation techniques or distraction before or during meals.
- Take antiemetic medication before therapy and every 4 to 6 hours after therapy. (Follow the physician's directions.)

—With alopecia, the onset and degree of hair loss will vary. (It may include all body hair.) Hair will grow back when therapy is completed, but it may grow back in a different color or texture.

- The patient may feel more comfortable wearing wigs, hats, scarves, or turbans.
- Hair loss can be prevented or minimized by using scalp constriction and/or scalp hypothermia. (The patient should ask the physician if this intervention may be used.)

—Stomatitis and mucositis may become apparent through changes in taste, sensation, or appearance of the oral cavity.

- Follow this mouth care regimen before and between meals: Use a soft toothbrush and rinse mouth for 2 minutes (swish and gargle) with hydrogen peroxide and water (1:4); hydrogen peroxide and saline solution (1:2); or salt and water (2 tsp:1,000 ml). Follow with plain water or saline rinse.
- Never use commercial mouthwashes; they contain alcohol, which dries the mucous membranes.
- Floss with unwaxed dental floss two or three times a day. Stop if pain, thrombocytopenia, or neutropenia is present.
- Moisten lips frequently.
- Avoid hot, spicy, or acidic foods.
- Increase fluid intake.
- Avoid tobacco and alcohol.
- Use a liquid analgesic before meals and as needed to decrease discomfort.
- Follow these guidelines if stomatitis/mucositis becomes severe: Increase frequency of mouth care, increase use of analgesic solution, use antifungal agents and antibiotics (dosage should be determined by the physician), and avoid wearing dentures.

—Diarrhea may require the following interventions:

- Increase fluid intake (avoid carbonated beverages).
- Avoid foods that irritate the gastrointestinal tract.
- Eat foods low in roughage but high in protein and calories.
- Avoid tobacco, alcohol, and caffeine.
- Eat small, frequent meals.
- Avoid very cold or very hot foods.
- Stay on a liquid diet if diarrhea is severe.
- Protect the skin in the rectal area by cleansing the

skin with warm water and a mild soap after each episode of diarrhea, gently patting it dry (never rub), and applying a soothing ointment to irritated skin.

• Sit in a tub of warm water, or take a sitz bath to ease discomfort.

• Take antidiarrheal medication(s), as ordered. (Dosage should be determined by the physician.)

—Constipation may be avoided or relieved by the following:

• Use a stool softener one or two times a day.

• Eat high-fiber foods.

• Avoid cheese products.

• Increase fluid intake.

• Increase physical activity, if possible.

• Use a laxative, suppository, or enema, as ordered by the physician.

—Infection is the result of bone marrow suppression. A reduced white blood cell count increases susceptibility to infection. (See *Preventing Infection*, p. 158.) To detect or prevent infection, the patient should do the following:

• Check his temperature daily or more often if other symptoms appear.

• Assess for signs of infection, such as increased warmth, redness, swelling, or tenderness, daily.

• Maintain good nutrition.

• Wash hands before eating, after using the toilet, and after blowing the nose.

• Avoid exposure to infection by avoiding crowds and persons with infections of any kind.

—Bleeding is the result of bone marrow suppression. A reduced platelet count increases the risk of bleeding and prolongs bleeding time. (See *Preventing Bleeding*, p. 159.) To detect or prevent bleeding, the patient should do the following:

• Assess skin and mucous membranes for signs of bleeding (petechiae). If present, notify the physician.

• Protect skin by using an electric razor; wearing gloves for washing dishes, raking, or gardening; wearing socks and shoes; and removing sharp objects (knives, scissors) on countertops or tables.

• Protect mucous membranes by using a soft toothbrush; avoiding dental floss; eating a soft diet; avoiding foods that are hot, spicy, acidic, and high in roughage; and blowing nose gently.

• Avoid medications that may cause or prolong bleeding (for example, aspirin), and ask the physician what medications can be taken.

• Eat foods high in protein.

• Check urine, stool, and sputum for blood.

• Apply pressure to the puncture site after having blood drawn or an I.V. line removed.

—Anorexia may require the following interventions:
- Eat in a pleasant environment.
- Eat small, frequent meals.
- Avoid drinking fluids during meals.
- Eat foods high in calories and protein.
- Cleanse mouth before eating.
- Take an analgesic at least 1 hour before eating if in pain.
- Use nutritional supplements to increase caloric intake.
- Take a daily multiple vitamin, after first checking with the physician.

RADIATION THERAPY

Patient objectives	Teaching plan content
1 Describe the procedure used in external radiation therapy.	In external radiation therapy, the patient should expect the following: —The physician will use an X-ray simulator to determine how to direct the radiation beam. —Special marks will be made on the patient's skin, using dyes or tattoos, to serve as guides for directing the radiation beam. The patient should be careful not to wash these marks off and not to use soaps or powders on them. If the marks are removed for any reason, he should not attempt to redraw them. —Shields will be used to protect surrounding normal tissue. —Although the patient will be alone during the procedure, someone will observe him through either a window or a video device. —The physician or radiation therapist will ask him to sit or lie in a certain position during treatment. He must remain motionless in this position during treatment and breathe normally. —He will not see, hear, or feel the radiation, but the machine administering the radiation may make a loud noise. —He must remove all metal objects (pens, buttons, jewelry) that may interfere with therapy. —He will not be radioactive and will not endanger those around him. —The treatment will take only a few minutes.
2 Discuss the types of internal radiation therapy.	Routes of administration of internal radiation therapy include the following: —Surgical implants: An implant is placed in the tumor, using tubes or needles that may or may not be re-

moved. The source of radiation is then inserted into the needles.

—Intracavity: Needles are placed in or near the tumor and the source of radiation is inserted into them to cause local destruction of cancer cells. Needles are removed when the treatment period is over.

—Interstitial: Tubes or needles are placed under the skin, and the source of radiation is then inserted into them. Needles and tubes are removed after the treatment period.

—Oral/parenteral: Radioactive isotopes are taken by mouth or injected into a vein. The body removes these isotopes through elimination.

3 **Explain patient guidelines for internal radiation therapy.**

During internal radiation therapy, the patient should expect the following:

—His activity will be limited while the radioactive material is in place.

—Visits will be limited to 30 minutes within a 24-hour period. (The family should know this.)

—No children or pregnant women will be allowed to visit.

—He will not be radioactive after the implanted material is removed or, in the case of seeds or pellets, has lost its radioactivity.

4 **Discuss the adverse effects of radiation therapy and the interventions used to manage them.**

The adverse effects of radiation therapy include skin reactions, nausea and vomiting, alopecia (hair loss), stomatitis and mucositis (inflammation of the mouth), diarrhea, infection, bleeding, fatigue, cystitis, and sexual dysfunction.

—Skin reactions may occur at radiation entrance and exit sites.

• The following are early signs of a skin reaction: localized dryness, mild-to-severe erythema, increased skin pigmentation, localized itching and peeling, localized hair loss.

• The following are late signs: localized dryness from permanently damaged sweat or sebaceous glands; increased pigmentation; leathery skin caused by decreased elasticity from fibrosis; epithelial thinning; telangiectasia (tissue reddening caused by capillary dilation); narrowing of small blood vessels; change in local hair pattern; open, raw skin.

—The patient should follow these steps to prevent skin reactions:

• Keep the skin dry.

• Do not use soaps, powders, perfumes, oils, or creams on affected skin without the approval of the physician. Products that may be used (with the physician's approval) include cornstarch, A and D Ointment, lanolin-based cream, hydrocortisone ointment, or Aquaphor.

- Use tepid water and mild soap to wash the affected area gently.
- Do not wear tight or rough-fiber clothing over the area.
- Do not rub or scratch the skin. (If scratching occurs during sleep, wear gloves or socks over hands at night.) Keep nails cut short.
- Do not shave the affected area.
- Avoid exposure to sun. If unavoidable, wear sunscreen.
- Do not use adhesive tape on the skin.

—Nausea and vomiting may require the following interventions:

- Eat small, frequent meals rather than three large meals a day.
- Avoid spicy or acidic foods. Bland foods are more tolerable.
- Select foods high in calories and protein.
- Eat in a pleasant environment. (Eliminate sights, sounds, or smells that stimulate nausea.)
- Cleanse mouth before eating.
- Drink clear liquids if unable to eat solid foods.
- If possible, sleep during periods of nausea.
- Use relaxation/distraction techniques before or during meals.
- Take antiemetic medication before and after therapy, if needed. (Follow the physician's directions.)

—Alopecia occurs only in the affected area and usually begins within 1 week after treatment.

- Hair may begin to regrow in the fourth or fifth week of treatment. (With high doses of radiation, hair loss may be permanent.)
- Hair may grow back in a different color or texture.
- The patient may feel more comfortable wearing wigs, hats, scarves, or turbans.

—Stomatitis and mucositis may become apparent through changes in taste, sensation, or appearance of oral cavity.

- Follow this mouth care regimen before and between meals: Use a soft toothbrush, and rinse mouth for 2 minutes (swish and gargle) with hydrogen peroxide and water (1:4); hydrogen peroxide and saline solution (1:2); or salt and water (2 tsp:1,000 ml). Follow with plain water or saline rinse.
- Never use commercial mouthwashes; they contain alcohol, which dries the mucous membranes.
- Moisten lips frequently.
- Avoid hot, spicy, or acidic foods.
- Increase fluid intake.
- Avoid tobacco and alcohol.

• Use a liquid analgesic before meals and as needed to decrease discomfort.

• Follow these guidelines if stomatitis/mucositis becomes severe: Increase the frequency of mouth care, increase use of analgesic solution, use antifungal agents and antibiotics (dosage should be determined by the physician), and avoid wearing dentures.

—Diarrhea may require the following interventions:

• Increase fluid intake (avoid carbonated beverages).

• Eat foods low in roughage but high in protein and calories.

• Eat small, frequent meals.

• Avoid very cold or very hot foods.

• Avoid tobacco, alcohol, and caffeine.

• Stay on a liquid diet if diarrhea is severe.

• Protect the skin in the rectal area by cleansing the skin with warm water and a mild soap after each episode of diarrhea, gently patting the skin dry (never rub), and applying a soothing ointment to irritated skin.

• Sit in a tub of warm water, or take a sitz bath to ease discomfort.

• Take antidiarrheal medications, as ordered. (Dosage should be determined by the physician.)

—Infection is the result of bone marrow suppression. A reduced white blood cell count increases susceptibility to infection. (See *Preventing Infection*, p. 158.) To prevent infection, the patient should do the following:

• Avoid exposure to infection (avoid crowds and people with any kind of infection).

• Wash hands before eating, after using the toilet, and after blowing the nose.

• Maintain good nutrition.

—Bleeding is the result of bone marrow suppression. A reduced platelet count increases the risk of bleeding and prolongs bleeding time. (See *Preventing Bleeding*, p. 159.) The patient should regularly check urine, stool, and sputum for blood. To prevent bleeding, he should do the following:

• Protect skin by using an electric razor and not shaving the affected area; wearing gloves for washing dishes, raking, or gardening; wearing socks and shoes; and removing sharp objects from countertops and tables.

• Protect mucous membranes by using a soft toothbrush; avoiding dental floss; eating a soft diet; avoiding hot, spicy, acidic, and high-roughage foods; and blowing the nose gently.

• Apply pressure to the puncture site after having blood drawn or an I.V. line removed.

—Fatigue requires the following interventions:
* Take frequent rests.
* Space activities to prevent becoming overtired.
—Cystitis requires the following interventions:
* Increase fluid intake to 3,000 ml/day.
* Void frequently.
* Avoid bladder-irritating substances, such as caffeine, alcohol, tobacco, and spices (pepper and curry).
* Drink cranberry juice to maintain acidic urine.
—Sexual dysfunction may occur in both sexes.
* In the female, irregular menstrual cycles are not unusual. Vaginal dryness can be reduced by using a water-based lubricant, and vaginal mucositis can be treated with tepid douches, as ordered by the physician. Intercourse should be avoided until the mucositis has been resolved. As a result of treatment, temporary or permanent sterility may occur.
* In the male, sterility may occur as a result of treatment. The patient may consider sperm banking before beginning therapy.

IMMUNOTHERAPY

Patient objectives	Teaching plan content
1 Discuss the purpose of immunotherapy in treating cancer.	Immunotherapy helps the body regain its defense mechanisms, since the immune systems of patients with cancer are not working as they should. Normal defense mechanisms act to reject tumors and abnormal cells.
2 Name the preparations used in the immunotherapy regimen and identify their adverse effects.	The adverse effects of preparations used in immunotherapy are as follows: —Bacille Calmette-Guérin (BCG) by intradermal injection can cause redness, swelling, or pain; and by intratumor injection can cause fever, chills, or hepatitis. —*Corynebacterium parvum (C. parvum)* can cause fever, headache, and hypertension. —Interferon can cause fever, pain at injection site, shivering, and fatigue. —Interleukin-2 can cause nausea, vomiting, muscular aches, chills, and fever. —Levamisole can cause neutropenia, evidenced by such signs of infection as fever and chills, nausea, insomnia, and alteration in taste and smell. —Monoclonal antibodies can cause fever, chills, hypotension, and allergic reactions.

Patient-Teaching Aid

WARNING SIGNS OF CANCER

Dear Patient:
Because early detection of cancer offers the best chance for cure, report any of these warning signs to your physician:

C	—Change in bowel or bladder habits
A	—A sore that does not heal
U	—Unusual bleeding or discharge
T	—Thickening or lump in breast, testicle, or elsewhere
I	—Indigestion or difficulty swallowing
O	—Obvious change in wart or mole
N	—Nagging cough or hoarseness.

Patient-Teaching Aid

PREVENTING POSTMASTECTOMY COMPLICATIONS

Dear Patient:
The removal of lymph nodes during your surgery may cause your arm to swell, and your body's ability to fight infection in that area will be greatly reduced. The following list of do's and don'ts will help you to prevent complications.

DO:

- Contact the physician if the affected arm becomes red, warm, or unusually hard or swollen.
- Protect the hand and arm on the affected side.
- Order and wear a Medic Alert tag engraved: *Caution—lymphedema arm—no tests—no injections.*
- Use a thimble when sewing.
- Wear loose rubber gloves when washing dishes.
- Stay out of strong sunlight.
- Apply lanolin hand cream several times a day.
- Elevate your arm if it feels heavy.

DON'T:

- Hold a cigarette in the affected hand.
- Injure cuticles or hangnails.
- Use strong detergents.
- Reach into a hot oven.
- Get cuts, bruises, or insect bites.
- Dig in the garden or work near thorny bushes.
- Have blood drawn or injections given.
- Wear jewelry or a wristwatch.
- Have a blood pressure cuff applied.
- Carry heavy bags or a purse.

![Clipboard icon] **Patient-Teaching Aid**

STRENGTHENING EXERCISES: AFTER YOUR MASTECTOMY

Dear Patient:
After your mastectomy, it is important that you exercise the involved arm and shoulder to prevent muscle shortening, to maintain muscle tone, and to improve blood and lymph circulation.

Wall climbing

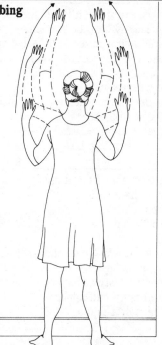

Stand facing a wall, with your toes as close to the wall as possible and your feet apart. Bending your elbows slightly, place your palms against the wall at shoulder level. Then, flexing your fingers, work your hands up the wall until your arms are fully extended. Work your hands back down to the starting point.

Pulley

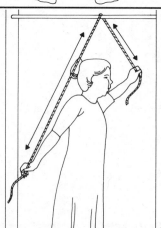

Toss a rope over your shower curtain rod and hold an end of the rope in each hand. Using a seesaw motion and with your arms outstretched, slide the rope up and down over the rod.

STRENGTHENING EXERCISES: AFTER YOUR MASTECTOMY—*continued*

Pendulum swing

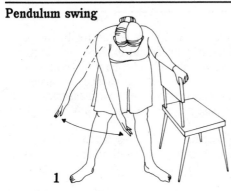

1

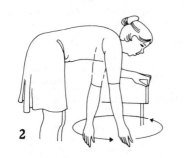

2

Place your uninvolved arm on the back of a chair. Let your involved arm hang loosely.
1. Swing your arm from left to right. Be sure the movement comes from your shoulder joint and not your elbow.
2. Swing your arm in small circles. Again, be sure the movement is coming from your shoulder joint. As your arm relaxes, the size of the circle will probably increase. Then circle in the opposite direction.
3. Swing your arm forward and backward from your shoulder, within the range of comfort.

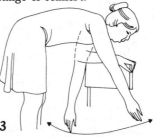

3

Rope turning

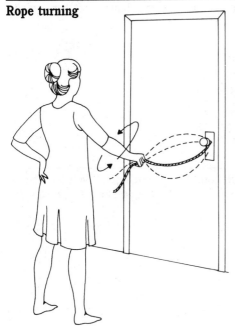

Stand facing the door. Take the free end of a rope in the hand of the operated side. Place your other hand on your hip. With your arm extended and held away from your body, turn the rope, making as wide a swing as possible. Start slowly, and increase your speed as your arm gets stronger.

Patient-Teaching Aid

BREAST SELF-EXAMINATION

Dear Patient:
Since 90% of breast cancers are discovered by the patients themselves, it is important to learn and practice self-examination. You should examine your breasts at least monthly. If you have not yet reached menopause, the best time is immediately after your menstrual period. If you are past menopause, choose any convenient day.

To examine your breasts: Undress to the waist, and sit or stand in front of a mirror, with your arms at your sides.

1

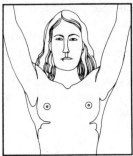

Carefully observe each breast for asymmetry of size or shape (some difference in size is not unusual); deviation or asymmetry of the nipple; retraction of the skin, nipple, or areola; edema or ulceration of the skin; and any other changes. Since you are most familiar with the structure of your own breasts, you should be the first to notice any changes. Repeat this visual inspection in the following two positions:

2

Raise your arms and press your hands together behind your head.

3

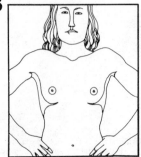

Press your palms firmly on your hips. If you see anything unusual, palpate the area carefully for any abnormality.

BREAST SELF-EXAMINATION—*continued*

 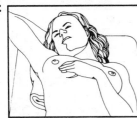

Next, lie flat on your back. This position flattens and spreads your breasts more evenly over the chest wall. Place a small pillow under your right shoulder, and put your right hand behind your head.

 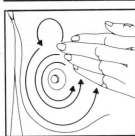

Examine your right breast with your left hand, using a circular motion and progressing clockwise, until you have examined every portion. You will notice a ridge of firm tissue in the lower curve of your breast; this is normal.

 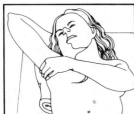

Check the area under your arm with your elbow slightly bent.

 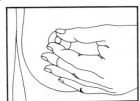

Then gently squeeze your nipple between your thumb and forefinger, and note any discharge. Repeat this examination on your left breast, using your right hand.

 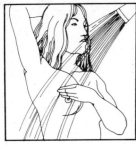

Now examine your breasts while in the shower, lubricating your breasts with soap and water. Using the same circular, clockwise motion, gently inspect both breasts with your fingertips. After you are toweled dry, squeeze each nipple gently, and note any discharge.

If you discover any abnormality, notify the physician immediately. Although self-examination is important, it is not a substitute for examination by your physician. Be sure to see your physician annually or biannually (if you are considered at special risk).

Patient-Teaching Aid

HOW TO STRENGTHEN YOUR MUSCLES AFTER LUNG SURGERY

Dear Patient:
The nurse has shown you exercises that will strengthen the arm, shoulder, and chest muscles affected by your surgery. Perform these exercises with your affected arm at least five times each day, and repeat each exercise at least three times.

1

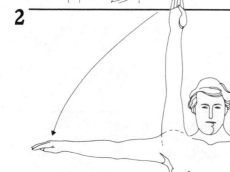

For your first exercise, lift your shoulders. Hunch your shoulders forward, as shown here, and then pull them back as far as possible.

2

Next, raise your elbow, bringing it as close to your ear as possible. Then extend your arm straight out at shoulder level.

3

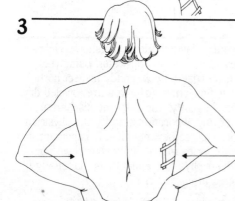

Now place your hands on the small of your back. Try to push your elbows and your shoulder blades toward one another.

HOW TO STRENGTHEN YOUR MUSCLES AFTER LUNG SURGERY—*continued*

4

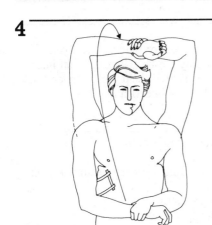

Bend your arm at your elbow, so the hand on your affected side rests on your abdomen. Use your opposite hand to grasp your wrist. Raise your arm off your abdomen and bring it directly over the top of your head, inhaling as you do so. As you exhale, lower your arm.

5

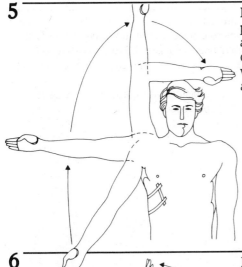

Place your arm at your side, with your palm facing forward. Then raise your arm to the side, bending it over the top of your head. Keep your palm facing forward. Again, inhale as you raise your arm and exhale as you lower it.

6

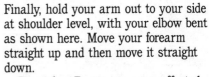

Finally, hold your arm out to your side at shoulder level, with your elbow bent as shown here. Move your forearm straight up and then move it straight down.

Remember: Try to use your affected arm in as many of your daily activities as possible.

Patient-Teaching Aid

Dear Patient:

Because of your disease and/or the treatment you are receiving, your body may not be able to fight off infection effectively. This guide will help you to understand the signs and symptoms of infection and how to prevent infection.

Signs and symptoms of infection
• Fever
• Warmth, redness, swelling, tenderness, and/or pain in any body area
• Persistent and/or productive cough
• Drainage from any open area.

Preventing infection
• Avoid crowds and people with any kind of infection.
• Examine your body and mouth daily for areas of warmth, redness, tenderness, swelling, and/or open tissue.
• Wash your hands before eating and after using the toilet or blowing your nose.

Patient-Teaching Aid

PREVENTING BLEEDING

Dear Patient:
Because of your disease and/or the treatment you are receiving, your body's blood-clotting ability may not be normal. This means that you may bleed more easily and that it will take longer for the bleeding to stop. This guide will help you to understand how to prevent bleeding.

DO:

- Use an electric razor.
- Wear gloves when washing dishes, raking, or gardening.
- Take your temperature only by mouth.
- Wear socks and shoes that fit properly.
- Check urine, stool, and sputum for blood.
- Apply pressure after having blood drawn or an I.V. line removed.
- Use a thimble while sewing.

DON'T:

- Use a straight-edged razor.
- Go barefoot.
- Leave knives, scissors, or other sharp objects on countertops or tables.

Patient-Teaching Aid

REVIEWING BREAST BASICS

Dear Patient:
This illustration will show you the anatomy of your breast so that you can better understand the type of cancer you have and how it affects your breast.

Mammary glands overlie the pectoral muscles. Each gland contains approximately 20 lobes, which are divided into lobules and alveoli. Ducts extend from the lobes through breast tissue and converge in the nipple.

Each mammary gland has an elaborate lymphatic system, which drains primarily into the axilla. This accounts for axillary node enlargement common in malignant breast disease.

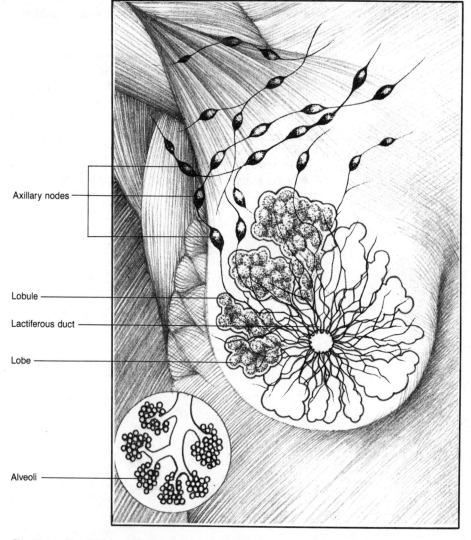

Axillary nodes

Lobule

Lactiferous duct

Lobe

Alveoli

EENT
Disorders

Patient-learner data base*

Areas of potential knowledge deficit
Risk factors for eye disorders
—Family history of eye disease
—Environmental irritants
—Allergies
—Eye stress
—Presence of other chronic diseases (e.g., diabetes mellitus)
—Presence of venereal disease (e.g., gonorrhea)
—History of traumatic eye injury
Risk factors for ear disorders
—Noise pollution
—Frequent use of earplugs, earphones, or earmuffs
—Cleaning ears with foreign objects
—History of traumatic injury to ear or head
Risk factors for nasal disorders
—Personal or family history of allergies
—Frequent forceful nose blowing
—History of traumatic injury to nose
—Chronic infections, including the common cold
—Smoking
Risk factors for throat disorders
—Chronic throat infections
—Chemical irritants
—Smoking
—Environmental irritants
—Excessive use of voice
Anatomy and physiology of EENT
Definition of the EENT disorder
Causes of the EENT disorder
Symptoms associated with the EENT disorder
Treatment of the EENT disorder

* A general assessment should be done for all patients. For general assessment guidelines, see Chapter 1, Principles of Patient Teaching.

Explaining diagnostic tests

TONOMETRY

Patient objectives	*Teaching plan content*
1 Define tonometry.	Tonometry is an indirect measurement of pressure within the eye (intraocular pressure).
2 State the purpose of tonometry.	The purpose of tonometry is to screen for early detection of glaucoma, an eye disorder characterized by elevated intraocular pressure.
3 Describe the procedure used in tonometry.	Tonometry is performed by placing an instrument (tonometer) on the cornea, the layer of transparent tissue covering the eye. —Topical anesthetic drops will be placed in the patient's eyes so that he will not feel the tonometer making contact with them. —After the eye drops are given, a nurse or physician will place the tonometer briefly on the cornea of each eye to register the intraocular pressure.
4 Discuss patient guidelines for tonometry.	Patient guidelines for tonometry are as follows: —The patient should relax, since anxiety may raise intraocular pressure. Verbalizing any concerns or questions before the test may help. —He should loosen or remove any restrictive clothing around his neck, which can also raise the pressure. —He should not cough or squeeze or close his eyelids during the procedure. —During the test, he will be asked to look down for the insertion of the eye drops and up when the tonometer is used. His eyes will be held open by the examiner's thumb and forefinger to prevent him from blinking. —If the patient wears contact lenses, he must remove them before the procedure and not reinsert them for 2 hours after the test. —To prevent scratching his eyes, he should not rub them for at least 20 minutes after the test.

FLUORESCEIN ANGIOGRAPHY

Patient objectives	*Teaching plan content*
1 Define fluorescein angiography.	Fluorescein angiography allows the physician to see the small blood vessels in the eye by means of a special camera.
2 State the purpose of fluorescein angiography.	The purpose of fluorescein angiography is to evaluate the circulation of blood in the eyes as an aid in diagnosing abnormalities such as tumors and circulatory or inflammatory disorders of the eye.
3 Describe the procedure used in fluorescein angiography.	During fluorescein angiography the patient can expect the following: —The test will be performed in a special room in the ophthalmology or X-ray department. —The patient will be asked to sit in a chair facing a camera. —Eye drops will be given, probably twice, to prepare the patient for the test. He will need to wait 15 to 40 minutes for the drops to work. —He will then be asked to place his chin in a chin rest and his forehead against a bar. —An I.V. line will be inserted in one of his arms. A few pictures may be taken of his eyes and then a dye will be injected through the I.V. line. As the dye passes through the circulation in his eye, 25 to 30 photographs will be taken in rapid sequence (1 second apart). The I.V. line will then be removed. —If more photographs are needed, he may need to wait an additional 20 minutes to 1 hour.
4 Discuss patient guidelines for fluorescein angiography.	Patient guidelines for fluorescein angiography are as follows: —He need not restrict foods or fluids before the test. —The procedure will take about 30 minutes. —He will be asked to sign a consent form. —If he has glaucoma (and if ordered), he should not use eye drops on the day of the test. —During the test, he will be instructed to keep his teeth together, open his eyes as widely as possible, stare straight ahead, and breathe and blink normally. —He should keep the arm with the I.V. line extended at all times. —He may experience nausea and a feeling of warmth when the dye is injected.

—His skin and urine will be slightly discolored for 24 to 48 hours after the test.
—His near vision will be blurred from the eye drops for 40 minutes to 2 hours.

OCULAR ULTRASONOGRAPHY

Patient objectives	Teaching plan content
1 Define ocular ultrasonography.	Ocular ultrasonography records images of the structures of the eye by directing harmless, high-frequency sound waves into the eye and converting the reflected echoes into a pattern of dots or waveforms on a display screen.
2 State the purpose of ocular ultrasonography.	The purpose of ocular ultrasonography is to evaluate the structures of the eye for abnormalities.
3 Describe the procedure used in ocular ultrasonography.	During ocular ultrasonography the patient can expect the following: —He will be placed supine on a table in the X-ray department. —A small transducer coated with jelly will be placed on his closed eyelid. The transducer will transmit high-frequency sound waves that will be reflected by the structures of the eye. As the structures reflect the waves, he will hear echoes. —At the completion of the test, the transducer and jelly will be removed from his eyelids.
4 Discuss patient guidelines for ocular ultrasonography.	Patient guidelines for ocular ultrasonography are as follows: —The patient need not restrict foods or fluids before the test. —The procedure is safe and painless and takes about 5 minutes. —During the test, he may be asked to move his eyes or change his gaze. —After the test, he may immediately resume his activities.

PURE TONE AUDIOMETRY

Patient objectives	Teaching plan content
1 Define pure tone audiometry.	Pure tone audiometry tests a person's ability to hear sounds.

2 State the purpose of pure tone audiometry.	The purpose of pure tone audiometry is to determine the presence and degree of hearing loss.
3 Describe the procedure used in pure tone audiometry.	During pure tone audiometry the patient can expect the following: —Each ear will be tested separately, starting with the one with better hearing. —The ear canal will be checked for wax buildup before the test. —The examiner will press a finger on the auricle (external ear) and then on the tragus (projection of cartilage at the entrance to the external ear canal) to rule out possible closure of the canal under pressure from the earphones. A small plastic tube may be inserted into the ear canal if the canal tends to close. —Earphones will be positioned to line up opposite the ear canals. A few test sounds will be presented to familiarize the patient with the procedure. —He will then hear tones at various intensities. He will be asked to give a signal or press a response button each time he hears the tone. —If bone conduction is to be checked, the earphones will be removed and a vibrator placed on a spot right behind his ear. He will be asked to signal when he first hears a tone and when he stops hearing it.
4 Discuss patient guidelines for pure tone audiometry.	Patient guidelines for pure tone audiometry are as follows: —The test takes about 20 minutes to perform. —The patient should signal when he hears a tone, even if the tone is faint. —He should avoid loud noises (loud enough to make face-to-face communication difficult) for at least 16 hours before the test.

ACOUSTIC IMMITTANCE TESTS

Patient objectives	*Teaching plan content*
1 Define acoustic immittance tests.	Acoustic immittance tests measure the flow of sound into the ear and the resistance to that flow.
2 State the purpose of acoustic immittance tests.	The purpose of acoustic immittance tests is to evaluate middle-ear function, nerve function (seventh and eighth cranial nerves), and eustachian tube function.
3 Describe the procedure used in acoustic immittance testing.	Acoustic immittance testing involves tympanometry and an acoustic reflexes test. —Before testing, the ear canal will be inspected for wax buildup.

—A probe will then be inserted into the ear canal and sealed in place with a puttylike substance.
—For tympanometry, air pressure in the middle ear will be changed via the probe, and measurements will be taken.
—For the acoustic reflexes test, loud tones will be presented for brief periods of time in one ear and the patient's reflexes to the sounds recorded.

4 **Discuss patient guidelines for acoustic immittance tests.**	Patient guidelines for acoustic immittance tests are as follows: —Each of the two tests takes approximately 2 to 3 minutes to perform. —The patient should not move, speak, or swallow while tympanometry is being recorded (he will be told when this is done) and should not be startled during the loud tone reflex-eliciting measurement. —Changes in ear canal pressure may cause transient vertigo. He should report any discomfort or dizziness. —Although the probe in the ear canal may cause discomfort, it will not harm the ear. —He may resume his usual activities immediately after the test.

DIRECT LARYNGOSCOPY

Patient objectives	Teaching plan content
1 **Define direct laryngoscopy.**	Direct laryngoscopy allows the physician to look at the voice box (larynx) and surrounding areas.
2 **State the purpose of direct laryngoscopy.**	The purpose of direct laryngoscopy is to detect laryngeal abnormalities.
3 **Describe the procedure used in direct laryngoscopy.**	During direct laryngoscopy the patient can expect the following: —The procedure will be performed in a dark operating room. —The patient will receive a sedative to help him relax, medication to reduce oral secretions, and, during the procedure, a general or local anesthetic to numb his throat. —His head will be positioned and held while the physician passes a tube through his mouth, down his throat, to his larynx. This will not obstruct his airway. —A specimen may be obtained at this time for future study, or polyps or nodules may be removed. —After the physician has inspected the area, the tube will be removed, and the patient will be returned to his room.

4 Discuss patient guidelines for direct laryngoscopy.	Patient guidelines for direct laryngoscopy are as follows: —The patient should fast for 6 to 8 hours before the test. —Just before the test, he should remove any dentures, contact lenses, or jewelry. He should also void at that time. —While in the operating room, he should lie still. —After the procedure, he will wear an ice collar to prevent or minimize swelling. —He should spit saliva into a basin rather than swallow it for the first 2 to 8 hours after the test. During that time, he should refrain from clearing his throat and coughing. —He may resume eating and drinking, beginning with sips of water, 2 to 8 hours after the procedure. —Voice loss, hoarseness, and sore throat are temporary.

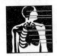 **Explaining disorders**

GLAUCOMA

Patient objectives	Teaching plan content
1 Define glaucoma.	Glaucoma is an eye disorder in which the pressure inside the eye (intraocular pressure) becomes abnormally high.
2 Identify the anatomical structures of the eye.	The structures of the eye include the cornea, sclera, choroid, iris, ciliary body, retina, and fovea. The two chambers of the eye are the anterior and posterior chambers. (An illustration can be used to demonstrate the location of these structures.)
3 Explain the cause of glaucoma.	Increased intraocular pressure results from excess production of fluid (called aqueous humor) in the eye or from an obstruction that blocks the drainage of this fluid. As the pressure builds, damage to the delicate structures of the eye can occur, resulting in impaired vision.
4 Identify the relevant type of glaucoma.	Glaucoma occurs in several forms: —Chronic open-angle glaucoma (the most common type) —Acute closed-angle (narrow-angle) glaucoma —Chronic closed-angle (narrow-angle) glaucoma.

5 Identify the signs and symptoms of glaucoma.

The signs and symptoms of glaucoma include the following:

—Chronic open-angle glaucoma usually affects both eyes and has a subtle onset and a slowly progressive course. Symptoms appear late in the disease and include mild aching in the eyes, loss of peripheral vision, visual perception of halos around lights, and reduced visual acuity (especially at night) that is uncorrectable with glasses.

—Acute closed-angle glaucoma typically has a rapid onset, constituting an emergency. Symptoms may include unilateral inflammation and pain, pressure over the eye, and visual disturbances such as blurred or decreased vision, visual perception of halos around lights, and sensitivity to light. Increased intraocular pressure may also cause nausea and vomiting.

—Chronic closed-angle glaucoma has a gradual onset. It usually produces no symptoms, although blurred vision and visual perception of halos around lights are possible. If untreated, this type of glaucoma progresses to absolute glaucoma, the final stage of this disease, producing pain and blindness.

6 Discuss the relevant treatment regimen for glaucoma.

Treatment regimens for glaucoma are as follows:

—In chronic open-angle glaucoma, medications are usually used. These may include both oral drugs such as epinephrine, timolol, or diuretics (to lower intraocular pressure) and eye drops such as pilocarpine (to aid the drainage of aqueous humor). Occasionally, these medications do not work. If this happens, intraocular pressure can be decreased by surgically creating an opening through which aqueous humor can drain.

—Acute closed-angle glaucoma requires emergency treatment. Drug therapy will be given to lower intraocular pressure. If the pressure does not decrease promptly, the patient is prepared for an emergency iridectomy. (See the "Iridectomy" teaching plan in this chapter.) A prophylactic iridectomy will be performed a few days later on the opposite eye to prevent an acute episode of glaucoma in the normal eye.

—If chronic closed-angle glaucoma occurs as a result of an acute closed-angle glaucoma attack, medication in the form of eye drops will be used to improve the outflow of aqueous humor and thereby decrease the intraocular pressure. If the medication is not effective, the pressure may be decreased by surgically creating an opening for aqueous humor drainage or performing a bilateral iridectomy to prevent further acute attacks.

7 Describe the medication regimen.

Some drugs commonly used for this disorder are atropine (ophthalmic), atropine injection, chlordiazepoxide, demecarium, dipivefrin, echothiophate iodide, epinephrine, isoflurophate, isosorbide, pilocarpine, and timolol. For specific medication instructions, refer to Chapter 10, Drug Therapy.

8 Demonstrate the use of eye drops.

Correct self-administration of eye drops is shown in *Giving Yourself Eye Drops*, pp. 186-187.

9 Discuss patient guidelines for daily living with glaucoma.

Patient guidelines for daily living with glaucoma include the following:
—The patient must comply meticulously with prescribed drug therapy. This is necessary to prevent eye changes that could result in the loss of vision.
—He should avoid activities that may increase intraocular pressure, such as weight lifting, push-ups, waterskiing, carrying heavy bundles, pulling a heavy golf cart, shoveling, moving furniture, mopping floors, opening stuck windows or jar lids, judo, and karate. If he is in doubt, the patient should have approval from his physician before performing an exercise.
—He should avoid excessive fluid intake and self-medication, which may be particularly hazardous because many over-the-counter medications contain ingredients that can increase intraocular pressure.
—He should inform any new physician about his eye condition, because many prescribed medications can also raise intraocular pressure.
—He should carry identification at all times that clearly indicates he has glaucoma. If an emergency should arise in which he is unable to speak or forgets to mention he has glaucoma, the identification card will alert the physician to avoid using certain drugs when providing emergency treatment.
—He should avoid stress and other emotionally upsetting situations as much as possible, because they may increase intraocular pressure.
—He should use safety precautions if his ability to see is impaired.
—He should keep follow-up appointments, have his intraocular pressure checked periodically, and seek medical attention immediately if eye pain or vision changes occur.

CATARACT

Patient objectives	Teaching plan content
1 Define cataract.	A cataract is a common disorder in which the lens or lens capsule gradually loses its transparency and becomes cloudy, thereby causing a loss in vision.
2 Identify the lens and lens capsule.	The lens is located behind the colored portion of the eye (the iris) and is enclosed in a transparent covering called the lens capsule. (An illustration can be used to demonstrate the location of these structures.)
3 State the function of the lens.	The lens enables the eye to focus on objects at different distances.
4 Discuss the cause of cataracts.	Cataracts have various causes: —Senile cataracts develop in the elderly, probably because of changes in the chemical state of lens proteins. —Congenital cataracts occur in newborns as genetic defects or because of maternal rubella during the first trimester. —Traumatic cataracts develop after a foreign body injures the lens. —Cataracts may occur as the result of other eye conditions and may also result from drug or chemical toxicity.
5 Identify the signs and symptoms associated with cataracts.	Typically, a patient with a cataract experiences painless, gradual blurring and loss of vision. As the cataract progresses, the normally black pupil turns milky white. —He may see halos around lights and blinding glare from headlights when driving at night. —He may have poor reading vision and experience an unpleasant glare and poor vision in bright sunlight. —Patients with central opacities can see better in dim light than in bright light.
6 Discuss the treatment of cataracts.	The only way to restore vision altered by a cataract is to remove the defective lens surgically and substitute an external or implantable lens for it. The cataract must "mature" before being removed; thus, surgery may be delayed if it is not fully developed. Contact lenses restore both central and peripheral vision; glasses restore only central vision. An implanted lens functions much as the natural lens does, but it must be placed in the eye surgically.

7 Describe the relevant surgical procedure.	One of the following surgical procedures may be used to remove the cataract: —Intracapsular cataract extraction removes the entire lens, leaving the lens capsule intact, by a technique called cryoextraction. In cryoextraction, the moist lens sticks to an extremely cold metal probe for easy and safe removal with gentle traction. —Extracapsular cataract extraction removes the cortex and lens and retains the posterior lens capsule. —Phacoemulsification fragments the lens with ultrasonic vibrations and aspirates the pieces. —Discission ruptures the lens capsule, allowing the aqueous humor access to the lens, which is slowly digested.
8 Explain what to expect before and after cataract surgery.	The patient should expect the general preparation and postoperative care given for any surgical procedure. (See Appendix B, *Preoperative and Postoperative Teaching,* for specific instructions.) In addition, he should expect the following: —The eye being operated on will be prepared by the frequent instillation of eye drops just before the patient is taken to the operating room. —After surgery, the eye will be patched, and eye drops will be instilled periodically. The patient will wear an eye shield at night to prevent accidental damage. —He will be checked frequently and will receive pain medication for discomfort. If he experiences sudden, acute pain, he should notify the nurse. —He should ring for the nurse rather than exert himself to take care of his needs. —He should not cough, sneeze, or move quickly for at least 4 weeks after surgery, because these maneuvers can increase intraocular pressure. —He should lie on the unaffected side to avoid exerting pressure on the eye. —Postoperative activity restrictions will depend on the number of sutures used and on the physician's preference.
9 Describe the medication regimen after surgery.	A drug commonly used is phenylephrine (ophthalmic). For specific medication instructions, see Chapter 10, Drug Therapy.
10 Demonstrate the use of eye drops.	Correct self-administration of eye drops is shown in *Giving Yourself Eye Drops,* pp. 186-187.

11 Discuss guidelines for daily living after cataract surgery.

Guidelines for daily living after cataract surgery include the following:
—In the first few weeks after a cataract extraction, the patient should wear dark glasses during the day to reduce glare and a Fox eye shield (a metal shield with perforations) at night to prevent accidental injury.
—He should avoid activities that increase intraocular pressure (bending, straining, or lying flat) until approved by his physician.
—He should notify his physician immediately if he experiences sharp eye pain.
—He should understand the importance of follow-up visits.

CONJUNCTIVITIS

Patient objectives	Teaching plan content

1 Define conjunctivitis.

Conjunctivitis is an inflammation of the conjunctiva.

2 Identify the conjunctiva.

The conjunctiva is the delicate mucous membrane that lines the eyelids and covers part of the eyeball.

3 Identify the causes of conjunctivitis.

The main causes of conjunctivitis fall into three categories: infection, allergy, and unknown causes.
—An infection can occur in the conjunctiva in response to bacterial agents, chlamydial agents, or viral agents. (The causative agent should be identified, especially if it is *Neisseria gonorrhoeae* or herpes simplex virus Type I, as further health teaching may be necessary.)
—Conjunctivitis may occur as an allergic reaction to pollen, grass, topical medications, air pollutants, smoke, occupational irritants, and unknown irritants.
—Conjunctivitis may occur without an apparent cause.

4 Discuss the signs and symptoms of conjunctivitis.

Because conjunctivitis can recur, the patient should know the following signs and symptoms and should seek prompt medical attention for them:
—Conjunctivitis generally produces redness, swelling, pain, tearing, and possibly a discharge.
—If the cornea is involved, a sensitivity to light may develop.
—Although it usually starts in one eye, it can quickly spread to the other eye by contamination of towels, washcloths, or the patient's hands.
—If it is caused by bacteria (usually referred to as pinkeye), the symptoms may last for about 2 weeks.
  • The patient may experience itching, burning, and the sensation of a foreign body in his eye.

• At the same time, he may notice a crust of sticky, puslike discharge on his eyelids or, if his conjunctivitis is caused by *N. gonorrhoeae,* a profuse, purulent (pus) discharge.
—Viral conjunctivitis produces copious tearing with minimal drainage. It may follow a chronic course, reappearing periodically, or may last for only 2 to 3 weeks.

---

5 Describe the treatment of conjunctivitis.

Treatment of conjunctivitis varies with the cause.
—For bacterial or viral infection, treatment consists of the application of ointments (type depending on the agent identified) to the conjunctiva. Occasionally, antibiotic eye drops may also be used to prevent secondary infection.
—For allergic conjunctivitis, treatment consists of medication to decrease redness and swelling and cold compresses to relieve itching. Occasionally, oral antihistamines may also be used to relieve the overall allergic reaction.

---

6 Demonstrate the correct use of eye drops and/or ointments, if appropriate.

Correct self-administration of eye drops is shown in *Giving Yourself Eye Drops,* pp. 186-187. Correct application of an ointment to the conjunctiva is shown in *How to Use Eye Ointment,* p. 185.

---

7 Discuss self-care guidelines for conjunctivitis.

Self-care guidelines for conjunctivitis are as follows:
—Proper handwashing technique should be used, since some forms of conjunctivitis are highly contagious. Hands should be washed before using medication. Clean washcloths or towels should be used to avoid infecting the other eye.
—Washcloths, towels, or pillows should not be shared. This can spread the infection to other persons.
—The affected eye should not be rubbed. This can spread the infection to the other eye and to other persons.
—The eye should never be irrigated, as this will also spread the infection.
—The physician should be notified if the condition worsens.

OTITIS EXTERNA

Patient objectives	*Teaching plan content*
1 Define otitis externa.	Otitis externa (often called swimmer's ear) is an inflammation of the skin of the external ear and ear canal.

2 Identify the causes of otitis externa.	Otitis externa may be caused by bacteria, fungi, or dermatologic conditions such as seborrhea or psoriasis.
3 Identify at least four predisposing factors for otitis externa.	Predisposing factors for otitis externa include the following: —Swimming in contaminated water may introduce a water-borne organism into the cerumen (earwax), which serves as a culture medium. —Cleaning the ear canal with a cotton swab, bobby pin, finger, or other foreign object may irritate the ear canal and introduce the infecting microorganism. —Exposure to dust, hair-care products, or other irritants may cause the patient to scratch his ear and break the skin. —Regular use of earphones, earplugs, or earmuffs traps moisture in the ear canal, creating a culture medium for infection. —Chronic drainage from a perforated tympanic membrane may lead to infection.
4 Discuss the signs and symptoms of otitis externa.	Because otitis externa can recur, the patient should know the following signs and symptoms and should seek prompt medical attention for them: —Fever, a foul-smelling drainage coming from the ear, redness, swelling, and partial hearing loss are common signs and symptoms. —In an acute episode, moderate to severe pain worsens when the external ear is moved or when the patient clenches his teeth, opens his mouth, or chews. —In chronic otitis externa, itching may lead to scaling and skin thickening.
5 Describe the treatment regimen for otitis externa.	With proper treatment, an acute episode usually subsides within 7 days, although otitis externa may become chronic and recur. Treatment consists of the following: —Heat therapy to the periauricular region in the form of a heat lamp; hot, wet compresses; or a heating pad —Pain medication —Cleansing of the ear and removal of debris —Antibiotic eardrops and/or creams, as well as other types of medicated creams. Treatment should be prompt to prevent perforation of the tympanic membrane.
6 Describe the medication regimen.	Some drugs commonly used for this disorder are acetic acid (otic), boric acid (otic), chloramphenecol (otic), dexamethasone (otic), hydrocortisone (otic), and poly-

myxin B sulfate (otic). See Chapter 10, Drug Therapy, for specific medication instructions.

7 Demonstrate the use of eardrops.	Correct self-administration of eardrops is shown in *Giving Yourself Eardrops,* p. 190.
8 Discuss patient guidelines to prevent otitis externa.	Patient guidelines to prevent otitis externa are as follows: —Use lamb's wool earplugs coated with petrolatum to keep water out of the ear when showering or shampooing. —Wear earplugs or keep the head above water when swimming. Also, instill two or three drops of 3% boric acid solution in 70% alcohol before and after swimming to toughen the skin of the external ear canal. —Do not clean the ears with cotton swabs, bobby pins, or other foreign objects.

OTITIS MEDIA

Patient objectives	*Teaching plan content*
1 Define otitis media.	Otitis media is an inflammation of the middle ear.
2 Describe the relevant type of otitis media.	There are three types of otitis media: —In serous otitis media, inflammation of the middle ear causes the eustachian tube to swell so that fluid and air cannot escape. —In acute otitis media, infection causes a change in the normal eardrum. —In chronic otitis media, repeated infection causes persistent tearing of the eardrum.
3 Identify at least three causes of otitis media.	Otitis media may be caused by any of the following: —Bacteria —Cold viruses —Allergies —Enlarged adenoids —Barotrauma (sudden descent in an airplane).
4 Identify at least three predisposing factors for otitis media.	Predisposing factors for otitis media include the following: —Misuse of nose drops —Indiscriminate use of nasal douching —Forceful nose blowing —Sneezing —Flying with an upper respiratory infection —Skull fracture (rare).

5 **Identify the signs and symptoms of otitis media.**	Children unable to verbalize signs and symptoms may exhibit excessive pulling on the ear, fussiness, tiredness, lack of appetite, or diarrhea. In serous otitis media, symptoms may be absent or may involve only a popping sensation when yawning, swallowing, or blowing the nose. However, the common signs and symptoms of otitis media include the following: —Ear pain —Fever —Decreased hearing —Ear noises —Sense of ear fullness —Headache —Loss of appetite —Nausea and vomiting —Foul-smelling discharge —Dizziness —Tinnitus (ringing in the ears).
6 **Describe the treatment regimen for otitis media.**	Treatment consists of the following: —Antibiotics to combat the infection —Antihistamines and/or decongestants to decrease swelling of the eustachian tube and promote fluid drainage from the ear —Eardrops for the relief of pain —Other medications if additional problems are present —Insertion of ear tubes in chronic otitis media, to provide adequate airflow from the ear —Use of the Valsalva maneuver in serous otitis media, to force air through blocked eustachian tubes. (The Valsalva maneuver is performed by pinching the nostrils shut, taking a deep breath, closing the lips, and vigorously blowing air against the cheeks and closed lips.)
7 **Describe the medication regimen.**	Some drugs commonly used for this disorder are acetaminophen, ampicillin, aspirin, co-trimoxazole, erythromycin, penicillin, and sulfisoxazole. See Chapter 10, Drug Therapy, for specific medication instructions.
8 **Demonstrate the use of eardrops.**	Correct self-administration of eardrops is shown in *Giving Yourself Eardrops*, p. 190.
9 **Discuss guidelines to prevent otitis media.**	Guidelines to prevent otitis media include the following: —Avoid cleaning the ears with cotton swabs, bobby pins, or other foreign objects. —Hold babies in an upright position during bottle feeding to keep milk from collecting at the opening of the eustachian tubes in the throat.

—Avoid contact with allergy-causing substances, if possible.
—Seek prompt treatment of colds.
—To prevent serous otitis media, chewing gum, sucking on hard candy (or a bottle for infants), and yawning or swallowing repeatedly during airplane descent may be helpful. Use of the Valsalva maneuver during air travel may also be helpful.

MÉNIÈRE'S DISEASE

Patient objectives	Teaching plan content
1 Define Ménière's disease.	Ménière's disease is a chronic degenerative disorder affecting the bony cochlea and vestibular labyrinths, organs within the inner ear responsible for hearing and equilibrium, respectively. (An illustration can be used to demonstrate the location of these organs.)
2 Explain how Ménière's disease develops.	In Ménière's disease, overproduction or decreased absorption of endolymph occurs. (Endolymph is the fluid that bathes and nourishes the cochlea and vestibular labyrinths.) Because endolymph is contained within a tube, the resulting accumulation of fluid will increase the pressure inside the tube. This in turn causes the endolymph to bathe the cochlea and vestibular labyrinths with greater force, which can damage the fragile hair cells of these delicate organs. Once they have been damaged, hearing and equilibrium become affected.
3 Explain the cause of Ménière's disease.	The cause of Ménière's disease is unknown, but it may result from an autonomic nervous system dysfunction that produces a temporary constriction of blood vessels in the inner ear, affecting endolymph production or absorption.
4 Identify the symptoms associated with Ménière's disease.	Ménière's disease produces three major symptoms: severe dizziness (vertigo), ringing in the ears (tinnitus), and sensorineural hearing loss. A full or blocked feeling in the ear is also common.
5 Describe the progression of Ménière's disease.	The clinical progression of Ménière's disease is as follows: —Severe dizziness, lasting from 10 minutes to several hours, may occur suddenly and without warning. —During an acute attack, other symptoms such as severe nausea, vomiting, sweating, and giddiness may occur. In addition, the patient may experience a loss of balance and may fall to the affected side.

—He may be asymptomatic between attacks, except for a residual ringing in the ears that worsens during an attack.

—Attacks may occur several times a year or be absent for several years. Eventually, the attacks will become less frequent as hearing loss progresses (usually only on one side), and they may cease when hearing loss is total.

---

6 Discuss the treatment measures used for Ménière's disease.

The treatment measures used for Ménière's disease are as follows:

—An acute attack may be stopped by a variety of medications. Long-term management includes a low-sodium diet and medication to decrease endolymphatic fluid.

—Medications called vasodilators may also be used to expand the blood vessels in the inner ear. Prophylactic antihistamines or mild sedatives may also be used.

—If Ménière's disease persists after more than 2 years of treatment or produces incapacitating dizziness, surgical destruction of the affected labyrinth may be necessary. Although this procedure permanently relieves symptoms, it is performed only in extreme cases because irreversible hearing loss results.

---

7 Describe the medication regimen.

Some drugs commonly used for this disorder are atropine injection, diazepam, diphenhydramine, epinephrine, phenobarbital, and scopolamine injection. For specific medication instructions, see Chapter 10, Drug Therapy.

---

8 Discuss guidelines for daily living with Ménière's disease.

Guidelines for daily living with Ménière's disease include the following:

—To minimize dizziness during an attack of Ménière's disease, avoid reading and exposure to glaring lights.

—To prevent falls, do not get out of bed or walk without assistance during an attack.

—Because such attacks are apt to begin quite rapidly, avoid sudden position changes and any tasks that vertigo makes hazardous, such as driving or operating machinery.

—Adhere to a low-sodium diet.

—Keep appointments for follow-up visits with the physician.

SINUSITIS

Patient objectives	Teaching plan content
1 Define sinusitis.	Sinusitis is an inflammatory condition of the paranasal sinuses. (An illustration can be used to demonstrate the location of these structures.)
2 Explain the cause of sinusitis.	Sinusitis usually results from a bacterial infection or, less commonly, from a viral infection. Bacterial invasion of the paranasal sinuses occurs when a cold spreads to the sinus passages. Excessive nose blowing forces infected material into the sinuses. The mucous lining of the affected sinuses then becomes inflamed and swells, blocking normal drainage from the area.
3 Identify the types of sinusitis.	Sinusitis occurs in a variety of forms: —Acute sinusitis follows the common cold. —Subacute sinusitis follows an acute episode. —Chronic sinusitis follows persistent bacterial infections. —Allergic sinusitis accompanies allergic rhinitis. —Hyperplastic sinusitis is a combination of acute, purulent sinusitis and allergic sinusitis.
4 Identify the signs and symptoms of sinusitis.	Symptoms of sinusitis include the following: —In acute sinusitis: nasal discharge (blood-tinged for 24 to 48 hours after onset, then becoming yellow-green), malaise, sore throat, headache, and low-grade fever (99° to 99.5° F. or 37.2° to 37.5° C.) —In subacute sinusitis: yellow-green nasal drainage that continues for longer than 3 weeks after an acute infection, stuffy nose, vague facial discomfort, fatigue, and nonproductive cough —In chronic sinusitis: symptoms like those of acute sinusitis except for a continuous mucoid, yellow-green nasal discharge —In allergic sinusitis: sneezing, frontal headache, watery nasal discharge, and stuffy, burning, itchy nose —In hyperplastic sinusitis: chronic nasal stuffiness and headache.
5 Discuss the treatment measures used for sinusitis.	Treatment measures used for sinusitis are as follows: —For acute sinusitis, pain medication to promote comfort is the primary treatment. Other measures that may be used include medications to decrease nasal secretions and combat persistent infections. Steam inhalation may be used to promote nasal drainage, while local applications of heat may help to relieve pain and congestion.

—For subacute sinusitis, medications to combat persistent infections, decrease nasal secretions, and promote comfort are used. After the infection subsides, sinus irrigation may be performed (needle puncture followed by saline [saltwater] wash). Occasionally, additional medications in the form of steroid therapy may be used to decrease inflammation.
—Allergic sinusitis occurs with allergic rhinitis, so treatment is geared toward both disorders. Antihistamine medication will be given, followed by identification of allergens by skin testing and desensitization by immunotherapy.
—Chronic sinusitis and hyperplastic sinusitis are treated in the same manner, using nasal irrigations to relieve pain and congestion. If irrigations fail to relieve symptoms, surgery may be done on one or more sinuses.

---

6 Describe the relevant surgical treatment of sinusitis.

For chronic or hyperplastic sinusitis requiring surgery, one of the following procedures may be used:
—The nasal window procedure creates an opening in the sinus, allowing secretions and pus to drain through the nose.
—The Caldwell-Luc procedure removes diseased mucosa in the maxillary sinus through an incision in the upper lip.
—Ethmoidectomy removes all infected tissue through an external or intranasal incision into the ethmoidal sinus.
—External ethmoidectomy removes infected ethmoidal sinus tissue through a crescent-shaped incision beginning under the inner eyebrow and extending along the side of the nose.
—Frontoethmoidectomy removes infected frontal sinus tissue through an extended external ethmoidectomy.
—An osteoplastic flap drains the sinuses through an incision across the skull, behind the hairline.

---

7 Describe the medication regimen.

Some drugs commonly used for this disorder are codeine, dexamethasone (nasal), epinephrine, meperidine, penicillin, and phenylephrine. For specific medication instructions, see Chapter 10, Drug Therapy.

---

8 Demonstrate the use of nasal medication.

Correct instillation of nasal medications is shown in *How to Use Nose Drops,* p. 191; *How to Use a Turbo-Inhaler,* pp. 192-193; and *How to Use an Atomizer,* p. 196.

---

9 Discuss self-care guidelines for sinusitis.

The patient should follow these guidelines for self-care:
—Stay in bed to get plenty of rest. While in bed, do not elevate the head on pillows higher than 30 degrees.

—Drink plenty of fluids to promote drainage.
—To relieve pain and promote drainage, apply warm compresses continuously, or four times daily for 2-hour intervals. If warm compresses are ineffective in relieving pain, try cold compresses. (See the "Heat Therapy" and "Cold Therapy" teaching plans in Chapter 2, Pain Management, for further instructions on application of warm and/or cold compresses.)
—Notify the physician immediately if vomiting, chills, fever, eyelid or forehead puffiness, blurred or double vision, and/or personality changes occur.
—Stop smoking.
—Blow the nose gently.
—Keep all follow-up appointments.

PHARYNGITIS

Patient objectives	*Teaching plan content*
1 Define pharyngitis.	Pharyngitis is a throat infection.
2 Identify two causes of pharyngitis.	Pharyngitis is most commonly caused by a virus. It may also be caused by bacteria. The most common bacterium causing pharyngitis is the streptococcus organism. If this organism is identified, the pharyngitis is often referred to as "strep throat."
3 Identify the symptoms of pharyngitis.	Symptoms of pharyngitis include the following: —Sore throat —Difficulty swallowing —Sensation of a lump in the throat —Associated symptoms such as fever, headache, and muscle and joint pain.
4 Identify the components of the treatment regimen for pharyngitis.	Treatment of pharyngitis includes the following: —Analgesics for pain relief —Antibiotics if the pharyngitis is caused by a bacteria —Warm saline gargles —Increased fluid intake —Rest.
5 Describe the medication regimen.	Some drugs commonly used for this disorder are aspirin and penicillin. For specific medication instructions, see Chapter 10, Drug Therapy.
6 Discuss self-care guidelines for pharyngitis.	Self-care guidelines for pharyngitis include the following: —Take medications as ordered. If an antibiotic has

been prescribed, complete the full course of therapy.
—Gargle with warm salt water frequently.
—For additional throat comfort, take throat lozenges containing a mild anesthetic (if not contraindicated) that can be purchased without a prescription.
—Drink at least 3 qt of fluid a day (if not contraindicated).
—Use a bedside humidifier to minimize sources of throat irritation in the environment.
—Do not smoke. (Smoking causes further throat irritation.)
—Obtain plenty of rest.
—Notify the physician if symptoms worsen or if new ones appear. (Symptoms should subside within 3 to 10 days.)

 # Explaining treatments

IRIDECTOMY

Patient objectives	Teaching plan content
1 State the purpose of iridectomy.	An iridectomy is done to relieve the elevated intraocular pressure caused by acute or chronic closed-angle (narrow-angle) glaucoma.
2 Explain the procedure used in an iridectomy.	The surgeon will excise a small part of the iris (the colored portion of the eye).
3 Describe the preoperative procedures.	The patient should expect the general preparation done for any surgical procedure. (See Appendix B, *Preoperative and Postoperative Teaching.*) In addition, the following preoperative procedures are performed for an iridectomy: —The eye that is being operated on will be prepared by the frequent instillation of eye drops just before going to the operating room. —If the patient has long hair, he will be asked to fix it so that it can be kept in place for several days postoperatively. —Occasionally, the surgeon may prescribe a bowel preparation to ensure lower-bowel evacuation the morning of surgery. This is done to prevent postoperative straining, because straining increases intraocular pressure.

4 Describe what to expect after an iridectomy.	After an iridectomy, the patient may expect the following: —An eye patch will be in place on the affected eye to collect drainage. It will be changed each time eye drops are given. —An eye shield may be used at night to prevent accidental damage to the eye. —The patient should lie on the unaffected side to avoid exerting pressure on the eye. Otherwise, he can move about without restriction. —He should ring for the nurse rather than strain to get out of bed or to reach for something. —He will receive pain medication for discomfort. —Nausea and vomiting commonly occur after this procedure. Vomiting needs to be avoided because it increases intraocular pressure. The patient should call the nurse at the first feeling of nausea.
5 Discuss patient guidelines to be followed after discharge.	The patient should receive specific guidelines about medications and activities from the physician. He or a family member should be able to administer his eye drops as well as apply an eye patch or shield (if needed).

HEARING AID

Patient objectives	*Teaching plan content*
1 State the purpose of a hearing aid.	A hearing aid is used to improve hearing ability, but it will not restore hearing to normal.
2 Discuss patient guidelines for adapting to a hearing aid.	The orientation period will critically affect the success of hearing rehabilitation. The following guidelines will help the patient to adapt: —Becoming accustomed to the hearing aid will require many hours of wear and much practice. —The patient should use it as much as possible. —He should wear the aid only for short periods; for instance, for 15 to 20 minutes the first 2 days and then for a half hour more each day until he is completely comfortable with it. He should turn off the aid and rest for a while if it makes him nervous or tired. —He should not turn the volume too high. Doing so will distort sounds and may cause a whistling or squealing sound. (NOTE: These sounds may also indicate a loose-fitting ear mold.) —He should ignore background noises when listening to conversations. Blocking out these distractions will require patience. If the background noise becomes too

annoying, he should turn down the volume on his hearing aid and closely watch the speaker's face.

—He should practice conversing with only one person at a time at first. He should then experiment with the aid in difficult situations; for example, when listening to a stereo or television set or with loud background noise.

—He should sit as close as possible to the speaker when in a large group.

—He should understand and follow instructions on wearing and caring for his aid. If he cannot maintain it, a family member should assist him.

—He should immediately contact the physician if he has pain or drainage in his ear, which could be caused by a skin or cartilage infection, a middle-ear infection, an ear tumor, or an improperly fitted ear mold.

---

3 Explain how to care for a hearing aid.

The patient can obtain long service from his hearing aid by caring for it correctly and referring to the instructions. In addition, he should follow these guidelines:

—Turn off the aid when it is not in use, and remove the battery. Leave the battery case open, and store the hearing aid in a properly identified container.

—Take care not to drop the aid on a hard surface. Work over a bed or a similar soft area when changing batteries or removing the aid from the ear.

—Turn off the hearing aid before replacing or inserting a battery.

—Clean the battery by gently rubbing it with a sharpened pencil eraser. This procedure removes corrosion. If the battery becomes damp, dry the contacts with a cotton swab.

—Store extra batteries in the freezer to lengthen shelf life. (NOTE: If the hearing aid is used 10 to 12 hours daily, the batteries will need to be replaced weekly.)

—Avoid getting moisture inside the hearing aid; for example, do not wear it in the rain, in the bathtub, or during activities that cause excessive perspiration. Steam from a vaporizer can also damage the hearing aid.

—Store the aid in an airtight container with a silica-gel packet, particularly in humid climates.

—Avoid applying any sprays on or near the head while wearing the aid to prevent clogging the microphone.

—Keep the hearing aid away from excessive heat or cold. Never place it near a stove or heater or on a sunny windowsill or wear it while using a hair dryer. Also, avoid wearing it for long periods outside in extremely hot or cold weather.

Patient-Teaching Aid

HOW TO USE EYE OINTMENT

Dear Patient:
To relieve your eye infection or irritation, your physician has prescribed eye ointment. Here is how to use it:

To instill eye ointment

- First, cleanse your eyelids and lashes with an irrigating solution.
- Then, remove the cap from the tube, taking care not to contaminate the applicator end by letting it touch anything.
- Squeeze a small ribbon of medication along the inside of your lower eyelid. (See illustration.)
- Keep your eyelids closed for 1 to 2 minutes after application to allow the medication to spread and be absorbed.

You may experience blurred vision for a few minutes after the ointment has been applied. This is normal.

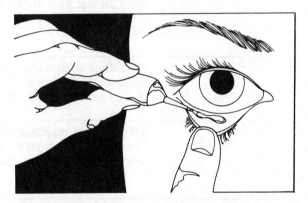

A final caution

Never put any medication in your eyes unless the label reads FOR OPHTHALMIC USE or FOR USE IN THE EYES. Call your physician immediately if you notice such adverse effects as decreased visual acuity, persistent blurred vision, or unusual redness or irritation when using medication.

Patient-Teaching Aid

GIVING YOURSELF EYE DROPS

Dear Patient:
To relieve your eye infection or irritation, your physician has prescribed these eye drops: _____

Use them exactly as directed on the label. Here is how:

1 Begin by washing your hands thoroughly.

2 Hold the bottle up to the light and examine it. If the medication is discolored or contains sediment, discard it immediately and have the prescription refilled. If it looks OK, warm the medication to room temperature by holding the bottle between your hands for 2 minutes.

3 Next, moisten a rayon ball or tissue with water, and clean all secretions from around your eyes. Use a fresh rayon ball or tissue for each eye, so you do not spread infection.

4 Now, stand or sit before a mirror, or lie on your back, whichever is most comfortable for you. Squeeze the bulb of the eyedropper to fill the dropper with medication.

5 Tilt your head slightly back and toward the eye you are treating. Pull down your lower eyelid. (Do not pull your upper eyelid, or you will put unnecessary pressure on your eye.)

6 Position the dropper over the conjunctival sac you have exposed between your lower lid and the white of your eye. Steady your hand by resting two fingers against your cheek or nose.

7 Look away from the dropper. Then, squeeze the prescribed number of drops into the sac. Do not drop the medication directly onto your eyeball. Take care not to touch the dropper to your eye or eyelashes. Wipe away excess medication with a clean tissue.

8 Repeat the procedure in the other eye, if the physician orders.

GIVING YOURSELF EYE DROPS—*continued*

9

Recap the medication. Store the bottle away from light and extreme heat.

IMPORTANT: Call your physician immediately if you notice any of these adverse effects: _____

And remember, never put any medication in your eyes unless the label reads FOR OPHTHALMIC USE or FOR USE IN THE EYES.

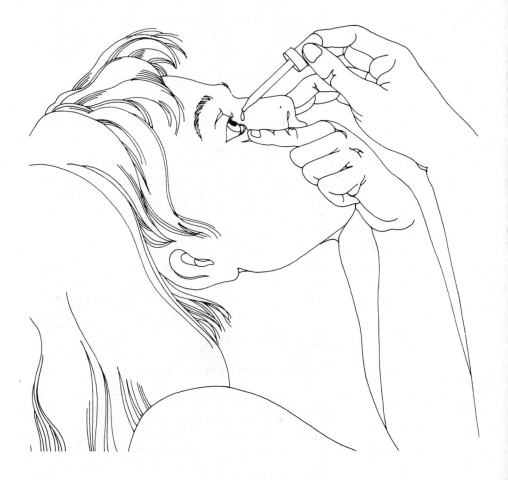

Patient-Teaching Aid

CONTACT LENSES

Dear Patient:
This comparison of the different types of contact lenses is intended only to give you a general idea of what is available. The eye specialist who prescribes your contacts will give you specific recommendations on the types of lenses best suited for you, including the cost and care involved.

Hard contact lenses

Advantages • Excellent vision correction, especially for astigmatism • Low costs, both in purchase price and infrequent replacements, compared to soft lenses • Can be changed slightly if prescription changes without needing a new pair • Easy to clean and don't require many special solutions • Can be tinted for cosmetic or identification purposes and to reduce light sensitivity and glare • Not affected by low humidity • Last an average of 10 years

Disadvantages • Sometimes lengthy adaptation period needed before they're comfortable to wear • Sometimes a feeling that something's in your eye when your eyelids rub against the lens' edges • Exact fit critical to prevent problems such as corneal swelling • Dirt and other foreign particles can float under the lens, causing tearing, redness, and pain • Daily wearing schedule (an average of 8 hours) must be followed or problems result. Wearing too long causes pain, redness, and blurred vision; if you don't wear them long enough, your eyes will have to readjust to wearing them longer again • When you remove your lenses, your vision is blurry until your corneas recover from having lenses molded over them (this "spectacle blur" may last for a few minutes or a few hours) • More likely to fall out or get scratched or chipped; must be handled carefully • Falling asleep with them in your eyes can cause corneal swelling and abrasion

Soft contact lenses

Advantages • Provide immediately comfortable wear • Adhere more closely to your cornea so are less likely to pop out or to let foreign particles slip under • Can be worn longer (an average of 14 hours or more) • Fewer cases of irritation or light sensitivity • No spectacle blur when you remove them

Disadvantages • Thirty to forty percent more expensive than hard lenses; lens solutions cost about $100 a year

CONTACT LENSES—*continued*

• Last an average of only 1 or 2 years • Need to be replaced with every prescription change • Can absorb unwanted substances, such as aerosol sprays, chlorine, cigarette smoke, eye drops, makeup, and oils • With every blink, tears wash under the lens and cause momentary wavy, blurred vision. • Conform to corneal irregularities so can't correct astigmatism, unless specially made to do so • Cleaning and handling are complicated and time consuming • In dry air, lenses can dry out at the edges and curl up, cause discomfort, or fall out

Gas-permeable lenses

Advantages • Sharp vision • Correct astigmatism better than soft but not as well as hard lenses • Last an average of 5 years • Easy to insert and remove • Reduced risk of overwear, corneal swelling, spectacle blur, irritation, or popping out • Have medical applications • Don't require a period of corneal adjustment

Disadvantages • Sometimes cause a scratchy feeling when inserted • Cost more than hard lenses • Susceptible to scratches, chips, and warping • Susceptible to deposits of protein, oils, and tears that can't always be removed by cleaning procedure

Extended-wear lenses

Advantages • More comfortable because of their thinness and absorbency • Good vision as soon as you open your eyes • Can be worn while sleeping and swimming (if you don't dive or open your eyes too wide) • Require little care and upkeep; more convenient • Reduced risk of allergic reactions to solutions

Disadvantages • High costs for lenses and follow-up visits • Less sharp vision (similar to soft lenses) • May have to be replaced twice a year • Absorbency makes them susceptible to sprays, vapors, and fumes and to deposits from your eyelids and tears • Difficult to handle • Discomfort caused by dry air or deposits on lens • May cause corneal problems, such as swelling, thickening, and infections • Possible grave side effects of overwear include scratches, inflammation, or ulcers of corneal surface (keratitis) or blood vessels on the cornea (neovascularization); these conditions should stop when lenses are removed

Patient-Teaching Aid

GIVING YOURSELF EARDROPS

Dear Patient:

To relieve your ear infection, your physician has prescribed these eardrops:

_____

Use them exactly as directed on the label. Here is how:

• Begin by washing your hands thoroughly.

• Examine the medication. If it is discolored or has sediment in it, notify the physician and get your prescription refilled. If nothing is wrong with the medication, proceed to the next step.

• For your own comfort, warm the medication by holding the bottle between your hands for 2 minutes.

• Shake the bottle, if directed, and open it.

• Fill the dropper; then, place the open bottle and dropper within easy reach.

• Lie on your side so the ear you are treating is exposed.

• Gently pull the top of your ear up and back, to straighten the ear canal.

• Position the dropper above your ear, taking care not to touch your ear with it. Squeeze the dropper's bulb to release one drop.

• Wait until you feel the drop in your ear. Then, if directed, squeeze the bulb again. Repeat this step until you have administered the prescribed number of drops.

• To keep the drops in your ear, continue to lie on your side for about 10 minutes.

• If you wish, plug your ear with cotton moistened with eardrops. Do not plug your ear with dry cotton, unless your physician directs. Dry cotton will absorb the drops.

• If your physician directs, repeat the procedure for the other ear.

• Recap the bottle. Store your drops away from light and extreme heat.

IMPORTANT: Call your physician immediately if you have any of these adverse effects: _____

_____

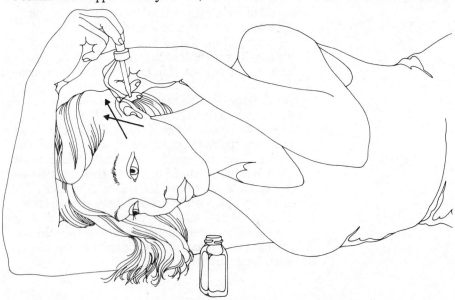

Patient-Teaching Aid

HOW TO USE NOSE DROPS

Dear Patient:
Your physician has prescribed nose drops for you to use at home. Here is what you will need to know:

To instill nose drops

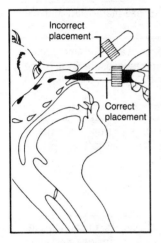

Incorrect placement

Correct placement

• Before you use your nose drops, look at the container to make sure you have the right medication and to check prescribed dosage.
• Position the dropper as shown in this illustration so the drops will flow down the back of your nose, not your throat.
• Squeeze the dropper bulb to instill the correct number of drops.
• Repeat the process in the other nostril, if indicated.
• Breathe through your mouth so you do not sniff the drops into your sinuses or aspirate them into your lungs.

Precautions to take

• Follow your physician's orders exactly. Do not overuse your nose drops.
• Because nose drops are easily contaminated, do not buy more than you will use in a short time. Discard nose drops that contain sediment or look discolored.
• Do not share your nose drops with family members. Doing so may spread infection.
• Call your physician if you notice any adverse effects.

Patient-Teaching Aid

HOW TO USE A TURBO-INHALER

Dear Patient:
Inhaling the medication in this whirly-bird inhalation device will help prevent asthma attacks. Use it exactly as your physician ordered at these times: _____

CAUTION: Never use more than four capsules a day.

1 Before you begin, wash and dry your hands. Unwrap one capsule so it is ready to use.

2 Hold the device so the white mouthpiece is on the bottom, like this. Slide the gray sleeve all the way to the top.

3 Open the mouthpiece by unscrewing its tip counterclockwise. Inside, you will see a small propeller on a stem.

4 Firmly press the colored end of your medication capsule into the center of the propeller, as shown here. Avoid overhandling the capsule, or it may soften.

5 Now, screw the device back together securely, and hold it with the mouthpiece at the bottom, as shown here. To puncture the capsule and release the medication, slide the gray sleeve all the way down. Then, slide it up again. Do this step one time only.

HOW TO USE A TURBO-INHALER—*continued*

6

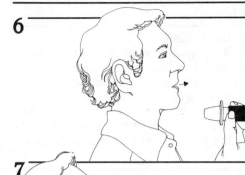

Make sure everything is secure. Then, hold the device away from your mouth, and exhale as much air as you can.

7

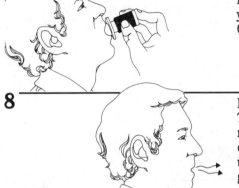

Now, tilt your head backward. Place the mouthpiece in your mouth, and close your lips around it, as shown here. Quickly inhale once, to fill your lungs.

8

Hold your breath for several seconds. Then, remove the device from your mouth, and exhale as much air as you can. Repeat steps 7 and 8 several times, until all the medication in the device is gone. Never exhale through the mouthpiece.

9

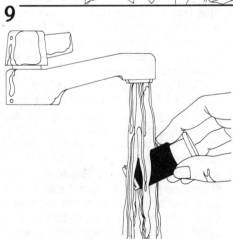

Discard the empty medication capsule. Then, place the entire device in its metal can, and screw on the lid. At least once a week, remove the device from the can, take it apart, and rinse it thoroughly with warm water. Make sure it is completely dry before reassembling it. Keep the capsules from deteriorating too rapidly by leaving them wrapped until needed.

IMPORTANT: Follow your physician's instructions exactly. Notify him at once if you have throat or chest irritation, coughing or choking, nasal congestion, dizziness, headache, or nausea.

Patient-Teaching Aid

HOW TO USE A NASAL INHALATION DEVICE

Dear Patient:
Your physician wants you to use a non-aerosol medicated spray, called _____, to relieve your runny nose. Carefully read the directions on the bottle's label, and use the spray exactly as your physician or nurse explained. The pictures on this page will remind you exactly what to do.

1

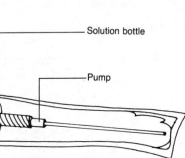

Adapter cover

Solution bottle

Pump

Adapter

First, take these pieces of equipment out of their box. As you can see, the pump is in a plastic bag to keep it clean.

2

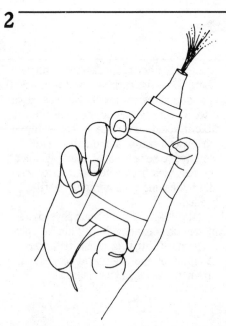

Next, take off the solution bottle's cap, and remove the pump from its bag. Tightly screw the pump into the bottle. Now, take the adapter, and remove its cover. Pointing the adapter *away* from you, slide the solution bottle into the bottom of the adapter. Make sure the solution bottle fits snugly.

Hold the adapter in your hand, as shown at left, and continue to point it away from you. Using a pumping motion, repeatedly push the bottle into the adapter with your thumb, until a fine spray mist appears. (You may have to pump five or six times.) This motion primes the pump. (You *do not* have to prime the pump each time you use the medication. But do prime the pump again after taking the equipment apart for cleaning. Also, you may need to prime the pump if you have not used this medication for 5 days or more.)

HOW TO USE A NASAL INHALATION DEVICE—*continued*

3

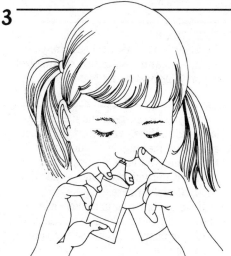

Gently blow your nose to clear your nostrils. (Or, clear your nostrils with medication your physician has given you.) Then, bend your head slightly forward, and put the tip of the adapter into one nostril. Press your other nostril closed with a finger, as shown here.

With one quick, firm motion, pump the solution bottle; sniff gently at the same time. Do this one more time, if your physician directs.

Then, repeat this step for the other nostril.

4

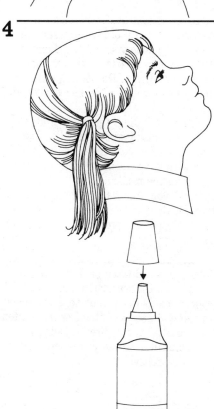

Now, remove the adapter tip from your nose, and tip your head slightly back for a moment. This allows the medication to spread across the back of your nose. Put the adapter cover back on the adapter tip.

Keep the adapter cover on the adapter tip when you are not using it. If the adapter tip becomes clogged, take the bottle out of the adapter, unscrew the pump from the bottle, and soak *only the pump* in warm water. Then, dry the pump, and put everything back together, as already shown on this page. Prime the pump again.

IMPORTANT: Do not use this equipment set for more than 5 months. Also, tell your physician if the medication does not help.

Patient-Teaching Aid

HOW TO USE AN ATOMIZER

Dear Patient:

To relieve your nasal congestion, your physician wants you to use an atomizer to spray medication into your nose. Here is how:

1

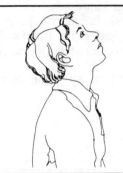

Before you begin, read the medication label carefully, so you know the exact amount of medication to administer. Make sure you have tissues handy. Then, sit upright, with your head tilted back, as shown here.

If that position is uncomfortable for you, lie on your back instead. Place a pillow under your shoulders, so your head tilts back.

2

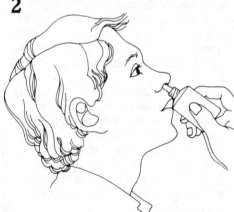

Now, place the tip of the atomizer about ½″ (1 cm) inside your nostril. Point it straight up your nose, toward the inner corner of your eye. Do not angle the atomizer downward, or the medication will run down your throat.

Without inhaling, squeeze the atomizer once, quickly and firmly. Use just enough force to coat the inside of your nose with medication. Too much force may send the medicine into your sinuses and give you a headache. Then, spray again, if the instructions on the label order it. Repeat the procedure in the other nostril.

3

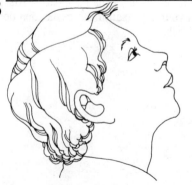

Keep your head tilted back for several minutes, so the medication has time to work. Avoid blowing your nose while you wait. Never use your atomizer more often than your physician directs. Doing so may actually increase your congestion instead of relieve it.

Musculo-skeletal Disorders

 Patient-learner data base*

Areas of potential knowledge deficit
Risk factors
—Advancing age
—Obesity
—Diet high in purine
—Improper use of body mechanics
—Poor posture
—Excessive and/or improperly performed exercise
—Family history of musculoskeletal disease
—Personal history of musculoskeletal injury/disease
Anatomy and physiology of the musculoskeletal system
Definition of the musculoskeletal disorder
Causes of the musculoskeletal disorder
Symptoms associated with the musculoskeletal disorder
Treatment of the musculoskeletal disorder: diet,
     medications, physiotherapy, other treatments used
Complications of the musculoskeletal disorder

 Explaining diagnostic tests

ORTHOPEDIC RADIOGRAPHY

Patient objectives	Teaching plan content
1 Define orthopedic radiography.	Orthopedic radiography is the process of taking an X-ray of a part of the skeletal system.

* A general assessment should be done for all patients. For general assessment guidelines, see Chapter 1, Principles of Patient Teaching.

2 **State the purpose of orthopedic radiography.**	Orthopedic radiography is used to detect and evaluate fractures, dislocations, degeneration, and deformities of bones and joints.
3 **Explain the procedure used in orthopedic radiography.**	This test requires no special preparation (although an analgesic may be given if pain is severe and extraneous material needs to be cleaned from any wound). During the procedure the patient can expect the following: —He will be placed on an X-ray table and instructed to assume different positions, depending on the bone or joint being X-rayed. —Changing positions may produce discomfort. —Radiographs are usually taken with the patient in the anteroposterior, lateral, or oblique (on a slant) position, or in a combination of these. —He will hear a thudding sound as each picture is taken.
4 **Discuss patient guidelines for orthopedic radiography.**	Patient guidelines for orthopedic radiography include the following: —The patient need not restrict foods or fluids before radiography. —He should know who will perform the test and where, that it may produce slight discomfort, and that it will take only a few minutes. —He will be asked to remove any jewelry or other metal objects that may distort the X-ray picture. —During the procedure, he will be asked to assume various positions (with assistance, as necessary) and then to remain still while the picture is taken. —He may be asked to remain in the X-ray department until the film is developed and checked for quality and to go through the procedure again if the film is not of good quality.

ARTHROGRAPHY

Patient objectives	*Teaching plan content*
1 **Define arthrography.**	Arthrography is the radiographic examination of a joint—usually the knee or shoulder—following the injection of air, a radiopaque contrast medium, or both into the joint space.
2 **State the purpose of arthrography.**	Arthrography is used to assess persistent, unexplained knee or shoulder discomfort. It is used to detect abnormalities of the cartilage and ligaments in the knee. It

is also used to detect shoulder abnormalities, such as a torn rotator cuff (the muscles and tendons that rotate the shoulder joint).

3 Explain the procedure used in arthrography.

After the area around the joint to be examined has been shaved, the patient will be taken to the X-ray department.

—For knee arthrography, the knee will be cleansed with an antiseptic solution, and the area around the puncture site anesthetized. (It is not usually necessary to anesthetize the joint space itself.)

• A 2″ (5-cm) needle will then be inserted into the joint space between the patella (kneecap) and femoral condyle (rounded projection of the thigh bone), and fluid will be aspirated. While the needle is still in place, the aspirating syringe will be removed and replaced with one containing dye. If fluoroscopic examination demonstrates correct placement of the needle, the dye will be injected into the joint space.

• The aspirated fluid will probably be sent to the laboratory for analysis.

• After the needle has been removed, the site will be rubbed with a sterile sponge to prevent air from escaping, and the wound may be sealed with collodion, a liquid that dries to form a clear dressing.

• The patient will be asked to walk a few steps or to move his knee through its range of motion, as directed, to distribute the dye in the joint space.

• A film series will be taken quickly—before the contrast medium can be absorbed by the joint tissue—with the knee held in various positions. If the films are of good quality and demonstrate proper dye placement, the knee will be bandaged.

—For shoulder arthrography, the skin will be prepared and a local anesthetic injected subcutaneously, just in front of the acromioclavicular joint (the joint formed between the shoulder blade and the collarbone). Additional anesthetic will be injected directly into the head of the humerus, the upper arm bone.

• The short lumbar puncture needle will then be inserted until the point is embedded in the joint cartilage. The stylet (rod) will be removed, a syringe of contrast medium will be attached, and, with fluoroscopic guidance, about 1 ml of dye will be injected into the joint space as the needle is withdrawn slightly. If fluoroscopic examination demonstrates correct placement of the needle, the remainder of the dye will be injected while the needle is withdrawn slowly and the site will be wiped with a sterile sponge.

• A film series will then be taken quickly to achieve maximum contrast.

4 Discuss patient guidelines for arthrography.	Patient guidelines for arthrography include the following: —The patient need not restrict foods or fluids before arthrography. —His cooperation in assuming various positions is vital, since films must be taken quickly to ensure optimum quality. —He should remain as still as possible during the procedure, except when following instructions to change position. —Although the joint area will be anesthetized, he may experience a tingling sensation or pressure in the joint on injection of the contrast medium.

BONE SCAN

Patient objectives	*Teaching plan content*
1 Define bone scan.	A bone scan permits imaging of the skeleton by a scanning camera after I.V. injection of a radioactive tracer compound. The tracer concentrates in bone tissue at sites of new bone formation or increased metabolism.
2 State the purpose of a bone scan.	A bone scan is primarily used to detect or rule out malignant bone lesions when X-ray findings are normal but cancer is confirmed or suspected. It is also used to detect occult (hidden) bone trauma due to pathologic fractures, to monitor degenerative bone disorders, and to detect bone infection. This test often detects abnormal skeletal pathology sooner than ordinary X-rays.
3 Explain the procedure used in a bone scan.	The procedure used in a bone scan is as follows: —After the patient has received an I.V. injection of the tracer compound and imaging agent, he will be asked to increase his fluid intake for the next 1 to 3 hours, to facilitate renal clearance of any tracer not picked up by the bone. —After this period, the patient will void and then be taken to the X-ray department and placed on a scanner table. —The scanner will then move back and forth over his body, detect low-level radiation emitted by the skeleton, and translate this into a film or chart, or both, to produce two-dimensional pictures of the area scanned. —As many views as needed to cover the specified area will be taken, and the patient may need to be repositioned many times during the test.

4 Discuss patient guidelines for a bone scan.

Patient guidelines for a bone scan are as follows:
—The patient should not drink large amounts of fluids before the test, as he will be required to drink several glasses of water or other fluid in the interval between injection of the tracer and the actual scanning.
—He should know who will perform the test and where, and that it will take about 1 hour.
—He must wear a hospital gown and sign a consent form.

ARTHROCENTESIS

Patient objectives	*Teaching plan content*
1 Define arthrocentesis.	In arthrocentesis, a specimen of synovial fluid is aspirated from a joint, most often the knee.
2 State the purpose of arthrocentesis.	Arthrocentesis aids in the differential diagnosis of arthritis and helps to identify the cause and nature of joint effusion (the excessive accumulation of synovial fluid). Arthrocentesis may also be used as a treatment procedure to relieve the pain and distention resulting from accumulation of fluid within a joint and to administer local drug therapy.
3 Explain the procedure used in arthrocentesis.	During arthrocentesis, the patient can expect the following: —He must assume a supine position with his knee fully extended and must maintain this position throughout the procedure. (For other joint aspirations, the physician will specify the required position.) —The skin over the puncture site will be cleansed with a surgical soap and alcohol and then painted with povidone-iodine solution. —A local anesthetic will be administered, and after it has taken effect, an aspiration needle will be quickly inserted into the joint space. —As much fluid as possible will be withdrawn into the syringe; a minimum of 10 to 15 ml should be obtained, although a lesser amount is usually adequate for analysis. (The joint, except for the puncture site, may be wrapped with an elastic bandage to compress the fluid and ensure maximal fluid collection.) —The needle will be withdrawn, the site wiped with alcohol, and pressure applied to prevent bleeding. A sterile dressing will then be applied to the site. —Ice or cold packs will be applied to the affected joint for 24 to 36 hours after aspiration to decrease pain and swelling.

—An elastic bandage may be wrapped around the joint to stabilize it if a large amount of fluid has been withdrawn.

—If medication is to be administered into the joint, the syringe on the aspiration needle will be detached, leaving the needle in the joint, and a syringe containing the medication will be attached. The medication will be injected and the needle withdrawn. The site will then be cleansed, pressure applied, and a sterile dressing placed over the site, as described previously.

4 Discuss patient guidelines for arthrocentesis.	Patient guidelines for arthrocentesis are as follows: —If glucose testing of synovial fluid has been ordered, the patient must fast for 6 to 12 hours before the test; otherwise, he need not restrict foods or fluids. —He must sign a consent form and put on a hospital gown before the procedure. —He may feel transient discomfort on insertion of the aspirating needle, despite the local anesthetic, but he should try to remain as still as possible. —He may resume usual activity after the procedure but should not use the joint excessively for a few days after the test.

ARTHROSCOPY

Patient objectives	*Teaching plan content*
1 Define arthroscopy.	Arthroscopy is the direct visualization of joint structures, using a specially designed fiber-optic endoscope.
2 State the purpose of arthroscopy.	Arthroscopy is usually performed to detect knee disorders—such as arthritis and traumatic injury—that are not readily revealed by radiography or arthrography. It may also be done to monitor the progression of joint disease or to perform joint surgery.
3 Explain the procedure used in arthroscopy.	Although arthroscopic techniques vary, depending on the surgeon and the type of endoscope used, for a typical knee arthroscopy the patient can expect the following: —His knee will be shaved the night before, and he will be taken to the operating room for the procedure. —This procedure is usually done under a local anesthetic, but it may be done under a general anesthetic if surgery is anticipated. —He will be placed on his back on the operating table, and a pneumatic tourniquet (similar to a blood pressure cuff) may be placed around his leg, but not tightened.

—His leg will be scrubbed, and a waterproof stockinette will be applied.

—His leg will then be elevated and wrapped from toe to thigh with an elastic bandage to drain as much blood as possible. The tourniquet will be inflated and the elastic bandage removed. (If a tourniquet is not used, 50 ml of a solution of lidocaine, epinephrine, and saline will be instilled into the knee just before insertion of the endoscope; this will help to distend the knee and reduce bleeding.)

—The foot of the table will be lowered so that the knee is bent at a 45-degree angle; the stockinette will be opened and a local anesthetic administered.

—The surgeon will then make a small (3 to 5 mm) incision in the knee, above the shinbone.

—A cannula (flexible tube) containing a pointed rod will be inserted into the joint capsule, and the endoscope will be inserted through it. Normal saline and epinephrine solutions will be infused into the joint through the endoscope to provide a viewing medium.

—At this point the endoscope may be moved into different joint spaces, or it may be held steady while the knee is bent, extended, and turned to aid visualization.

—Although the whole joint may be visualized from one puncture site, an obstruction may necessitate additional punctures.

—A camera may be attached to the endoscope and pictures taken for later study.

—After the surgeon has examined the joint structures, a synovial biopsy or appropriate surgery may be performed.

—When the examination has been completed, the endoscope will be removed, the joint irrigated with saline solution through the cannula, the cannula removed, and gentle pressure applied to the knee to help remove the saline solution. An adhesive strip and compression dressing will then be applied over the incision site.

—The patient will be returned to his room and allowed to walk as soon as he feels comfortable, but he should avoid excessive use of the joint for a few days.

4 Discuss patient guidelines for arthroscopy.

Patient guidelines for arthroscopy are as follows:

—The patient should fast after midnight before the procedure.

—He must sign a consent form and put on a hospital gown before the procedure.

—He may be given a sedative before the procedure.

—He must lie still during the procedure.

—He may experience transient discomfort from the injection of the local anesthetic.

SYNOVIAL MEMBRANE BIOPSY

Patient objectives	*Teaching plan content*
1 Define synovial membrane biopsy.	Synovial membrane biopsy is needle excision of a tissue specimen for histologic examination of the thin lining of the joint capsule.
2 State the purpose of synovial membrane biopsy.	Synovial membrane biopsy is performed to diagnose joint disorders, such as gout and rheumatoid arthritis, and infections. It may also be done to monitor joint disorders.
3 Explain the procedure used in synovial membrane biopsy.	During the procedure, the patient can expect the following: —The physician will instruct him to assume the proper position, depending on which joint is involved. —The area will be cleansed and draped. —A local anesthetic will be injected into the joint space, and a trocar (a sharp, pointed rod in a thin tube) will be inserted. —The biopsy needle will then be passed through the trocar and suction applied with a 50-ml syringe. The biopsy needle will be twisted to cut off a small tissue segment, and then withdrawn. Several specimens may be obtained by changing the angle of the biopsy needle each time. —When all specimens have been taken, the trocar will be removed, the biopsy site cleansed, and a pressure dressing applied.
4 Discuss patient guidelines for synovial membrane biopsy.	Patient guidelines for synovial membrane biopsy are as follows: —The patient need not restrict foods or fluids before the procedure. —He must sign a consent form and put on a hospital gown. —He may receive a sedative. —He should know who will perform the test and where, and that it will take about 30 minutes. —He must remain still during the procedure. —He should rest the involved joint for 1 day before resuming normal activity.

BONE BIOPSY

Patient objectives	*Teaching plan content*
1 Define bone biopsy.	A bone biopsy is the removal of a piece or core of bone for histologic examination.
2 State the purpose of bone biopsy.	A bone biopsy is performed to distinguish between benign and malignant bone tumors.
3 Explain the procedure used in bone biopsy.	This procedure is performed with a special drill needle under a local anesthetic (drill biopsy) or by surgical excision under a general anesthetic (open biopsy). —For a drill biopsy, the biopsy site will be shaved and meticulously cleansed after the patient is properly positioned on the operating table. • The physician will inject a local anesthetic at the site. • When it has taken effect, he will make a small incision and insert the biopsy needle into the bone. • Once in the bone, the needle will be rotated 180 degrees while the physician applies continuous pressure. • When the bone core has been obtained, the needle will be removed by reversing the drilling motion, and pressure will be applied to the site. —For an open biopsy, the site will be shaved, cleansed with surgical soap, and disinfected with iodine and alcohol after the patient has been anesthetized. • The physician will make an incision, remove a piece of bone, and send it to the laboratory for immediate analysis. • Further surgery may be performed at that time, as indicated by specimen findings.
4 Discuss patient guidelines for bone biopsy.	Patient guidelines for bone biopsy are as follows: —If the patient is to have a local anesthetic, he need not restrict foods or fluids beforehand. He must remain very still during the procedure. —If he is to receive a general anesthetic, he should fast overnight before the test. —He should know who will perform the test and where, and that it will take no longer than 30 minutes, unless further surgery is needed. —Before the procedure, he should sign a consent form and put on a hospital gown.

Explaining disorders

GOUT

Patient objectives	Teaching plan content
1 Define gout.	Gout is a metabolic disease in which urates (salts of uric acid, usually found in urine) are deposited in the joints, causing swelling and pain. It can strike any joint, but favors those in the feet and legs. Gout may be primary, occurring in men over age 30 and in post-menopausal women; or secondary, occurring in the elderly.
2 Explain what causes gout.	In both types of gout, increased concentration of uric acid leads to urate deposits (called tophi) in joints or tissues, causing local necrosis or fibrosis. —The exact cause of primary gout is not known, but it results from the overproduction of uric acid (hyperuricemia), retention of uric acid, or both. This may be linked to a genetic defect in the metabolism of purine (purines are nitrogen compounds found in many foods and drugs). —Secondary gout develops during the course of another disease that produces hyperuricemia. It can also follow drug therapy that interferes with the excretion of urates.
3 Discuss the signs and symptoms of gout.	Gout follows an intermittent course and leaves many sufferers totally free of symptoms for years between attacks. It develops in four stages: asymptomatic, acute, intercritical, and chronic. —Asymptomatic gout produces no symptoms. —Acute gout produces sudden, extreme pain in the affected joints; the joints may be hot, tender, inflamed, and dusky red, or they may be cyanotic. The great toe is usually affected first. Other symptoms may include a low-grade fever, headache, rapid heartbeat, malaise, and loss of appetite. Mild attacks of acute gout subside quickly and recur at irregular intervals. Severe attacks may persist for days or weeks. —The intercritical period or stage is the symptom-free period between attacks. This period often lasts for 6 months to 2 years but may last for 5 to 10 years. —The final stage, chronic gout, is marked by persistent pain in many joints. Large, subcutaneous tophi or nodules develop in cartilage, synovial membranes, tendons,

and soft tissue. The skin over these tophi may ulcerate and release an exudate. Chronic inflammation and these tophi may cause further joint degeneration, resulting in deformity and disability.

4 Identify the components of the treatment regimen for gout.	The treatment regimen may consist of the following: —Bed rest and joint immobilization during an acute attack —Dietary restrictions —Medication to terminate an acute attack, relieve pain, and prevent recurrence —Surgery to improve joint function or correct deformities —Hemodialysis, if renal impairment is severe.
5 Discuss dietary restrictions used in the management of gout.	Dietary restrictions for gout are as follows: —Drink plenty of fluids (2 to 3 liters/day) to prevent the formation of kidney stones. —Restrict the purine content in the diet. Avoid such foods as anchovies, liver, sardines, kidneys, sweetbreads, lentils, and alcoholic beverages (especially beer and wine), which raise the urate level. —Obese patients should know the principles of a gradual weight-reduction diet (moderate protein and very little fat intake).
6 Describe the medication regimen.	Some drugs commonly used for this disorder are allopurinol, colchicine, and probenecid. See Chapter 10, Drug Therapy, for specific medication instructions.

OSTEOARTHRITIS

Patient objectives	*Teaching plan content*
1 Define osteoarthritis.	Osteoarthritis, the most common form of arthritis, is a chronic, progressive disorder that causes deterioration of the joint cartilage and formation of new bone in the area.
2 Explain what causes osteoarthritis.	Osteoarthritis may be a normal part of aging and result from a genetic predisposition, or it may result from joint damage as a result of trauma, infection, stress, metabolic disorders, or underlying joint disease.
3 Discuss the signs and symptoms of osteoarthritis.	The most common symptom of osteoarthritis is joint pain, particularly after exercise or weight bearing. The pain is usually relieved by rest. —Other common symptoms may include the following:

- Morning stiffness
- Aching during changes in the weather
- Grating of the joint during motion
- Limitation of movement
- Pain at rest due to muscle spasm
- Contractures of the hip and knee.

—Bony enlargement may be seen in the affected joints. Outgrowths of bone and cartilage may develop in the distal joints of the fingers (Heberden's nodes) or in the proximal joints of the fingers (Bouchard's nodes). These nodes are painless at first but may become red, swollen, and tender, causing numbness and loss of dexterity.

---

4 Identify the components of the treatment program for osteoarthritis.

Osteoarthritis progresses slowly, and with adequate treatment, joint function may be maintained more effectively than with other types of arthritis. Treatment may include the following:

—Weight reduction (if appropriate) to relieve stress on affected joints

—Medications to relieve pain, joint inflammation, and muscle spasm

—Reduction of stress on affected joints by using crutches, braces, a cane, a walker, a cervical collar, or traction

—Physical therapy, such as massage, moist heat applications, paraffin dips, and prescribed exercises to help relax muscles and relieve aching and stiffness

—Surgery to reduce abnormal stresses within joints, delay progression of early disease, correct joint instability or misalignment, remove loose bodies or torn cartilage, and replace or fuse severely affected joints.

---

5 Describe the medication regimen.

Some drugs commonly used for this disorder are aspirin, ibuprofen, indomethacin, naproxen, and phenylbutazone. See Chapter 10, Drug Therapy, for specific medication instructions.

---

6 Demonstrate the use of walking aids, if applicable.

See the "Walkers," "Crutches," and "Canes" teaching plans in this chapter.

---

7 Discuss the principles of traction, if applicable.

See the "Traction" teaching plan in this chapter.

---

8 Demonstrate recommended exercises.

See the "Active Range-of-Motion (ROM) Exercises" teaching plan in this chapter; *Exercises for Your Joints,* pp. 232-234; *Exercises to Ease Your Aching Shoulder,* pp. 236-237; and *How to Strengthen Your Muscles and Joints,* pp. 238-241.

9 **Discuss recommended surgery.**	See the "Total Hip Replacement" teaching plan in this chapter.

10 **Discuss ways to minimize the long-term effects of osteoarthritis.**	The long-term effects of osteoarthritis may be minimized in the following ways: —The patient should receive emotional support and reassurance to help him cope with his limited mobility and its effect on his daily activities. —He should get adequate rest during the day, particularly after exertion, and at night. He should pace his activities—moderation is the key—and avoid overexertion. —He should stand and walk correctly, minimize weight-bearing activities, and be especially careful when stooping or picking up objects. —He should wear well-fitting, supportive shoes and not allow the heels to become too worn down. —He should install safety aids at home, such as guardrails in the bathroom, as necessary. —He should do prescribed exercises and take his medications as prescribed. —He should maintain proper body weight to lessen the strain on joints.

RHEUMATOID ARTHRITIS

Patient objectives	*Teaching plan content*
1 **Define rheumatoid arthritis.**	Rheumatoid arthritis is a chronic, systemic disease in which inflammatory changes occur throughout the body's connective tissues. It primarily affects the peripheral joints and surrounding muscles, tendons, ligaments, and blood vessels.
2 **Explain what causes rheumatoid arthritis.**	The exact cause is unknown, but several theories are under investigation. These theories propose that rheumatoid arthritis may result from impairment of the autoimmune system, an unknown virus, or metabolic disturbances. There may be a genetic predisposition to rheumatoid arthritis.
3 **Explain how rheumatoid arthritis results in musculoskeletal dysfunction.**	The joint and surrounding tissues are progressively destroyed by chronic inflammation and replaced with scar tissue. As the joint is destroyed, the patient experiences pain, stiffness, and swelling.

4 Identify the signs and symptoms of rheumatoid arthritis.

Rheumatoid arthritis develops gradually and initially produces nonspecific symptoms, such as fatigue, malaise, anorexia (loss of appetite), persistent low-grade fever, weight loss, enlarged lymph nodes, and vague joint symptoms. The following signs and symptoms occur in later stages of the disease:
—The joints stiffen after inactivity; this is especially noticeable upon rising in the morning.
—The fingers may assume a spindle shape from marked edema in the joints.
—The joints become tender and painful during movement and at rest. They may feel warm to the patient. Joint deformities are inevitable if active disease progresses.
—Rheumatoid nodules—round or oval subcutaneous, nontender masses—gradually appear, usually on the elbows.
—Numbness and tingling in the feet or weakness and loss of sensation in the fingers may occur.
—Stiff, weak, or painful muscles are common.
—Periodic exacerbations and remissions of symptoms are common. Emotional stress may cause an exacerbation.

5 Identify the components of the treatment regimen for rheumatoid arthritis.

The treatment regimen may include the following:
—Medication to relieve pain and reduce inflammation
—Supportive measures, such as plenty of sleep at night, frequent rest periods during the day between activities, and splinting or traction to rest inflamed joints
—Physical therapy to maintain joint function and mobility, including range-of-motion exercises, carefully individualized exercises prescribed by the physician, application of heat or ice, paraffin baths, and whirlpool treatments
—Surgery, including joint replacement, arthrodesis (joint fusion) to stabilize the joint and relieve pain, synovectomy (removal of destructive, proliferating synovia) to halt or delay the course of the disease, osteotomy (cutting of bone or excision of a wedge of bone) to realign joint surfaces and redistribute stress, or tendon transfers to prevent deformities or relieve contractures.

6 Discuss the medication regimen.

Some drugs commonly used for this disorder are aspirin, gold salts, ibuprofen, indomethacin, naproxen, and prednisone. See Chapter 10, Drug Therapy, for specific medication instructions.

7 **Demonstrate recommended exercises.**	See the "Active Range-of-Motion (ROM) Exercises" teaching plan in this chapter and *Exercises for Rheumatoid Arthritis*, pp. 250-251.
8 **Discuss recommended surgery.**	See the "Total Hip Replacement" teaching plan in this chapter.
9 **Discuss guidelines for daily living with rheumatoid arthritis.**	Rheumatoid arthritis is a chronic, systemic disease that requires major changes in life-style. —The patient should know how to stand and walk correctly and should sit upright and erect. He should wear shoes that provide proper support and should sit in chairs with high seats and armrests. —He will find it easier to get up from a chair if his knees are lower than his hips. If the patient does not own a chair with a high seat, he can put blocks of wood under the legs of a favorite chair. The use of an elevated toilet seat is suggested. —The patient should carefully pace daily activities, resting for 5 to 10 minutes of each hour and alternating sitting and standing tasks. Adequate sleep and correct sleeping posture are important. The patient should sleep on his back on a firm mattress, using a small pillow. He should avoid placing a pillow under his knees; this encourages flexion deformity. —The patient should avoid putting undue stress on joints, use the largest joint available for a given task, support weak or painful joints as much as possible, avoid positions of flexion and favor positions of extension, hold objects parallel to the knuckles as briefly as possible, always use his hands toward the center of his body, and slide—not lift—objects whenever possible. —The patient should consider using helpful household items, such as easy-to-open drawers, a hand-held shower nozzle, handrails, and grab bars. (An occupational therapist can show him how to simplify activities and protect arthritic joints.) —The patient should consider using dressing aids, such as a long-handled shoehorn, a reacher, elastic shoelaces, a zipper-pull, and a buttonhook. The patient who has trouble maneuvering fingers into gloves should wear mittens. —He should dress in a sitting position as much as possible. —For more information on coping with rheumatoid arthritis, the patient should contact the Arthritis Foundation.

HERNIATED DISK (Slipped disk)

Patient objectives	Teaching plan content
1 Define herniated disk.	A herniated disk occurs in the lumbar or lumbosacral part of the spine when all or part of the nucleus pulposus (the soft, mucoid, central portion of an intervertebral disk) is forced through the disk's weakened or torn outer ring. This impinges on spinal nerve roots and results in back pain.
2 Explain what causes a herniated disk.	A herniated disk results from severe trauma or strain or may be related to intervertebral joint degeneration as a result of aging.
3 Identify the signs and symptoms of a herniated disk.	The major symptom of a herniated disk is severe low back pain that may radiate to the buttocks, legs, and feet, usually unilaterally. —When herniation follows trauma, the pain may begin suddenly, subside in a few days, and then recur at shorter intervals and with progressive intensity. Sciatic pain follows, beginning as a dull pain in the buttocks. Valsalva's maneuver (bearing down while holding one's breath), coughing, sneezing, and bending intensify the pain, which is often accompanied by muscle spasms. —A herniated disk may also cause sensory and motor loss in the area innervated by the compressed spinal nerve root and, in later stages, weakness and atrophy of leg muscles.
4 Identify the components of the treatment regimen for a herniated disk.	The treatment for a herniated disk may include the following: —Bed rest, possibly with pelvic traction if pain is severe —Heat application to the area to decrease pain and relieve muscle spasms. (See *How to Relieve Muscle Spasm*, p. 235.) —An individually prescribed exercise program to strengthen back muscles. (See *Exercises for Chronic Low Back Pain*, p. 252.) —Medications to decrease pain, inflammation, and muscle spasms —Surgery to remove the protruding portion of the disk (laminectomy) and/or stabilize the weakened area of the spine (spinal fusion).
5 Discuss the principles of traction, if applicable.	See the "Traction" teaching plan in this chapter.

6 **Discuss the medication regimen.**	Some drugs commonly used for this disorder are aspirin, diazepam, ibuprofen, indomethacin, naproxen, and prednisone. See Chapter 10, Drug Therapy, for specific medication instructions.
7 **Discuss recommended surgery.**	See the "Laminectomy" teaching plan in this chapter, if applicable, and *After a Laminectomy: How to Care for Yourself*, pp. 254-255.
8 **Discuss patient guidelines to prevent a herniated disk or minimize recurrence.**	Patient guidelines include the following: —The patient should avoid putting too much stress on his back. He should use good body mechanics—bend at the knees and hips (never at the waist) and stand straight and carry objects close to his body. —He should lie down when tired and sleep on his side (never on his abdomen) on an extra-firm mattress or a bed board. —He should maintain proper body weight to prevent lordosis (swayback) caused by obesity.

ANKYLOSING SPONDYLITIS

Patient objectives	*Teaching plan content*
1 **Define ankylosing spondylitis.**	Ankylosing spondylitis is a chronic, progressive disease that affects the joints. It primarily affects the sacroiliac, apophyseal, and costovertebral joints and adjacent soft tissue. Affecting mostly young men, it usually begins in the sacroiliac joints and progresses to the lumbar, thoracic, and cervical regions of the spine.
2 **Explain what causes ankylosing spondylitis.**	The exact cause of ankylosing spondylitis is unknown, but a genetic predisposition exists.
3 **Identify the signs and symptoms of ankylosing spondylitis.**	The first indication of ankylosing spondylitis is intermittent low back pain. This pain is usually severest in the morning or after a period of inactivity and is not relieved by rest. Other symptoms depend on the stage of the disease, which progresses unpredictably and can go into sudden remission, exacerbation, or arrest at any stage. They may include the following: —Stiffness and limited motion of the lumbar spine —Pain and limited expansion of the chest due to involvement of the thoracic spine —Peripheral arthritis pain involving shoulders, hips, and knees —Kyphosis (hunchback) in advanced stages, caused by chronic stooping to relieve symptoms

—Tenderness over the site of inflammation
—Mild fatigue, fever, anorexia, or loss of weight
—Occasional iritis (inflammation of the iris of the eye).

4 Identify the components of the treatment regimen for ankylosing spondylitis.	Treatment does not stop the progression of this disease, but it can delay deformity and promote comfort. Treatment may include the following: —Medications to reduce inflammation and control pain —Supportive measures, such as local heat applications and massage to relieve pain —Exercises and maintenance of good posture to delay and minimize deformities —Surgery, such as total hip replacement, to relieve pain and disability.
5 Discuss the medication regimen.	Some drugs commonly used for this disorder are aspirin, indomethacin, and phenylbutazone. See Chapter 10, Drug Therapy, for specific medication instructions.
6 Discuss patient guidelines to minimize deformities.	Deformities may be minimized in the following ways: —Avoid any physical activity that places undue stress on the back, such as lifting heavy objects. —Stand upright. —Sit upright in a high, straight chair. —Avoid leaning over a desk. —Sleep in a prone position on a firm mattress, and avoid using pillows under the neck or knees. —Avoid prolonged walking, standing, sitting, or driving. —Perform regular stretching and deep-breathing exercises. —Swim regularly, if possible. —Have height measured every 3 to 4 months to detect any tendency to lean forward. —Seek vocational counseling if work requires standing or prolonged sitting at a desk.
7 Demonstrate recommended exercises.	See *Exercises for Ankylosing Spondylitis*, p. 253.
8 Discuss recommended surgery.	See the "Total Hip Replacement" teaching plan in this chapter.

FRACTURED HIP

Patient objectives	*Teaching plan content*
1 Define fractured hip.	A fractured hip is a fracture of the head, neck, or trochanter region of the femur.

2 **Identify the relevant type of hip fracture.**	There are two major types of hip fracture. —Intracapsular fractures are fractures of the neck of the femur. —Extracapsular fractures are fractures of the trochanter region (between the base of the neck and the lesser trochanter of the femur) or subtrochanter region.
3 **Identify the components of the treatment regimen for a hip fracture.**	Treatment for a fractured hip usually includes the following: —Surgery to treat the fracture and maintain alignment, using internal fixation devices (nails and plates) to replace the head of the femur with a prosthesis, or total hip replacement —Temporary preoperative traction (skin traction) to maintain alignment and relieve pain until surgical fixation can be performed —Postoperative exercises to strengthen muscles in preparation for using a walking aid, such as a walker, a cane, or crutches; to prevent complications of immobilization, such as venous stasis or thromboembolism; and to increase endurance, strength, and mobility (including range-of-motion exercises, isometric exercises, coughing and deep-breathing exercises, and calf-pumping exercises) —Medications (preoperatively and postoperatively) to relieve pain and to prevent thromboembolism —Frequent skin care and changes of position (postoperatively) to prevent skin breakdown —Use of ambulation aids, such as a walker, a cane, or crutches, to assist in early mobilization after surgery and restoration of the ambulatory function of the hip joint.
4 **Discuss recommended surgery.**	See the "Total Hip Replacement" teaching plan in this chapter.
5 **Discuss principles of traction.**	See the "Traction" teaching plan in this chapter.
6 **Demonstrate recommended exercises.**	See the "Active Range-of-Motion (ROM) Exercises" teaching plan in this chapter; *How to Perform Active Range-of-Motion Exercises,* pp. 248-249; and *How to Do Isometric Exercises,* p. 231.
7 **Describe the medication regimen.**	Some drugs commonly used for this disorder are acetaminophen, aspirin, codeine, meperidine, morphine, pentazocine, and propoxyphene. See Chapter 10, Drug Therapy, for specific medication instructions.

8 Demonstrate the use of walking aids, if applicable.	See the "Walkers," "Crutches," and "Canes" teaching plans in this chapter; *How to Use Crutches,* pp. 242-244; and *Going Home with a Cane,* pp. 246-247.
9 Discuss patient guidelines for safe walking at home.	In addition to learning how to use his walking aid, the patient should know the specific problems he may confront in his home environment. —He should be especially careful when walking on thick shag wall-to-wall carpeting, which may adversely affect his balance. —Any loose area rugs should be removed. —Hardwood, tile, and linoleum floors provide the best walking surfaces for using a walking aid. —The patient should avoid walking on slippery, waxed, or wet floors or on uneven surfaces, such as gravel- or dirt-covered driveways. —Furniture should be rearranged temporarily so that wide, uncluttered pathways are available for walking. —The patient may rent a raised toilet seat or commode. —A ramp leading into the house may be helpful.

SYSTEMIC LUPUS ERYTHEMATOSUS (S.L.E.)

Patient objectives	*Teaching plan content*
1 Define SLE.	SLE is a chronic, systemic, inflammatory disease of the connective tissues that involves multiple organ systems. It is characterized by remissions and exacerbations of symptoms.
2 Explain what causes SLE.	The exact cause of SLE is unknown. It may be an autoimmune disorder, and there may be a genetic predisposition to the disease. Certain drugs, such as hydralazine and procainamide, may cause a lupuslike syndrome, often called "drug-induced lupus." Discontinuation of the drug resolves the condition.
3 Identify the signs and symptoms of SLE.	The primary clinical features include the following: —The first and most common symptom is joint pain and stiffness, which is seldom deforming and usually involves the hands, feet, and large joints. Joints may show redness, warmth, tenderness, and synovial effusions (escape of synovial fluid into the tissues), with associated muscle weakness and tenderness. —Rashes may appear, especially in exposed areas. Ultraviolet rays often provoke or aggravate skin erup-

tions. Perhaps the most distinctive feature of SLE is the "butterfly rash" that appears across the nose and cheeks in about 40% of patients. Discoid lesions (plaques) appear most commonly on the face, neck, and scalp.

—Vasculitis (inflammation of the blood vessels) can occur, especially in the digits, possibly leading to infarctive lesions (necrosis due to obstruction), necrotic leg ulcers, or digital gangrene.

—Raynaud's phenomenon appears in about 20% of patients.

—Patchy alopecia (loss of hair) and ulcers of the mucous membranes are common.

—Constitutional symptoms of SLE include aching, malaise, fatigue, low-grade or spiking fever, chills, loss of appetite, and weight loss.

—Lymph node enlargement (diffuse or local, and nontender), abdominal pain, nausea, vomiting, diarrhea, and constipation may occur.

—Women may experience irregular menstrual periods or amenorrhea, particularly during the active phase of this disease.

—About 50% of SLE patients develop signs of cardiopulmonary abnormalities, such as dyspnea; rapid heartbeat may occur.

—Renal effects include hematuria (blood in urine), proteinuria (protein in urine), urine sediment, and cellular casts. Renal failure may result. Urinary tract infections may result from a heightened susceptibility to infection.

—Central nervous system involvement may produce emotional instability, psychosis, and organic brain syndrome. Headaches, irritability, and depression are especially common.

—Convulsive disorders and mental dysfunction may indicate neurologic damage.

---

4 Identify factors that can exacerbate symptoms of SLE.

Sunlight, ultraviolet light, physical stress, and emotional stress can initiate a flare-up of symptoms. These should be avoided if possible.

---

5 Identify the components of the treatment regimen for SLE.

Treatment for SLE may include the following:
—Medications to decrease inflammation and control arthritic symptoms
—Supportive measures, such as local heat application and massage to relieve joint pain
—Plasmapheresis (the removal of blood, separation of the plasma by centrifugation, and reinjection of the packed cells into the patient) to remove immune complexes from the blood.

6 Discuss the medication regimen.	Some drugs commonly used for this disorder are dexamethasone, hydrocortisone, ibuprofen, indomethacin, and prednisone. See Chapter 10, Drug Therapy, for specific medication instructions.
7 Discuss patient guidelines for coping with the long-term effects of SLE.	Patient guidelines for coping with the long-term effects of SLE include the following: —To maintain skin integrity and promote comfort and relief of itching, the patient should take cool baths and avoid powders or other irritants. —He should wear protective clothing (hat, sunglasses, long sleeves, slacks) when out in the sun and use a screening agent containing para-aminobenzoic acid (PABA). —He should rest often during the day to combat fatigue and weakness. —He should get 10 to 12 hours of sleep each night, if possible. —He should exercise regularly and in moderation, as tolerated, to maintain full range of motion in joints and prevent contractures. —The patient should know some practical tips on personal grooming to support his self-image. —He should use assistive devices for household activities and dressing if joint involvement is severe. (See the "Rheumatoid Arthritis" teaching plan in this chapter.) —He should purchase medications in quantity, if possible, and should avoid "miracle drugs" for relief of arthritic symptoms. —The patient should receive emotional support to help him accept his illness. —He should be referred to the Lupus Foundation of America and the Arthritis Foundation for additional information on coping with his condition.

 Explaining treatments

TRACTION

Patient objectives	*Teaching plan content*
1 Describe traction.	Traction exerts a pulling force on a part of the body—usually the spine, the pelvis, or the long bones of the arms and legs.

2 **State the purpose of traction.**	Traction is used for the following purposes: —To treat fractures and dislocations —To correct or prevent deformities —To improve or correct contractures —To decrease muscle spasms —To temporarily maintain bone alignment and prevent further soft-tissue damage before surgery is performed to treat a fracture —To reduce stress on joints affected by osteoarthritis.
3 **Identify the relevant type of traction.**	The two major types of traction are skin traction and skeletal traction. —Skin traction is ordered when a light, temporary, or noncontinuous pull is required. It is applied directly to the skin and thus indirectly to the bone. —In skeletal traction, an orthopedist inserts a pin or wire through the bone and attaches the traction equipment to the pin or wire to exert a direct, constant, longitudinal pull.
4 **Discuss patient guidelines for maintaining traction.**	Patient guidelines for maintaining traction are as follows: —The patient should maintain correct body alignment and position while in traction. —He should know the type of traction being used and should not remove it unless specifically ordered to do so by his physician. —He should report such symptoms as pain, burning, tingling, or numbness immediately, as these may indicate circulatory compromise from improperly applied traction. —He should put every joint (except those immediately above and below fractures) through full range of motion several times a day. —He should perform deep-breathing and abdomen-setting exercises. —He should perform prescribed exercises as ordered by his physician. —The patient should do as much of his personal care as possible to provide stimulation and exercise.

ACTIVE RANGE-OF-MOTION (R.O.M.) EXERCISES

Patient objectives	*Teaching plan content*
1 **Define active ROM exercises.**	Active ROM exercises are performed to maintain joint mobility and prevent contractures. They may also help prepare the patient for walking.

2 Describe the relevant active ROM exercises.	Active ROM exercises include the following: —For the neck, move the head backward and forward as far as possible, as if nodding "yes." —For the shoulders, raise the shoulders and move them forward in a circular motion. Then, move them backward in a circular motion. —For the elbows, straighten the arm, then bend the elbow and touch the shoulder with the hand. Then, straighten the arm slowly. Repeat the pattern with the other arm. —For the wrist and hand, rest the forearms on the arms of a chair, palms down, and bend the wrists slowly up and down. —For the hips and knees, lie in bed, keeping one knee bent and foot flat on the bed, and bend the other leg, bringing it as close as possible to the chest. Slowly stretch this leg out again, straightening the knee and hip. Relax. Repeat the pattern with the other leg. —For the ankle, make a circle with the foot, moving first clockwise and then counterclockwise. Repeat with the other foot.
3 Discuss patient guidelines for active ROM exercises.	The patient should exercise slowly and repeat each exercise three to five times at first, adding repetitions gradually as his tolerance increases. He should stop immediately if he experiences pain. He should receive instructions for home use, in accord with hospital policy. (See *How to Perform Active Range-of-Motion Exercises,* pp. 248-249.)

CASTS

Patient objectives	*Teaching plan content*
1 Describe a cast.	A cast is a stiff dressing that fits around a body part, usually an extremity, and immobilizes it without discomfort.
2 State the purpose of a cast.	A cast is used for the following: —To immobilize —To correct deformities —To promote healing after surgery.
3 Discuss the procedure used in applying a cast.	With the application of a cast, the patient can expect the following: —The nurse will gently support the limb while the physician applies a tubular stockinette and then wraps sheet wadding around the limb, starting at the distal end.

—The physician will then apply the plaster rolls, which will be wet, around the limb. Before he wraps the last roll, he will pull the end of the stockinette over the cast edge to create padded edges, prevent crumbling, and reduce skin irritation. He will then use the final plaster roll to keep the ends of the stockinette in place.
—Heat will build under the cast because of a chemical reaction between the water and the plaster.
—Some aspects of proper cast care will be explained.
—Vascular status will be checked by palpating distal pulses and assessing the color and temperature of the fingers or toes. The limb will then be elevated with pillows or blankets (with the pressure evenly distributed under the cast) above the level of the heart to promote venous return and to reduce edema.
—An X-ray may be taken to ensure proper positioning.
—The cast will be dry and hard within 24 to 48 hours.

---

4 Discuss patient guidelines for cast care.

Patient guidelines for cast care are as follows:
—It is important to report such signs and symptoms as pain, tightness, numbness, tingling, burning, or a change in the color of the visible part of the extremity, as these may indicate improper cast application.
—The patient should know the correct position to maintain.
—He should perform the exercises prescribed by his physician.
—He should receive instructions on cast care, in accord with hospital policy. (See *Do's and Don'ts of Cast Care*, p. 259, and *Caring for Your Cast at Home*, pp. 256-258.)

LAMINECTOMY

Patient objectives	*Teaching plan content*
1 Define laminectomy.	Laminectomy is the removal of a portion of the vertebral arch (lamina) and excision of the protruding part of the vertebral disk.
2 State the purpose of a laminectomy.	A laminectomy is performed to relieve pain and pressure on spinal nerve roots.
3 Briefly explain the surgical procedure used in a laminectomy.	A small incision will be made in the patient's back in the area of the herniated disk. The lamina of the vertebral disk and the affected portion of the disk will be removed. (An illustration can be used to demonstrate the procedure.)

4 Describe the preoperative procedures for a laminectomy.	In addition to the routine procedures (see Appendix B, *Preoperative and Postoperative Teaching*), preoperative procedures for a laminectomy are as follows: —Along with routine preoperative tests, a myelogram will be performed to locate the exact area of irritation. —The area on the patient's back will be shaved and cleansed with antiseptic solution. —The patient will be taught to turn himself as a unit (logrolling) and to perform deep-breathing, coughing, and muscle-setting exercises. —He will need to restrict fluids and foods as ordered.
5 Describe the postoperative procedures for a laminectomy.	Postoperative procedures for a laminectomy are as follows: —The patient will be positioned in bed with a pillow under his head and a knee rest slightly elevated to relax the muscles of the back. —A dressing will be in place over the site, and it will be checked frequently, along with the patient's vital signs. —Sensation and motor strength in the extremities will be assessed periodically, along with the color of the patient's legs. —He will be encouraged to move from side to side to relieve pressure. When he is on his side, a pillow will be placed between his legs, and he will be logrolled without twisting his back. —He may experience varying degrees of pain and sensory manifestations in the legs. These will be temporary, and medications will be given to relieve pain. —Early ambulation will be encouraged, and he will receive instructions for self-care, in accord with hospital policy. (See *After a Laminectomy: How to Care for Yourself*, pp. 254-255.)

TOTAL HIP REPLACEMENT

Patient objectives	*Teaching plan content*
1 Define total hip replacement.	Total hip replacement is the replacement of a severely damaged hip with artificial parts (prostheses).
2 State the purpose of total hip replacement.	Total hip replacement is performed to relieve pain, return mobility and stability to the joint, and permit walking.
3 Briefly explain the surgical procedure.	The femoral head and the acetabulum are both replaced by prostheses in total hip replacement. The prostheses are then cemented into the bone. (An illustration can be used to demonstrate the procedure.)

4 Describe the preoperative procedures for total hip replacement.

In addition to the routine procedures (see Appendix B, *Preoperative and Postoperative Teaching*), preoperative procedures for total hip replacement are as follows:
—X-rays may be taken.
—The patient may need to remain on his back for several days and learn how to use a trapeze correctly to lift himself for back care.
—He will be taught to perform postoperative exercises, such as quadriceps-setting exercises, gluteus-setting exercises, and isometric hip extension and abduction exercises.
—The area will be scrubbed carefully with soap and an antiseptic solution, and antibiotics may be administered prophylactically.

5 Describe the postoperative procedures for total hip replacement.

Postoperative procedures for total hip replacement are as follows:
—The patient will be placed flat in bed with the affected extremity held in abduction by a splint or pillow. This will prevent dislocation of the prosthesis. The head of the bed may be elevated 45 degrees for comfort.
—A dressing will be in place over the incision, and a drainage device may be in place for a couple of days.
—He should be assisted in turning to his unaffected side with a pillow between his legs. A knee sling may be placed on the bed for support of the affected leg.
—Exercises will begin the following day, and coughing and deep-breathing exercises should begin immediately after surgery and be continued.
—The patient will be helped out of bed, usually on the second postoperative day, with the splint or pillows kept between his legs.
—He will gradually increase his activity until he is able to use a walker, a cane, or crutches.
—He will receive antibiotics and pain medications and will resume his diet as tolerated.
—He will receive instructions on hip positioning for use at home, as well as discharge instructions, in accord with hospital policy. (See *How to Position Your Leg after Total Hip Replacement*, p. 245.)

WALKERS

Patient objectives	*Teaching plan content*
1 State the purpose of a walker.	The use of a walker provides stability and aids in maintaining balance during ambulation.

2 Demonstrate walking with a walker.

The patient should use a reciprocal walker, if possible, because it is more stable than a stationary walker. Reciprocal walkers are also recommended for patients with decreased arm strength and balance.
—For the two-point gait, a transfer belt is placed around the patient's waist.
• He then stands with his weight evenly distributed between his legs and the walker. The nurse stands behind him, slightly to one side.
• He simultaneously advances the walker's right side and his left foot. Next, he advances the walker's left side and his right foot. He continues in this manner.
—For the four-point gait, a transfer belt is placed around the patient's waist.
• He distributes his weight evenly between his legs and the walker. The nurse stands behind him and slightly to one side.
• He moves the right side of the walker and then his left foot forward. Then he moves the left side of the walker and then his right foot forward. He continues in this manner.
—To use a stationary walker, the patient stands within the walker and holds the handgrips firmly and equally.
• If the patient has one-sided leg weakness, he advances the walker 6″ to 8″ (15 to 20 cm), steps forward with the affected leg (supporting himself with his arms), and follows with the unaffected leg.
• If he has equal strength in both legs, he advances the walker 6″ to 8″ and steps forward with either leg.
• If he cannot use one leg, he advances the walker 6″ to 8″ and swings into it, supporting his weight with his hands.

3 Demonstrate sitting and rising with a walker.

The patient should follow these guidelines for sitting down and rising from a chair:
—To sit down, the patient stands with the back of his stronger leg against the front of a chair with armrests, with his weaker leg slightly off the floor, and the walker directly in front.
• He grasps the armrest with the hand on his weaker side and then shifts his weight to the stronger leg and the hand grasping the armrest.
• He lowers himself into the chair and slides backward. After he is seated, he should place the walker beside the chair.
—To get up, the patient brings the walker to the front of his chair and slides forward.
• He places the back of his stronger leg against the

seat and then advances the weaker leg.
• Next, placing both hands on the armrests, he can push himself to a standing position.
• He supports his weight with the stronger leg and the opposite hand, then grasps the walker's handgrip with his free hand.
• Next, he grasps the free handgrip with his other hand and begins walking.

CRUTCHES

Patient objectives	Teaching plan content
1 State the purpose of crutches.	The use of crutches will reduce or eliminate the amount of weight the patient places on his lower extremity(ies) or joint(s).
2 Discuss patient guidelines for walking with crutches.	Patient guidelines include the following: —Before walking with crutches, the patient should make sure they are ready to use. He will need rubber suction cups placed over the wooden crutch tips to prevent sliding. He will also need rubber pads on the underarm pieces to make them more comfortable. He may also pad the hand supports. —When he is standing with the crutch tips 6″ (15 cm) from the sides of his feet, underarm pieces should be about 1″ to 1½″ (two finger widths; 2.5 to 4 cm) below his armpits. If they touch his armpits, the length should be adjusted. When he grasps the hand supports, his arms should be slightly bent—never straight. —Walking with crutches requires practice. The patient should not get discouraged if he has difficulty at first. —He should always use his arms, not the top part of the crutches, to support his weight. If he feels any tingling or numbness in his upper torso, he is probably using the crutches incorrectly. Or they may be the wrong size. —Before he attempts walking with his crutches, he should lean his body slightly forward. For added psychological support, a transfer or walking belt may be placed around the patient's waist. He should always keep the crutches in front of him. Doing so will ensure better balance.
3 Demonstrate the relevant gait for walking with crutches.	Four gaits are used with crutches. The three-point gait is used when the patient must avoid placing weight on an affected leg, the three-point-and-one gait when he can place partial weight on it, and the two-point or four-point gait when he can place weight on both legs.

—For a three-point gait, the patient should place all of his weight on his unaffected leg and his crutches. He should put a supportive, nonskid shoe on his unaffected foot.

• The patient sits on the edge of the bed and holds both crutches in the hand on the affected side. He leans forward and brings his unaffected foot slightly ahead of his affected foot. Then he places his free hand on the side of the bed and pushes himself up, using that hand and the crutches for support. He should not place any weight on his affected foot.

• After he is standing, he transfers one crutch to his unaffected side and grasps it firmly. He positions his unaffected foot so it is even with the crutch tips. His affected knee is slightly flexed and his affected foot is on the floor. He should put pressure on the hand supports, not on the crutch tops, when he walks.

• Then, with his balance maintained, he leans his body slightly forward, supporting his weight on his unaffected foot and the crutches. He should put all of his weight on his unaffected leg, maintain his balance, and move both crutches forward. Next, he swings his affected leg forward, keeping all weight off his affected foot.

• The patient balances his weight on both crutches as he swings his unaffected foot forward. Then, he moves both crutches and his affected foot forward and repeats the procedure.

• As the patient's balance and strength improve, he can perform the swing-through three-point gait. To do this, he advances his unaffected foot beyond the crutches. Then he advances both crutches and his affected leg past his unaffected foot.

—For the two-point gait, a transfer belt is placed around the patient's waist. Then, he stands with his weight evenly distributed between both legs and crutches. He shifts his weight to his right crutch and left foot as he moves his left crutch and right foot about 8″ (20 cm) forward. Next, he shifts his weight to his left crutch and right foot as he moves his right crutch and left foot approximately 8″ forward. He repeats these steps.

—For the four-point gait, the patient stands with his weight evenly distributed between both legs and the crutches.

• Then, he moves his left crutch about 8″ forward. As he does, he shifts his weight so it is distributed evenly between his right crutch and both legs.

• Next, he moves his right foot approximately 8″ forward, so it is even with the left crutch. Then, he

moves his right crutch about 8″ forward as he shifts his weight onto his left crutch and both legs.
- He moves his left foot 8″ forward, even with his right crutch.
- He repeats this procedure—moving each crutch forward, then moving the opposite foot.

—For the three-point-and-one gait, the patient distributes most of his weight between the handgrips of the crutches and his unaffected leg, with some of his weight supported by his affected leg.
- He moves both crutches forward. Then, he moves his affected leg up to the crutches.
- Next, he puts some weight on the affected leg and his crutches, as he moves his unaffected leg about 8″ ahead of the crutches. Again, he moves the crutches and then his affected leg forward.
- The patient continues in this manner.

4 Demonstrate sitting and rising with crutches.

The patient should follow these guidelines for sitting down and rising from a chair:

—To sit down, the patient approaches the chair so his unaffected leg is close to the front of the chair seat.
- He grasps both crutches, using his affected hand. Then, he puts the hand on his unaffected side on the same side of the chair. He places the crutches against the chair's armrest.
- Next, he pivots on his unaffected foot until the back of his unaffected leg is against the seat of the chair. He places his hand on the affected side on the same side of the chair.
- Then, as he supports his weight with his hands, he lowers himself into the chair, keeping his weight off his affected foot.

—To get up, the patient slides forward, keeping his unaffected foot slightly under the chair. He should not put any weight on his affected foot.
- He presses down on the armrests. Then, he supports his weight on his hands and unaffected foot as he lifts himself out of the chair.
- Next, he pivots on his unaffected foot, while grasping the armrest with his unaffected hand. With his hand on the affected side, he can grasp the crutches.
- Then, he places both crutches under his arm on the affected side. As soon as he feels steady, he shifts one crutch to his unaffected arm. He is now ready to walk.

5 Demonstrate picking up objects while using crutches.

The patient should follow these guidelines:
—First, he pushes the object over to a chair with the crutch on his unaffected side.

—He shifts his crutches to his affected hand and places them against the armrest.
—Then, he sits down in the chair, following the procedure described above.
—Next, he leans forward in the chair, reaches down, and picks up the object with the hand on his unaffected side.
—Grasping the crutches with the hand on his affected side, he pushes himself off the chair with the hand on his unaffected side while holding on to the object.
—Finally, he transfers one crutch to his hand on the affected side, which is the side holding the object, after he has risen and balanced himself.

6 Demonstrate using stairs with crutches.

The patient should follow these guidelines:
—To go up stairs, the patient stands at the bottom of the stairs, shifts his crutch on the unaffected side to his other hand, and grasps the banister with the unaffected hand. He supports his weight on both crutches and his unaffected leg.
• Then, he pushes down on his crutches and hops onto the first step with his unaffected foot. His other leg will move up onto the step at the same time.
• Next, he swings his crutches up onto the step, alongside his feet, and hops onto the second step with his unaffected leg.
• He repeats this procedure, advancing his unaffected leg first, until he reaches the top of the stairs.
—To go down stairs, the patient stands with his unaffected leg closest to the banister, shifts his unaffected crutch to his other hand, and grasps the banister.
• Then, he lowers his crutch tips to the step below him and lowers his unaffected foot onto the step. As he does, his other leg will follow.
• He repeats this procedure, advancing the crutches first.

CANES

Patient objectives | *Teaching plan content*

1 State the purpose of a cane.

The use of a cane will aid in maintaining balance when weight can be placed on the affected extremity or joint or when an extremity or joint is weakened.

2 Discuss guidelines for the use of a cane.

The patient should wear nonskid shoes. He should look ahead when he walks, instead of looking at his feet. When his family comes to visit, they should be shown the proper procedure for walking with a cane.

3 **Demonstrate walking with a cane.**

The patient should follow these guidelines:
—He slides to the edge of the bed and places his feet flat on the floor 6″ (15 cm) apart. He is helped into a standing position.
—He holds the cane in the hand on his unaffected side, with the tip about 4″ (10 cm) to the side of his unaffected foot.
—He distributes his weight evenly between his feet and the cane, keeping the cane's rubber tip on the floor at all times.
—Then, he shifts his weight to his unaffected leg as he moves the cane forward about 4″. He supports his weight on his unaffected leg and the cane.
—Then, he moves his affected foot forward, parallel with the cane.
—Then, with his weight supported on his affected leg and the cane, he moves his unaffected leg forward ahead of the cane. If he does this correctly, his heel will be slightly beyond the tip of the cane.
—He moves his affected foot forward so it is even with his unaffected foot. Then, he moves his cane forward.

4 **Demonstrate sitting and rising with a cane.**

The patient should follow these guidelines for sitting down and rising from a chair, with a transfer belt around his waist:
—To sit down, he steadies himself with his cane as he stands with the backs of his legs against the chair's seat.
• He then moves his cane out from his side and reaches back with both hands to grasp the chair's armrests.
• He supports his weight on the armrests and lowers himself onto the seat. Then, he hooks the cane on the armrest or chair back.
—To get up, the patient unhooks the cane from the armrest or chair back and holds it in his unaffected hand as he grasps the armrests.
• Next, he places his unaffected foot slightly forward. He leans slightly forward and pushes against the armrests to raise himself upright.
• He steadies himself by placing the cane's tip about 4″ to the side of his unaffected foot.

5 **Demonstrate using stairs with a cane.**

The patient should always check that stairs are safe, clean, dry, and well-lighted. He should follow these guidelines for using stairs, with a transfer belt around his waist:

—To go up stairs, he stands at the bottom of the stairs with his feet about 6″ apart. His unaffected side is next to the banister.

• He grasps the banister with his unaffected hand about 4″ from the end. As he does, he transfers the cane to his other hand.

• Then, he hooks the cane over his arm or belt or, if he is using a broad-based cane, places the cane on the step ahead of him, so his hand is free to grasp the banister.

• He looks ahead, not at his feet.

• He holds onto the banister firmly as he shifts his weight to his weak leg. He pulls himself forward with his unaffected hand, using the banister, as he lifts his unaffected foot to the first step.

• He shifts his weight to the unaffected leg. Then, he uses the banister to pull himself forward with his unaffected hand as he lifts his affected foot to the first step.

—To go down stairs, the patient lowers his affected foot and then his unaffected foot to each step while he grasps the banister with his unaffected hand to balance himself. He handles his cane as he did in going up stairs.

—If the patient is going up stairs with only one banister on his affected side, he will have to go up the stairs backward. He stands with his back to the stairs and his unaffected side next to the banister. He lifts his unaffected foot and then his affected foot to each step, following the procedure previously described.

—If the patient is going down stairs with only one banister on his affected side, he should go down the stairs backward. He stands with his back to the stairs and his unaffected side next to the banister. He lowers his affected foot and then his unaffected foot to each step, following the same procedure.

Patient-Teaching Aid

HOW TO DO ISOMETRIC EXERCISES

Dear Patient:

After you leave the hospital, the physician wants you to continue the isometric exercises you have learned to help you strengthen and tone your muscles. By performing these exercises regularly, you will find it easier to carry out your day-to-day activities. Work this isometric program into your daily routine, repeating each exercise three times and the entire program at least five times a day. Use the following instructions as a guide:

1

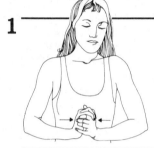

First, strengthen your arm muscles. Hold your arms in front of you, with your palms together. As you breathe slowly and deeply, press your hands together firmly, or grasp a ball in each hand for 3 to 5 seconds. Now relax. Remember, increased arm strength will make it easier for you to transfer, move in bed, or propel a wheelchair.

2

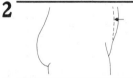

Next, strengthen the muscles in your abdomen. To do this, pull your abdominal muscles in as tightly as you can for 3 to 5 seconds. Breathe slowly and deeply. Then, relax the muscles gradually.

3

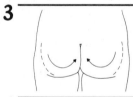

Now, exercise the muscles in your buttocks. As you breathe slowly and deeply, tighten your buttocks' muscles for 3 to 5 seconds. Then, relax them. Strengthening these muscles will help you stay balanced when you are seated.

4

Then, strengthen your leg muscles. Lie on your back and bend your left leg at the knee. Keeping your left foot flat on the floor, raise your right leg 3″ (8 cm), and hold it there for 5 seconds. Then, lower it. Relax your legs. Repeat the exercise, raising your left leg.

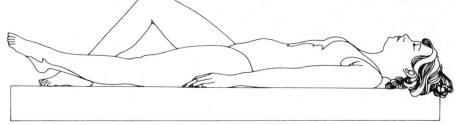

Patient-Teaching Aid

EXERCISES FOR YOUR JOINTS

Dear Patient:

Now that you are ready to return home, you will need to keep affected joints active and strengthen the muscles around them. Performing everyday activities such as cooking and cleaning is a start. But you will also need some form of regular exercise, such as daily walking, swimming, or joint exercises, to make sure you work out *all* joints.

The following exercises should help increase joint movement and reduce stiffness and pain. Follow the exact directions for performing these exercises. Make sure you complete the number of repetitions required. If you cannot, notify the physician. He may prescribe a different exercise.

IMPORTANT: If you feel severe pain when performing any of these exercises, stop immediately. If the pain continues, notify your physician. Never force or overstretch a muscle or joint, or you may cause further damage.

To get the most out of this program, try to work the exercises into your daily routine; for example, exercise as you bathe or while you are sitting in a chair watching television. Begin each exercise session by briefly limbering up and stretching, and pause between exercises to relax. Perform each exercise slowly and carefully.

NOTE: If you are performing the exercises in a bed or chair with wheels, make sure the wheels are locked before you begin.

For your fingers

While either sitting or standing, extend both arms out in front of you at shoulder level, with your palms down. Spread your fingers apart as much as possible; then bring them back together. Perform this exercise five times.

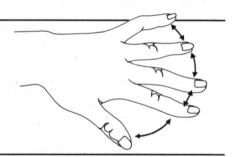

For your wrists and hands

While either sitting or standing, extend one arm out in front of you, keeping it slightly bent at the elbow, with your palm down. Using your other hand, gently push your fingers back toward your forearm. Then, push your fingers down, as shown. Perform this exercise five times. Then, switch hands and repeat the exercise five times.

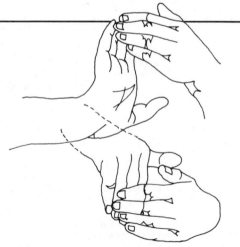

EXERCISES FOR YOUR JOINTS—*continued*

For your shoulders and arms

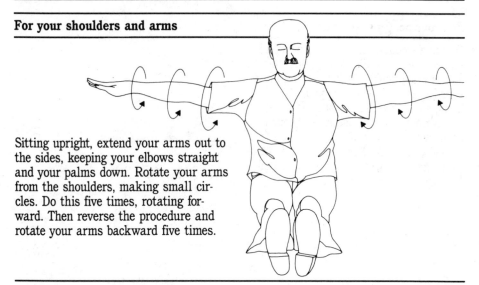

Sitting upright, extend your arms out to the sides, keeping your elbows straight and your palms down. Rotate your arms from the shoulders, making small circles. Do this five times, rotating forward. Then reverse the procedure and rotate your arms backward five times.

For your neck

While either sitting or standing, slowly move your head back as far as possible. Then move it to the right, toward your shoulder. From that position, lower your chin toward your chest (as shown here). Then, complete the exercise by moving your head toward your left shoulder and then back to starting position. Perform this exercise five times; then change direction, and perform it five times.

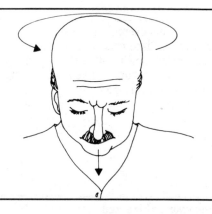

For your hips

Perform this exercise while lying flat on your back. Place your arms at your side, palms down. Then, use your hands and arms to lift your hips a maximum of 6" (15 cm) off the bed. Hold this position momentarily; then relax. Perform this exercise five times.

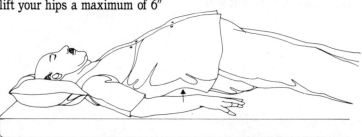

EXERCISES FOR YOUR JOINTS—*continued*

For your posture and back

Obtain a wooden stick (for example, a broom or mop handle) long enough for you to grasp with both hands. Hold it in your hands, and rest it on your lap. Then, slowly extend the stick straight out in front of you, raise it over your head (with arms straight), and place it behind your neck. Next, return the stick to its starting position in your lap. Perform this exercise five times.

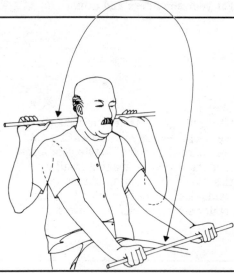

For your hips and legs

Perform this exercise while lying flat on your back. Place your arms at your sides, palms down. Lift both legs and slowly pump them, as if you were riding a bicycle. Do this exercise five times.

For your ankles and feet

Sit in a rocking chair and rock back and forth. The constant pushing movement of your feet and ankles will stimulate blood circulation and reduce joint stiffness.

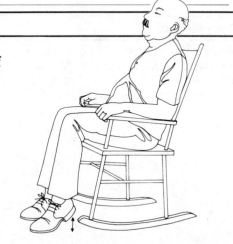

Patient-Teaching Aid

HOW TO RELIEVE MUSCLE SPASM

Dear Patient:

To relieve your muscle spasm, apply moist heat to the painful area. Moist heat is less drying to the skin, is less likely to burn, does not cause sweating with excessive fluid and salt loss, and penetrates more deeply than dry heat. Apply heat for 20 to 30 minutes, as follows:

• Place a moist towel over the painful area.

• Cover the towel with a hot-water bottle.

• Remove the hot-water bottle and wet pack after 20 to 30 minutes. Never continue application for longer than 30 minutes, at which point therapeutic value decreases.

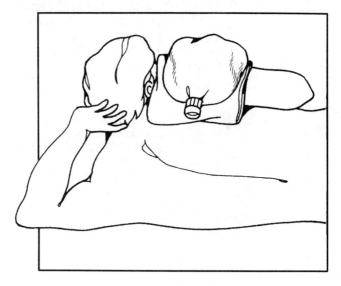

Patient-Teaching Aid

EXERCISES TO EASE YOUR ACHING SHOULDER

1

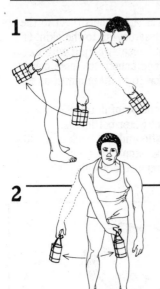

Dear Patient:
Holding a weight with your hand on the affected side, bend from your hips and swing your arm backward and forward at your side. To retain your balance, you may hold onto a counter or the back of a chair with your other hand. The weight should be from 2 to 5 lb (1 to 2 kg). For a 2- to 2½-lb weight, put two large cans of beans or half a brick in a string bag. For a 5-lb weight, use an old-fashioned flatiron or a bag of sugar in a string bag. Do *not* use a weight of more than 5 lb.

2

Then, swing the weight across the front of your body. As your range of motion increases, swing your arm in a large circle in front of you, first clockwise, then counterclockwise, while bending from your hips.

3

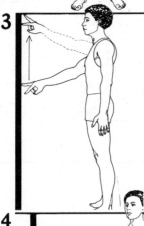

Stand facing a wall, an arm's length away. Slowly walk your index and middle fingers up the wall as high as you can.

4

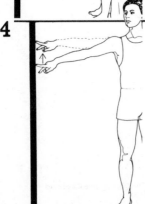

Then, stand at a right angle to the wall and repeat the exercise. As your hand gets higher, step closer to the wall to allow your shoulder the maximum range of motion.

EXERCISES TO EASE YOUR ACHING SHOULDER—*continued*

5

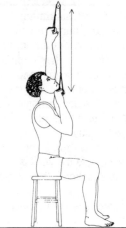

Have someone attach a pulley and rope in a doorway and sit directly underneath the pulley. Holding the ends of the rope in each hand, use your unaffected arm to gently pull the affected arm as high as possible. Then, allow the affected arm to drop slowly down.

6

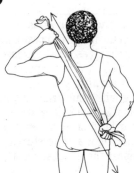

Grasp the ends of a large bath towel behind your back. Then, simulate the motion of drying your back, reaching and pulling as far as possible. Reverse the position of your arms and repeat the exercise.

7

Grasp a broomstick with both hands at your hip level and raise it up over your head. Then, lower it behind your head to the back of your neck.

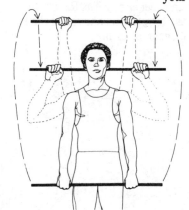

Patient-Teaching Aid

HOW TO STRENGTHEN YOUR MUSCLES AND JOINTS

Dear Patient:
Now that you are ready to return home, you will need to continue strengthening and toning your muscles. By exercising twice a day, you will find it easier to carry out your day-to-day activities. Repeat each exercise five times on the muscle or joint being strengthened.

IMPORTANT: If you feel severe pain when performing any of these exercises, stop immediately. If pain persists, notify your physician. Never force or overstretch a muscle, as you may cause further damage.

And remember, to get maximum benefit out of this program, perform each exercise slowly and gently. Try performing all the exercises the nurse has circled on these sheets in the morning and again before dinner. Work the exercises into your daily routine; for example, exercise as you bathe or while sitting in a chair watching television.

NOTE: If you are performing the exercises in a bed or chair with wheels, make sure they are locked before you begin.

Use these instructions as a guide:

Shoulder exercises

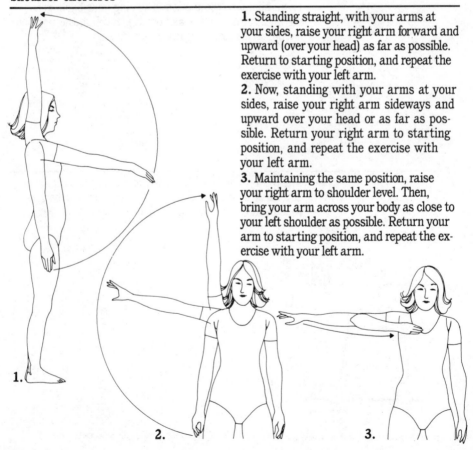

1. Standing straight, with your arms at your sides, raise your right arm forward and upward (over your head) as far as possible. Return to starting position, and repeat the exercise with your left arm.
2. Now, standing with your arms at your sides, raise your right arm sideways and upward over your head or as far as possible. Return your right arm to starting position, and repeat the exercise with your left arm.
3. Maintaining the same position, raise your right arm to shoulder level. Then, bring your arm across your body as close to your left shoulder as possible. Return your arm to starting position, and repeat the exercise with your left arm.

HOW TO STRENGTHEN YOUR MUSCLES AND JOINTS—*continued*

Neck exercises

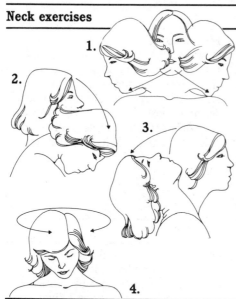

1. Keeping your shoulders level, touch your chin to your right shoulder or as close to it as possible. Then, touch your chin to your left shoulder or as close to it as possible. Do not raise your shoulder to your chin. Return to starting position.

2. Now, touch your chin to your chest or as close to it as possible. Raise your chin to starting position.

3. Next, bend your head and neck backward as far as possible. Return your head to starting position.

4. Rotate your head and neck clockwise. Then, rotate your head and neck counterclockwise.

Trunk exercises

1. Sit on a chair so your legs are straight and your arms hang loosely at your sides. Bend forward as far as possible. Return to starting position.

2. Now, maintaining the same position, bend to the right side, making sure you bend from the waist. Then, bend to the left. Return to starting position.

3. Next, stand with your feet 2″ (5 cm) apart. Let your arms hang loosely at your sides and—without bending your knees—bend backward as far as possible. Return to starting position.

4. Keeping your hips facing straight ahead, twist your upper body to the right as far as possible. Then, twist your body to the left as far as possible. Return to starting position.

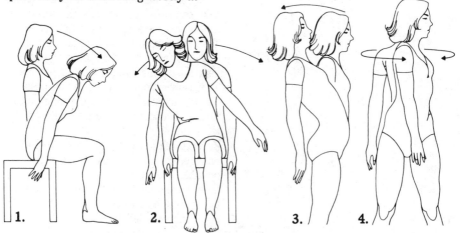

HOW TO STRENGTHEN YOUR MUSCLES AND JOINTS—*continued*

Elbow exercise

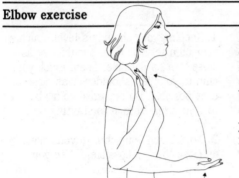

For this exercise, you can sit in a chair or stand, whichever is most comfortable. Let your arms hang loosely at your sides. Then, bending your right elbow, bring your fingertips to your right shoulder or as close to it as possible. Return your right arm to starting position, and repeat the exercise with your left arm.

Forearm exercise

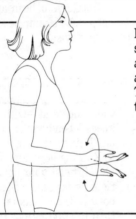

Keeping your upper right arm at your side, bend your elbow so your forearm is at a 90-degree angle to your upper arm and your palm is facing the ceiling. Turn your palm down, then up. Repeat the exercise with your left hand.

Wrist exercises

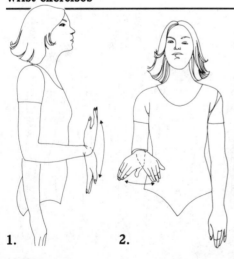

1. Keeping your upper right arm at your side, bend your elbow so your forearm is at a 90-degree angle to your upper arm. Turn your palm up so it is facing the ceiling. Now, without bending your elbow, raise your hand as far as possible. Then, lower your hand as far as possible. Return your hand to starting position, and repeat the exercise with your left hand.

2. Next, maintaining the same position, move your hand as close to your body as possible. Then, move your hand as far away from your body as possible. Return to starting position, and repeat the exercise with your left hand.

1.   **2.**

HOW TO STRENGTHEN YOUR MUSCLES AND JOINTS—*continued*

Knee exercise

For this exercise, you can sit on the bed with your legs straight ahead of you or lie on your abdomen with your legs extended. Bend your right knee as much as possible. Return to starting position, and repeat the exercise with your left knee.

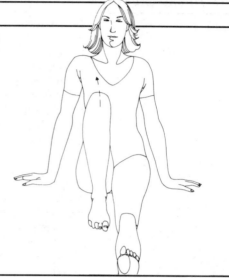

Hip exercises

1. Lie on your back and bend your right knee. Bring your knee as close to your chest as possible. Return your knee to starting position, and repeat the exercise with your left knee.

2. Next, keeping your knee and hip straight and toes pointed upwards, move your right leg to the right as far as possible. Return to starting position, and repeat the exercise with your left leg.

3. Bend your hip and knee so the bottom of your right foot is flat on the bed. Roll your leg inward as far as possible. Return to starting position, and repeat the exercise with the left leg.

4. Now, maintaining the same position with your back and hips flat on the bed, raise your right leg upward as far as possible. Return your right leg to starting position, and repeat the exercise with your left leg.

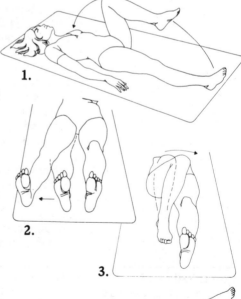

Patient-Teaching Aid

HOW TO USE CRUTCHES

Dear Patient:
Has the physician given you crutches? If used properly, these crutches will help you reduce or eliminate the amount of weight you put on your injured leg or foot.

But first, find out if the crutches are right for you. Check them out by following these guidelines:
• Make sure the crutches are ready to use. You will need rubber suction cups placed over the wooden crutch tips to prevent sliding. You will also need rubber pads on the underarm pieces to make them more comfortable. You may also ask the nurse to pad the hand supports.
• Are the crutches the right size? When you are standing—with the crutch tips 6" (15 cm) from the sides of your feet—underarm pieces should be about 1" to 1½" (two finger widths, or 2.5 to 4 cm) *below* your armpits. If they touch your armpits, ask the nurse to adjust the length.
• Check the placement of the hand supports. When you grasp them, your arms should be slightly bent—*never* straight. When you are certain the crutches are the right size and properly padded, let the nurse show you how to use them. But remember, walking with crutches requires practice. Do not get discouraged if you have difficulty at first.

Here are some hints to help you get started:
• Always use your *arms,* not the top part of the crutch, to support your weight. If you feel any tingling or numbness in your upper torso, you are probably using the crutches incorrectly. Or they may be the wrong size.
• Before you attempt walking with your crutches, lean your body slightly forward.
• Always keep the crutches in front of you. Doing so will ensure better balance. Now, study the instructions with the illustrations on these pages to find out how to use your crutches.

How to walk with crutches, using the three-point gait	If the physician says you can put no weight on your injured leg, he will probably want you to walk with a three-point gait. Read the captions with these illustrations to discover how to do this. NOTE: Depending on the type of injury you have, the physician may also want you to learn a three-point-and-one, a two-point, and a four-point gait. (Ask the nurse about these.)

HOW TO USE CRUTCHES—*continued*

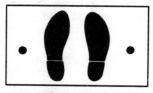

With the crutches in place, stand straight, with your shoulders relaxed and your arms slightly bent. Use your hands to support your weight.

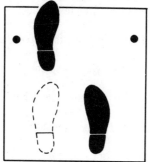

Now, swing your injured leg in front of you at the same time that you move the crutches forward. Maintain your balance by placing some weight on your uninjured leg.

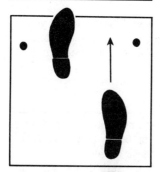

Balance your weight on both crutches as you swing your uninjured leg forward.

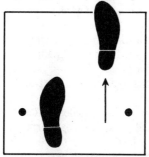

Advance your uninjured leg to the position shown here. Put your weight on this leg as you bring your crutches forward.

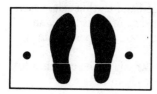

Then, advance your injured leg to the first position, and repeat the procedure.

HOW TO USE CRUTCHES—*continued*

How to use your crutches on stairs

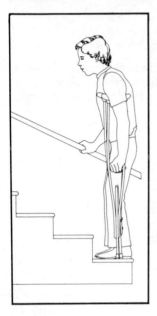

Sooner or later, you will have to get up and down stairs using your crutches. Assuming the banister is on the right, here is how to proceed:
• First, stand at the bottom of the stairs, and shift your crutches to your left hand.
• Grasp the banister firmly with your right hand. Using your left hand, carefully support your weight on the crutches.
• Now, hop up onto the first step with your uninjured leg.
• Support your weight on that leg as you grasp the banister tightly.
• Swing your crutches up onto the first step (see illustration).
• Now, hop up onto the second step with your uninjured leg.
• Continue the procedure as before, but go slowly to avoid losing your balance.
    To get down the stairs, reverse the guidelines you have just learned. But, when you do, remember that you always advance the crutches and your uninjured leg first.

Getting in and out of a chair

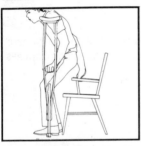

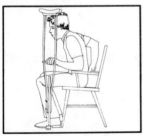

If you are on crutches, you will need practice getting in and out of a chair. Before you begin, study the illustrations at left. Then, follow these guidelines:
• Select the chair carefully. Make sure it is sturdy and has arms. Never attempt to sit in a chair that is on casters.
• Now, stand with your back toward the chair. Slowly move backward until you feel the back of your knees touch the front edge of the chair.
• Transfer both crutches to the hand that is next to your *injured* leg.
• As you support your weight on the crutches, reach back with your other hand and grasp the chair arm. Lower yourself into the chair slowly.
• To get up from the chair, bring both crutches alongside your injured leg. With the hand on this side, grasp the hand supports of the crutches firmly. Place your other hand on the arm of the chair, and push yourself up.
• Once you are upright, transfer one of the crutches to your uninjured side, and get ready to walk.

Patient-Teaching Aid

HOW TO POSITION YOUR LEG AFTER TOTAL HIP REPLACEMENT

Dear Patient:

Because you have had hip surgery, you will need to be particularly careful about leg movements. For the next 3 months, observe the following *do's* and *don'ts:*

• Do not cross your legs, whether you are lying, sitting, or standing.

• Do place a pillow between your legs when you lie on your unaffected side, with your affected leg uppermost.

• Do not sit on low stools, low chairs, or low toilets. You may need to use firm cushions to raise chair seats. Also, consider renting or buying a raised toilet seat or special commode.

• Do sit only in chairs with arms. You will need chair arms to help you stand up.

• Do move to the edge of your chair before getting up. Place your affected leg in front of your other leg, which should be well under the chair. Keep your affected leg in front while getting up.

• Do not reach down to the end of your bed to pull up your covers. This flexes your hip too much.

• Do not bend down to pick up things from the floor or to reach into lower cupboards or drawers.

• Do keep your affected leg facing front at all times, whether you are sitting, lying, or walking. Never turn your hip or knee inward or outward.

Patient-Teaching Aid

GOING HOME WITH A CANE

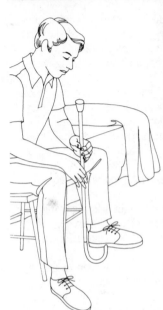

Dear Patient:
Your physician says you are ready to return home. But he wants you to use a cane to help you put full weight on your affected leg as you walk. Below we give guidelines for a person with an affected *left* leg. If your *right* leg is affected, start with the cane on your left side, and adapt the instructions. You may want to draw the patterns for yourself.

Before you begin, be sure you have nonskid, flat-soled, supportive shoes on, and check that they are buckled or tied securely. Avoid wearing slip-on shoes, such as loafers or clogs, as they do not support your weight properly. In addition, check your cane's rubber tip to be sure it is without cracks or tears and is wearing evenly. Also, make sure the tip fits securely on the cane's end.

If possible, remove throw rugs and avoid walking on slippery, wet, or waxed floors or gravel driveways. Also, try to walk close to a wall, so you have something to lean against if you drop your cane.

1

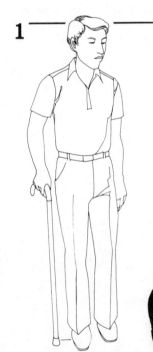

Now, position the cane about 4″ (10 cm) to the side of your unaffected leg, as shown in this illustration. Distribute your weight between your feet and your cane.

GOING HOME WITH A CANE—*continued*

2

● Next, shift your weight to your unaffected leg and move the cane about 4″ in front of you.

3

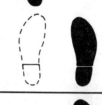

Now, you are ready to move your affected foot forward so it is parallel with the cane.

4

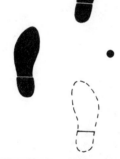

Shift your weight to your affected leg and the cane. Now, move your unaffected foot forward, ahead of the cane. If you have done this step correctly, your heel will be slightly beyond the tip of the cane.

5

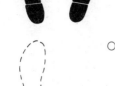

● Next, move your affected foot forward, so it is even with your unaffected foot. Then, move your cane in front of you about 4″.

Repeat these steps. As you proceed, remember to keep your head erect, shoulders back, back straight, abdomen in, and knees slightly flexed.

Patient-Teaching Aid

HOW TO PERFORM ACTIVE RANGE-OF-MOTION EXERCISES

Dear Patient:
Your physician has prescribed active range-of-motion exercises to help you maintain joint mobility and prevent contractures. You can do these exercises while lying down, sitting, or standing. Repeat each exercise three to five times at first, increasing the number gradually as your activity tolerance increases. Remember to exercise slowly.

Neck

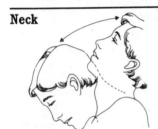

Move your head backward and forward as far as possible, as if you were nodding "yes."

Shoulders

Raise your shoulders and move them forward in a circular motion. Then, move them backward in a circular motion.

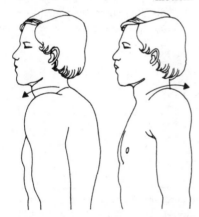

Ankles

Make a circle with your foot, moving first clockwise and then counterclockwise. Repeat with the other foot.

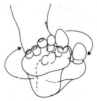

HOW TO PERFORM ACTIVE RANGE-OF-MOTION EXERCISES—*continued*

Elbows

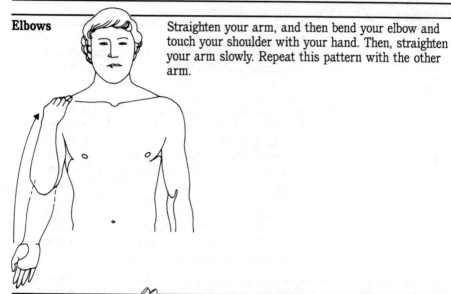

Straighten your arm, and then bend your elbow and touch your shoulder with your hand. Then, straighten your arm slowly. Repeat this pattern with the other arm.

Wrists and hands

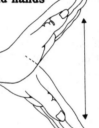

With your forearms resting on the arms of a chair, palms down, bend your wrists slowly up and down.

Hips and knees

Keeping one foot flat on the bed and knee bent, bend the other leg, bringing it as far as possible toward your chest. Slowly stretch this leg out again, straightening the knee and hip. Relax. Repeat the pattern with the other leg.

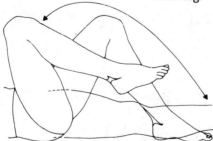

Patient-Teaching Aid

EXERCISES FOR RHEUMATOID ARTHRITIS

Dear Patient:

By exercising regularly, you can help manage your rheumatoid arthritis. Among other things, exercise will:

- improve your circulation
- rebuild your strength and then maintain it
- keep your joints limber, enabling them to move through their full range.

A good way to start is with the six sets of exercises shown here. If possible, run through them two or three times daily, for about 5 to 10 minutes each time.

During the first few days, you will probably develop some sore spots. But do not worry: that is normal when you first begin moving long-unused ligaments and muscles. Just take it easy and chances are, within a week or two the soreness will disappear.

Exercising the elbow

Raise one elbow, then bend it, as shown in A. Then straighten the elbow and turn your wrist slowly back and forth, as though turning a doorknob.

Next, place the same elbow at your side, then bend it 90 degrees (B). Again, turn your wrist slowly back and forth, but do not move your elbow from your side.

Repeat for the other elbow.

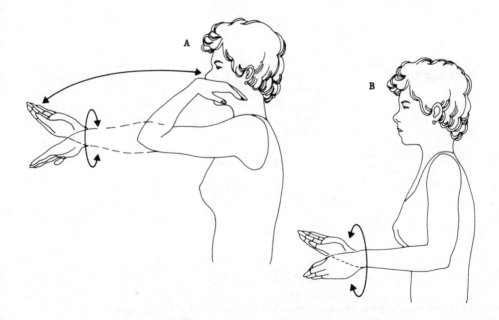

EXERCISES FOR RHEUMATOID ARTHRITIS—*continued*

Exercising the shoulder

Lie on your back with your legs straight and arms at your sides. Raise one arm upward and as far back as it will go, swing it out to the side, then bring it back down to your side, as in A.

Next, with your arms at your sides, palms toward body, raise the same arm sideways as far as possible, then bring it back to your side (B).

Now, raise the arm forward and as far upward as it will go; return it to your side (C).

Finally, as shown in D, sit or stand with your arm extended to the side. Make increasingly larger circles with your hand, keeping your elbow still as you move your shoulder.

Repeat for the other shoulder.

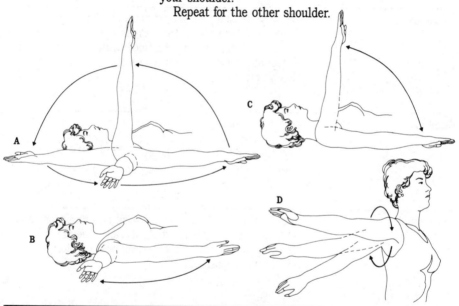

Exercising the wrist

Hold one hand with thumb upward, then move the hand up and down (A).

Next, hold your hand palm down, then bend your wrist forward and backward as far as possible (B).

Repeat for the other wrist.

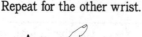
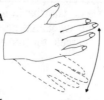
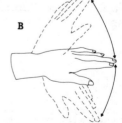

Patient-Teaching Aid

EXERCISES FOR CHRONIC LOW BACK PAIN

Dear Patient:
If you have chronic low back pain, the exercises illustrated here may help relieve your discomfort and prevent further lumbar deterioration. When you perform these exercises, keep in mind the following points:
• Breathe slowly, inhaling through your nose and exhaling completely through pursed lips.
• Begin gradually, performing each exercise only once per day and progressing to 10 repetitions.
• Exercise moderately; expect mild discomfort, but stop if you experience severe pain.

Back press

Lie on your back, with your arms on your chest or abdomen and your knees bent. Press the small (lower portion) of your back to the floor while tightening your abdominal muscles and buttocks. Count to 10, then slowly relax.

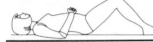

Knee grasp

Lie on your back, with your knees bent. Bring one knee to your chest, grasping it firmly with both hands; lower your knee. Repeat with the other knee—then with *both* knees, as shown here.

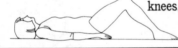

Knee bend

Stand with your hands on the back of a chair for support. Keeping your back straight, slowly bend your knees until you are in a squatting position. Return to your starting position.

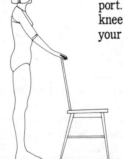

Sit-up

Lie on your back, with your arms at your sides. Using your abdominal muscles, slowly sit up and reach for your toes, touching them if you can.

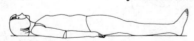

Patient-Teaching Aid

EXERCISES FOR ANKYLOSING SPONDYLITIS

Dear Patient:
The following exercises can help maintain muscle strength and prevent deformity.

Spine extension exercises

• *Pelvic tilt:* Stand with legs slightly apart and back against the wall. Take a deep breath and pull abdomen in and up, flattening the small of your back against the wall. Hold for four counts and exhale.
• *Bridging:* Lie on your back with knees bent and soles on the floor. Keeping arms at your sides, arch your back and place weight on forearms, shoulders, and soles. Hold for six counts.
• Stand with arms tightly against your sides. Bend elbows, bringing forearms to the front of your body. Take a deep breath, and rotate forearms toward the back, keeping elbows tightly against your body. Hold for four counts and exhale.
• Stand and face the corner of the room. Place one hand on each wall at shoulder level. Bend elbows slightly, and pull abdomen in slowly, while leaning forward, forcing your chest toward the corner. Hold for six counts, and return to starting position. Repeat 10 to 20 times. •

Chest-expanding exercises

• While lying on your back, clasp hands behind your head, pulling elbows toward each other. Push elbows to the bed while breathing in deeply. Hold that breath for 10 counts; then exhale and relax.
• Lie on your back with arms at your sides. Take a deep breath while raising arms over your head. As you let the breath out slowly with a hissing noise, bring arms back to your sides.
• Stand with hands clasped behind your head. While keeping your head erect, extend elbows as far as possible toward your back.
• Stand with feet slightly apart. Hold your left arm at your side, and extend your right arm over your head. Bend your body to the left. Repeat this exercise on the opposite side.

Breathing exercise (for diaphragm)

• Lie on your back, and rest your hands on your abdomen. On inspiration you will feel your abdomen swell, and on expiration you will feel it flatten. Repeat this exercise while standing and sitting.

Patient-Teaching Aid

AFTER A LAMINECTOMY: HOW TO CARE FOR YOURSELF

Dear Patient:

Because you have just had back surgery, you must take special precautions to help speed your recovery. Above all, never overexert yourself. In addition, your nurse has filled in the physician's specific instructions on the following list. Read it carefully. If you have questions, talk to your nurse. Then, when you go home, make a special effort to follow the guidelines listed here:

• Restrict your activities. For example, you may go up and down the stairs _____ times a day. Ride in a car as little as possible during the first weeks, because the vehicle motion may create back pain. Also, wait at least _____ weeks before driving a car.

• Do not lift or carry anything that is heavier than 5 lb (2 kg) for _____ weeks. Do not engage in strenuous physical activity for at least _____ weeks or you will experience back pain.

• Avoid sexual activity for _____ weeks after surgery.

• Take a shower _____ days after surgery. But before taking a tub bath, get your physician's approval.

• Spend at least _____ hours a day in a bed with a firm mattress. When lying on your back, elevate your legs on pillows. If you prefer lying on your side, bend your knees. Position a small pillow under your head and neck to avoid straining your neck, shoulders, and arms. *Never lie on your stomach.*

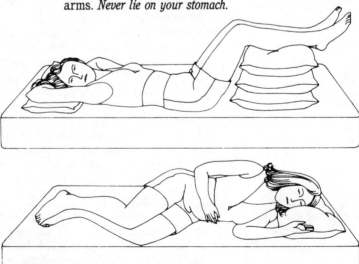

AFTER A LAMINECTOMY: HOW TO CARE FOR YOURSELF—*continued*

● Ask a family member to check your incision site once a day. If he notices drainage or redness or if you notice increased incisional pain, call your physician.
● To strengthen your arm and leg muscles, continue the exercises you learned in the hospital.
● When stooping down, bend your knees, keeping your back straight.

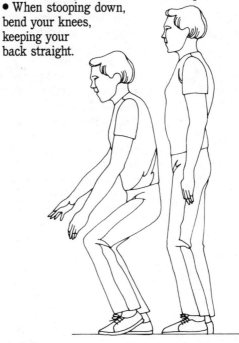

● When sitting, support your feet on a footstool with your knees at hip level or higher.

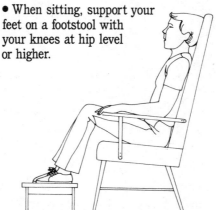

● Remember to return to your physician for a checkup.

Patient-Teaching Aid

CARING FOR YOUR CAST AT HOME

Dear Patient:
As you know, the physician has immobilized your injury site with a cast. Of course, proper healing depends on your cooperation.

Contact your physician immediately or return to the emergency department at once if you note any of the following in your casted arm or leg:
- Increasing pain
- Pain unrelieved by prescribed medication
- Swelling unrelieved by elevating the cast above heart level for 1 hour
- A change in sensation
- Numbness, tingling, or burning
- Decreased movement or loss of movement in your fingers or toes
- A change in skin color above or below the cast
- A bad smell coming from inside the cast
- A warm area or fresh stain on the cast
- An object dropped into or stuck in the cast
- A weakened, cracked, loose, or tight cast.

To care for your casted arm or leg, follow these guidelines:

1

To prevent excess swelling, keep your casted arm or leg elevated on pillows, above chest level, as much as possible (see the illustration). Check for swelling above and below the cast several times a day. To do this, compare your casted arm or leg with your other arm or leg. Consider a little swelling normal. Apply ice to swollen areas.

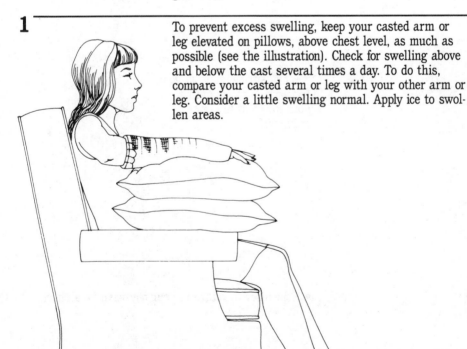

CARING FOR YOUR CAST AT HOME—*continued*

2

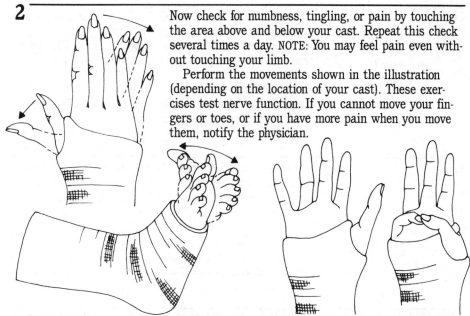

Now check for numbness, tingling, or pain by touching the area above and below your cast. Repeat this check several times a day. NOTE: You may feel pain even without touching your limb.

Perform the movements shown in the illustration (depending on the location of your cast). These exercises test nerve function. If you cannot move your fingers or toes, or if you have more pain when you move them, notify the physician.

3

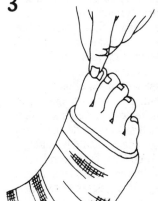

To check your circulation, press briefly on your middle fingernail (on a casted arm) or large toenail (on a casted leg) until it turns white. Then, let go. If normal pink color does not return quickly, notify your physician at once. Repeat this check at least three times a day.

If your fingers or toes are cold, cover them. If that does not warm them, notify the physician.

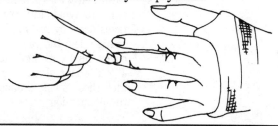

4 ☐

If the nurse has checked this box, you are wearing a plaster cast. That means that if you are planning to bathe or go out in wet weather, you will need to encase your cast in a plastic bag, such as a garbage bag. Tie the bag securely above the cast. Do not use rubber bands.

IMPORTANT: Do not let a plaster cast get wet. Moisture will weaken or destroy it. If the cast does become wet, allow it to dry naturally, for example, by sitting in the sun. Do not cover the cast until it is thoroughly dry.

CARING FOR YOUR CAST AT HOME—*continued*

5

If the nurse has checked this box, your cast is made of one of the new casting materials. Check with your physician to find out if you may shower or swim with your cast. He will also give specific instructions about drying it.

He will probably want you to let your wet cast dry naturally in the air. Because your cast dries from the inside out, a hair dryer or fan will not hasten the drying.

6

When your cast becomes soiled, clean it with a damp cloth and dry cleanser, such as Comet. Be sure to wipe off any excess moisture. Or follow these special instructions: _____

_____

_____

_____

_____

7

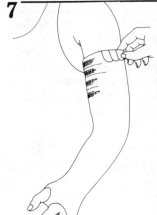

Wash the skin along the edges of your cast with mild soap and water every day. First, protect the cast edge with plastic wrap. Then, use a damp cloth to clean the skin you can reach inside the cast. Take care not to get the cast wet when you wash. Dry your skin thoroughly with a towel. Then, massage the skin at the cast edges and under the cast with a towel or a pad saturated with rubbing alcohol. This helps toughen the skin. To avoid skin irritation, remove loose plaster particles daily by reaching an inch or two inside the cast.

Also, feel the cast for rough edges each day, and cover them with moleskin. To do this, cut several $2'' \times 4''$ strips of moleskin and round their edges. Attach these strips around the cast edges, as shown in the illustration.

8

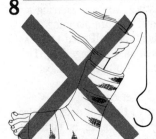

Occasionally, the skin under your cast will feel itchy. *Do not insert any object into the cast to try to relieve the itching (or for any other reason).* Doing so could damage your skin and lead to infection.

Finally, return to your physician on the following date to have your cast removed:

_____

Do not ever try to trim or remove the cast yourself.

Patient-Teaching Aid

DO'S AND DON'TS OF CAST CARE

Dear Patient:
To care for your casted arm or leg, follow these guidelines:

DO'S

- *DO* keep your casted limb elevated above heart level whenever possible to prevent excess swelling. For example, if your leg is in a cast, lie down and elevate your leg with pillows. If your arm is in a cast, prop the arm so your hand and elbow are higher than your shoulder.
- *DO* call your physician if your fingers or toes become numb or tingle or if you have difficulty moving them. These signs could indicate a developing infection.
- *DO* call your physician if you develop a fever, experience unusual pain, or notice a foul odor coming from the cast. These signs could indicate a developing infection.
- *DO* any exercises you have been taught by your physician, nurses, or physical therapist to maintain your muscle strength.
- *DO* call your physician if your cast needs to be repaired (for example, if it becomes loose and slides) or if you have *any* questions at all about caring for it.

DON'TS

- *DON'T* get your plaster cast wet; moisture will weaken or destroy it. If your cast is fiberglass, ask your physician if moisture will affect it.
- *DON'T* insert anything, such as a back scratcher, into your cast to relieve an itch. You could damage your skin and cause an infection.
- *DON'T* put powder, liquid, or lotion in your cast. Use alcohol only on the skin at the cast edges.
- *DON'T* chip, crush, cut, or otherwise break your cast.
- *DON'T* bear weight on your cast unless your physician tells you to do so.

Obstetric Disorders

Patient-learner data base*

Areas of potential knowledge deficit
Anatomy and physiology of the female reproductive
    system
Menstrual cycle
Personal hygiene
Definition, causes, and symptoms of obstetric disorder
Treatment of obstetric disorder: medications, surgery,
    guidelines for daily living, prevention of complica-
    tions, coping strategies (for both patient and family)
Other treatments used
Presence of factors that affect attitudes toward
    learning
—Age
—Religion
—Cultural standards
—Self-esteem
—Psychological stress

Explaining diagnostic tests

PREGNANCY TESTS

Patient objectives	Teaching plan content
1 Define pregnancy tests.	Pregnancy tests identify the hormone human chorionic gonadotropin (HCG) in a woman's blood or urine. This hormone is produced by the placenta when pregnancy has occurred.

*A general assessment should be done for all patients. For general assessment guidelines, see Chapter 1, Principles
of Patient Teaching.

2 State the purpose of pregnancy tests.	Pregnancy tests help confirm or disprove the diagnosis of fertilization and implantation of an ovum (pregnancy).
3 Discuss the relevant type of pregnancy test.	There are two types of pregnancy tests: —One type requires a tube of blood from the patient and identifies levels of HCG in the serum. —The other type is done on maternal urine to identify the antigenic property of HCG; that is, whether it does or does not cause clumping of the test cells. When HCG is present in the urine, *no* clumping occurs.
4 Discuss patient guidelines for pregnancy testing.	Patient guidelines for pregnancy testing are as follows: —If the test for HCG is to be done using a sample of her blood, she will not have to restrict her food or fluids. A tube of blood will be drawn by her physician or a laboratory technician. The results of the test will be given to her by her physician. The time it takes to obtain these results will depend on where the test is done and how long it takes the laboratory to complete the process of testing and reporting—usually, 24 to 48 hours. —If a test on maternal urine is used, usually a clean-catch specimen of the first voided urine of the day will be collected in a specimen container supplied by her physician or the laboratory. Usually, these results can be obtained within a short time. —These tests are approximately 95% accurate in diagnosing pregnancy and 98% accurate in diagnosing absence of pregnancy. —Over-the-counter pregnancy tests are similar and use maternal urine.

PELVIC ULTRASONOGRAPHY

Patient objectives	*Teaching plan content*
1 Define pelvic ultrasonography.	In pelvic ultrasonography, high-frequency sound waves are directed into the pelvic area and reflected to a transducer, which in turn converts sound energy into electrical energy and forms images of the interior pelvic area on a display screen.
2 State the purpose of pelvic ultrasonography.	Pelvic ultrasonography in obstetrics permits assessment of fetal growth, the amount of amniotic fluid, and the condition and position of the placenta during pregnancy. It may be ordered for a patient with a history or signs of fetal anomalies (malformations) or multiple pregnancy, a history of

bleeding, inconsistency between fetal size and conception date, or indications for amniocentesis.

3 **Describe the procedure used in pelvic ultrasonography.**	During pelvic ultrasonography, the patient can expect the following: —She will be placed on her back, and her pelvic and abdominal areas will be coated with mineral oil or water-soluble jelly to increase sound-wave conduction. —The transducer crystal will be guided over the area, images observed on the screen, and a good image photographed.
4 **Discuss patient guidelines for pelvic ultrasonography.**	Patient guidelines for pelvic ultrasonography are as follows: —The day of the test, the patient will need to drink a large amount of fluid. A full bladder is needed as a landmark during testing. —She is not to urinate before the test. —It is important for her to lie still during the test. —The only discomfort she will experience will be from her full bladder, which she may empty immediately after the test. —Repeat testing may be ordered to check on the fetus or on her condition.

AMNIOCENTESIS

Patient objectives	*Teaching plan content*
1 **Define amniocentesis.**	Amniocentesis is the withdrawal of fluid from the amniotic sac with a sterile needle.
2 **State the purposes of amniocentesis.**	The purposes of amniocentesis include the following: —To detect abnormalities in the formation of the fetal nervous system —To detect chromosomal and genetic defects —To determine the sex and health of the fetus —To evaluate fetal lung maturity during the last trimester of pregnancy.
3 **Describe the procedure used in amniocentesis.**	During amniocentesis, the patient can expect the following: —She will be asked to lie on her back on a table with her hands crossed on her chest. —The nurse will take her pulse, her respiratory rate, her blood pressure, and the fetal heart rate. —An ultrasound scan will be done to identify the fetus and placenta (see the "Pelvic Ultrasonography" teach-

ing plan in this chapter).
—The physician will then prepare her abdomen by washing it with antiseptic solution.
—She then may be injected with a local anesthetic at the needle insertion site.
—The physician will insert a very thin, long needle with a stylet (wire) through the abdominal and uterine walls, into the amniotic sac.
—The stylet will then be removed from the inside of the needle and, when a drop of amniotic fluid appears, the physician will attach a glass syringe to the needle and aspirate some amniotic fluid.
—The physician will then remove the needle and place an adhesive bandage over the insertion site.

---

4 Discuss patient guidelines for amniocentesis.

Patient guidelines for amniocentesis are as follows:
—She will be asked to empty her bladder and put on a hospital gown before the test.
—She will be asked to sign a consent form.
—She will be asked to lie as still as possible.
—A support person may accompany her during the test.
—When the test is over, she may be asked to lie on her side for 15 to 30 minutes and rest while the nurse periodically checks her pulse, respirations, and blood pressure and the fetal heart rate.
—She will be asked to report any vaginal discharge of fluid or blood, decreased fetal movement, contractions, or fever or chills to her physician.

ESTRIOL MEASUREMENT TEST (Urine placental estriol test)

Patient objectives	*Teaching plan content*
1 Define estriol measurement test.	The estriol measurement test monitors fetal viability by measuring urine levels of placental estriol, the predominant estrogen excreted in urine during pregnancy.
2 State the purpose of an estriol measurement test.	An estriol measurement test assesses fetoplacental status, especially in high-risk pregnancy.
3 Describe the procedure for an estriol measurement test.	The patient will collect a 24-hour urine specimen. (The laboratory will provide her with a bottle that will contain a preservative.) She need not restrict food or fluids, but she should tell the physician what (if any) medications she is taking. Serial tests will be needed for comparison, because a rise or fall in estriol levels indicates fetal condition.

4 Discuss patient guidelines for an estriol measurement test.	Patient guidelines for an estriol measurement test include the following: —The patient should discard her first-voided urine specimen the morning she starts the test. —After her first specimen, all other urine specimens are to be put in the special collection bottle provided by the laboratory. —This bottle is to be kept refrigerated during the collection period. —She should discard toilet tissue separately and avoid mixing fecal matter with the specimen. —After her first-voided urine on the second day, the test is terminated, and the bottle should be returned to the laboratory as soon as possible on that day.

ANTEPARTAL NONSTRESS TEST (N.S.T.)

Patient objectives	*Teaching plan content*
1 Define NST.	The NST records fetal heart rate acceleration, which indicates fetal well-being.
2 State the purpose of NST.	The NST evaluates fetal well-being by measuring fetal response to spontaneous uterine contractions or fetal movements; such contractions or movements produce transient accelerations in the heart rate of a healthy fetus.
3 Describe the procedure used in an NST.	For an NST, the patient can expect the following: —She will be placed in a semi-Fowler's position (head and chest raised at about a 45-degree angle) in a quiet area. —A tocotransducer (instrument for recording uterine contractions) and a fetal heart rate transducer (instrument for recording the fetal heartbeat) will be strapped to her abdomen; conductive jelly will be applied under both transducers for good conduction of the waves. —Baseline maternal pulse, respiration, and blood pressure will be taken. —She will be given a button to push every time she feels the baby move. This button will prompt the monitor to mark an arrow on the monitor tape to signify fetal movement. This will allow correlation between fetal heart rate and fetal movement. —The monitor will then be allowed to run for approximately 30 to 40 minutes. —If no fetal activity is recorded within 20 minutes, external stimulation, such as a loud noise or movement of

the patient's abdomen, may be used to stir the fetus. Fetuses go through 20-minute periods of rest and activity.
—If no fetal movement is recorded in 30 to 40 minutes, the patient may be asked to eat a light meal (or drink glucose) and then to return for repeat testing. Fetal movements may increase in response to an increase in blood glucose or fullness of the patient's stomach.

4 **Discuss patient guidelines for an NST.**	Patient guidelines for an NST are as follows: —The patient should schedule her appointment for a time when she will not be rushed, since the test itself may take 30 to 40 minutes and may have to be repeated if the fetus does not exhibit sufficient movement. —She will not have to restrict food or fluids on the day of the test. —She should wear comfortable clothing. —She should empty her bladder right before the test starts, since she will have to lie still for almost an hour.

OXYTOCIN CHALLENGE TEST (O.C.T.) (Stress test)

Patient objectives	*Teaching plan content*
1 **Define oxytocin challenge test (OCT).**	The OCT uses indirect electronic monitoring to measure fetal heart response (in the form of late deceleration of the fetal heart rate) to spontaneous or oxytocin-induced uterine contractions.
2 **State the purpose of an OCT.**	The OCT evaluates placental function and identifies the fetus that will be unable to withstand the stress of labor.
3 **Describe the procedure used in an OCT.**	For an OCT, the patient can expect the following: —She will be placed in a semi-Fowler's position (head and chest raised at about a 45-degree angle). —Baseline maternal pulse, respirations, and blood pressure will be obtained. —A tocotransducer (instrument used to record uterine contractions) and a fetal heart rate transducer (instrument used to record the fetal heart rate) will be strapped to her abdomen after the application of conductive jelly. —Baseline uterine contractions, fetal heart rate, and fetal movement will be measured for 20 minutes. —If three spontaneous uterine contractions are recorded within a 10-minute period, the fetal heart response will be evaluated, and the test will be concluded.

—If no contractions occur, the physician will order intravenous oxytocin to be started or breast self-stimulation (BSS) done. In BSS, the patient's nipples are stimulated by warm washcloths and then by manual rolling of one nipple. BSS causes the body to produce internal oxytocin.

—After a recording of three contractions, the oxytocin drip or BSS will be terminated.

—Tracings will be continued until they return to preoxytocin or pre-BSS status. The patient's vital signs (heart rate, respirations, and blood pressure) will be checked frequently during the test and afterward.

—When all parameters have returned to pre-test status, the patient may be allowed to return home.

—A negative test (absence of late decelerations of fetal heart rate with uterine contractions) suggests fetal tolerance to labor due to adequate placental functioning.

—A positive test (presence of late decelerations of fetal heart rate with more than 50% of the uterine contractions) must be interpreted by the physician using other parameters, as false positives are possible; then a decision will be made by the physician and patient to induce labor or do a cesarean delivery.

---

4 Discuss patient guidelines for an OCT.

Patient guidelines for an OCT are as follows:

—Depending on her physician's instructions or the protocol of the institution, the patient may be asked to refrain from eating breakfast the morning of the test.

—If the institution requires it, she will have to sign a consent form.

—The test will be performed on an outpatient basis near or on the labor floor.

—She will be asked to empty her bladder before the test, since it takes about 1½ to 2 hours.

—She will be asked to empty her bladder and to change into a hospital gown before the test.

—During the recording of baseline information on the patient and the fetus, she will have to lie as still as possible.

—If BSS is to be done, she will have to roll one of her nipples between her thumb and fingers until a contraction occurs.

—If intravenous oxytocin is to be administered, she will have to lie still while the I.V. needle is inserted.

—She should report to the nurse or physician any unusual feelings during the test and any discomfort or problems after the test.

CHORIONIC VILLI SAMPLING

Patient objectives	Teaching plan content
1 **Define chorionic villi sampling.**	Chorionic villi sampling is the collection of cells from a membrane surrounding the fetus. These cells can be analyzed for fetal abnormalities.
2 **State the purpose of chorionic villi sampling.**	Chorionic villi sampling, or biopsy, is a new and somewhat experimental prenatal test for detection of fetal chromosomal and biochemical disorders. The test is safe and may someday replace amniocentesis.
3 **Describe the procedure used in chorionic villi sampling.**	This test is done between the 8th and 10th weeks of pregnancy. The patient can expect the following: —She will be placed in the lithotomy position (lying on her back, with her legs up in stirrups). —The physician will check the placement of her uterus manually. —A vaginal speculum will be inserted, and her cervix will be cleansed with a cotton-tipped applicator and antiseptic solution. —Guided by ultrasonography (see the "Pelvic Ultrasonography" teaching plan in this chapter), the physician will insert a cannula and pass a catheter through it and into the cervix and uterus. —Suction will then be applied to the catheter and a small amount of tissue removed from the fetal membrane. —The sample will be withdrawn and placed in a Petri dish (a container filled with nutrients to promote growth of the fetal cells). —Part of the specimen will be grown for further testing, while other parts will be examined through a microscope.
4 **Discuss patient guidelines for chorionic villi sampling.**	Patient guidelines for chorionic villi sampling are as follows: —The patient will be asked to disrobe from the waist down. A sheet will be provided for her privacy. —She will be asked to lie still during the test. —During the test, she will experience minimal discomfort as the cannula and catheter are passed through her cervical opening. —After the test, she will be asked to report any bleeding, cramping, or fever (signs of infection) to the physician.

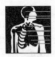 **Explaining disorders**

SPONTANEOUS ABORTION

Patient objectives	*Teaching plan content*
1 Define abortion.	Abortion is the spontaneous or induced (therapeutic) expulsion of the products of conception from the uterus before fetal viability (before fetal weight of 500 g and gestation of 20 weeks).
2 Discuss the cause of spontaneous abortion.	Spontaneous abortion may result from fetal, placental, or maternal factors. —Fetal factors usually cause such abortions between 9 and 12 weeks of gestation. They include defective embryologic development due to abnormal chromosome division (the most common cause of fetal death); faulty implantation of the fertilized ovum; and failure of the inner lining of the uterus to accept the fertilized ovum. —Placental factors usually cause abortion around the 14th week of gestation, when the placenta takes over the hormone production necessary to maintain the pregnancy. They include premature separation of the normally implanted placenta; abnormal placental implantation; and abnormal platelet function. —Maternal factors usually cause abortion between 11 and 19 weeks of gestation. They include maternal infection or severe malnutrition; abnormalities of the reproductive organs (especially incompetent cervix, in which the cervix dilates painlessly and bloodlessly in the second trimester); endocrine problems, such as thyroid dysfunction or lowered estriol secretion; trauma, including any type of surgery that necessitates manipulation of the pelvic organs; blood group incompatibility and Rh isoimmunization; and drug ingestion.
3 Describe the symptoms of spontaneous abortion.	Early symptoms of spontaneous abortion may include spotting (a pink discharge for several days or a scant brown discharge for several weeks) before onset of cramps and increased vaginal bleeding. For a few hours, the cramps intensify and occur more frequently; then the cervix dilates for expulsion of uterine contents. If the entire contents are expelled, cramps and bleeding subside. However, if any contents remain, cramps and bleeding continue.

4 Explain how the diagnosis of spontaneous abortion is made.	Diagnosis of spontaneous abortion is based on clinical evidence of expulsion of uterine contents, pelvic examination, and laboratory studies. Human chorionic gonadotropin in the blood or urine confirms pregnancy. (See the "Pregnancy Tests" teaching plan in this chapter.) Pelvic examination determines the size of the uterus and whether this size is consistent with the length of the pregnancy. Examination of the tissue that was expelled can indicate products of conception. Decreased blood cell count reflects the blood loss at the time of the abortion.
5 Discuss the difference between therapeutic and spontaneous abortion.	The goal of therapeutic abortion is to preserve the mother's mental or physical health in cases of rape, unplanned pregnancy, or medical conditions such as moderate or severe cardiac dysfunction. —Dilatation and extraction (D&E) is used in first-trimester therapeutic abortions. —In second-trimester therapeutic abortions, an injection of hypertonic saline solution into the amniotic sac or a prostaglandin vaginal suppository induces expulsion.
6 Describe the treatment for spontaneous abortion.	An accurate evaluation of uterine contents is necessary before planning treatment. Spontaneous abortion usually requires the following: —The patient should have bed rest for 24 hours after spotting or complete bed rest for as long as spotting continues. The progression of spontaneous abortion cannot be prevented, except in those cases caused by an incompetent cervix. —Hospitalization is necessary to control severe hemorrhage. Severe bleeding requires transfusion with packed red blood cells or whole blood. —Intravenous administration of oxytocin may be started to stimulate uterine contractions and help empty the uterus of any retained products of conception. —If any contents remain in the uterus, dilatation and curettage (D&C) or dilatation and extraction (D&E) should be performed (see the "Dilatation and Curettage" and "Dilatation and Vacuum Extraction" teaching plans in this chapter). —If the patient has Rh-negative blood, she will receive an injection of $Rh_o(D)$ immune human globulin (RhoGAM) to prevent problems with future pregnancies. (This is also done in therapeutic abortion.) —If the patient has an incompetent cervix, resulting in

habitual abortions, treatment will involve surgical intervention for reinforcement of the cervix. This is called a Shirodkar-Barter procedure, and it is done at the 14th to 16th week after her last menstrual period.

7 **Discuss guidelines for self-care after a spontaneous abortion.**	Patient guidelines include the following: —The patient should expect vaginal bleeding or spotting and should immediately report bleeding that lasts longer than 8 to 10 days or excessive bright red blood. —She should watch for signs of infection, such as a temperature higher than 100° F. (37.8° C.) and a foul-smelling vaginal discharge. —Daily activities should be gradually increased to include whatever tasks the patient feels comfortable doing (cooking, sewing, cleaning, for example), as long as these activities do not increase vaginal bleeding or cause fatigue. Most patients return to work within 2 to 4 weeks. —The patient should abstain from intercourse for 2 to 3 weeks and should avoid using tampons for 2 to 4 weeks.
8 **Describe the medication regimen.**	Some drugs used for this disorder are oxytocin and $Rh_o(D)$ immune human globulin. For specific medication instructions, see Chapter 10, Drug Therapy.
9 **Explain the importance of routine medical follow-up.**	Follow-up care is needed to assess the patient's treatment. If a D&C or a D&E was performed, a postoperative checkup may be required by her physician after 2 to 4 weeks.

ECTOPIC PREGNANCY

Patient objectives	*Teaching plan content*
1 **Define ectopic pregnancy.**	Ectopic pregnancy is the implantation of a fertilized egg outside the uterine cavity.
2 **Identify at least three causes of ectopic pregnancy.**	Conditions that prevent or retard the passage of the fertilized egg through the fallopian tube and into the uterine cavity cause ectopic pregnancy. These include the following: —Inflammation of the folds of the tubal mucosa (lining), causing the tube to narrow —Formation of blind pouches that cause tubal abnormalities —Tumors pressing against the tube —Previous surgery on the tubes, or adhesions from ab-

dominal or pelvic surgery
—Migration of the egg from the ovary to the opposite tube
—Present or past use of an intrauterine device (IUD), which stops the egg from implanting in the uterine lining, making the fallopian tube a more favorable spot
—Rarely, congenital defects in the reproductive tract.

3 Discuss the signs and symptoms of an ectopic pregnancy.	Ectopic pregnancy sometimes produces symptoms of normal pregnancy or no symptoms other than mild abdominal pain (the latter is especially likely in abdominal pregnancy), making diagnosis difficult. Characteristic signs and symptoms after fallopian tube implantation include the following:

—The patient experiences amenorrhea (absence of menses) or abnormal menses, followed by slight vaginal bleeding and unilateral pelvic pain over the mass.
—Rupture of the tube causes life-threatening complications, including hemorrhage, shock, and peritonitis (inflammation of the peritoneal cavity).
—The patient experiences sharp lower abdominal pain, possibly radiating to the shoulders and neck, often precipitated by an activity that increases abdominal pressure, such as a bowel movement.
—She feels extreme pain on motion of the cervix and palpation of the adnexa (related structures in the area) during a pelvic examination.
—She has a tender, spongy uterus.

4 Explain how the diagnosis of ectopic pregnancy is made.	Diagnosis of ectopic pregnancy is based on a patient history, presenting signs and symptoms, and a pelvic examination. The following tests may also be done to confirm the diagnosis:

—Serum pregnancy test to detect the presence of human chorionic gonadotropin (see the "Pregnancy Tests" teaching plan in this chapter)
—Ultrasonography, if the pregnancy test is positive, to determine intrauterine pregnancy or ovarian cyst (see the "Pelvic Ultrasonography" teaching plan in this chapter)
—Fluid aspiration from the vaginal cul-de-sac (the area behind the vagina and in front of the rectum) to detect any free blood in the peritoneum (the membrane that covers the entire abdominal wall)
—Laparoscopy to observe any problems via a fiber-optic tube inserted through the abdominal wall
—Exploratory laparotomy to confirm the ectopic pregnancy. (This surgical procedure is also used for treatment.)

5 Describe the treatment of ectopic pregnancy.	Treatment of ectopic pregnancy is determined by the site. Most often, the affected tube or ovary is removed to prevent rupture and possible hemorrhage. —This is usually done during exploratory laparotomy, which requires a general anesthetic. An incision is made in the abdomen, and an exploration of the abdominal organs is conducted. If an ectopic pregnancy is confirmed, the affected fallopian tube and/or ovary is removed, and procedures for controlling bleeding are performed. —An interstitial ectopic pregnancy (one in the area where the tube and uterus meet) may require a hysterectomy (removal of the uterus). —Supportive treatment includes transfusion of whole blood or packed red blood cells to counter excessive blood loss and broad-spectrum antibiotics I.V. for septic infection. —The patient receives supplemental iron P.O. or I.M. and a diet high in protein.
6 Discuss the prevention of ectopic pregnancy.	Pelvic infections should be treated promptly to prevent diseases of the fallopian tube. Patients who have undergone surgery involving the fallopian tubes and those with confirmed pelvic inflammatory disease are at increased risk of ectopic pregnancy. The patient who is vulnerable to ectopic pregnancy should delay using an IUD until after she has completed her family.
7 Describe the medication regimen.	Some drugs used for this disorder are ampicillin, penicillin, and $Rh_o(D)$ immune human globulin. For specific medication instructions, see Chapter 10, Drug Therapy.
8 Explain the importance of routine medical follow-up.	If the patient has had surgical intervention for her ectopic pregnancy, the physician will probably want to see her in approximately 2 weeks. The physician will assess her treatment and will discuss her future childbearing plans at that time.

HYPEREMESIS GRAVIDARUM

Patient objectives	*Teaching plan content*
1 Define hyperemesis gravidarum.	Unlike the transient nausea and vomiting normally experienced between the 6th and 12th weeks of pregnancy, hyperemesis gravidarum is severe and unremitting nausea and vomiting that persist beyond the first trimester.

2 **Discuss the cause of hyperemesis gravidarum.**

Although its cause is unknown, hyperemesis gravidarum often affects pregnant women with conditions that produce high levels of human chorionic gonadotropin (a hormone produced during pregnancy), such as hydatidiform mole (an intrauterine mass of grapelike, enlarged chorionic villi) or multiple pregnancy. This disorder may also be a symptom of pancreatitis (inflammation of the pancreas). It may also be seen in liver disease, drug toxicity, inflammatory obstructive bowel disease, and vitamin deficiency (especially of vitamin B_6). In some patients, hyperemesis gravidarum may be related to psychological factors, such as ambivalence toward pregnancy.

3 **Discuss the signs and symptoms associated with hyperemesis gravidarum.**

The signs and symptoms associated with hyperemesis gravidarum are as follows:
—The outstanding symptoms are unremitting nausea and vomiting. The vomitus initially contains undigested food, mucus, and small amounts of bile; later, only bile and mucus; and finally, blood and what resembles coffee grounds.
—Persistent vomiting causes the patient to lose a substantial amount of weight and eventually to become emaciated.
—Her skin may turn pale, dry, and waxy and may appear jaundiced (yellow); her temperature may be subnormal or elevated; and her pulse may become rapid. Her breath may have a fruity odor.
—If the vomiting persists, she may become confused or delirious or may experience headaches, stupor, sleepiness, and possibly coma.

4 **Explain how the diagnosis of hyperemesis gravidarum is made.**

The diagnosis of hyperemesis gravidarum is made by taking a detailed history and by observing characteristic clinical features.
—The certain distinguishing facts about her history are uncontrolled nausea and vomiting that persist beyond the first trimester and evidence of substantial weight loss.
—The diagnosis may be confirmed by laboratory tests to detect the following:
  • Ketones and protein in her urine (due to the body using fat for fuel)
  • Decreased protein, chloride, sodium, and potassium levels (those elements lost from the body during extended bouts of vomiting)
  • Increased hemoglobin and white blood cell count.
—Diagnosis must rule out other conditions with similar clinical effects.

5 Describe the treatment of hyperemesis gravidarum.	Treatment of hyperemesis gravidarum may necessitate hospitalization to correct electrolyte imbalance and prevent starvation. —I.V. infusions will be given until the patient can tolerate oral feedings. She will progress slowly from a clear liquid diet to a full liquid diet and finally to small, frequent meals of high-protein solid foods. A midnight snack will help stabilize blood glucose levels; vitamin B supplements will help correct vitamin deficiency. —If vomiting continues, she may be placed on drug therapy to reduce gastrointestinal spasms, but this is controversial because of potential teratogenic effects on the developing embryo. The safest possible drug will be used in the lowest possible dose to minimize any harmful effects on the fetus. —When vomiting has stopped and electrolyte balance has been restored, the pregnancy usually continues without recurrence of hyperemesis gravidarum. —The patient should begin to feel better as she regains normal weight. —If she continues to vomit throughout her pregnancy, extended treatment will be required, and she may benefit from consultations with a clinical nurse specialist, a psychologist, or a psychiatrist.
6 Explain the importance of routine medical follow-up.	The patient should follow her nutritional instructions. She should return to her physician for prenatal visits so that he may observe how her pregnancy is advancing.

PREGNANCY-INDUCED HYPERTENSION (P.I.H.)

Patient objectives	*Teaching plan content*
1 Define pregnancy-induced hypertension.	Pregnancy-induced hypertension, a potentially life-threatening disorder, elevates blood pressure to dangerous levels. It usually develops late in the second trimester or in the third trimester. There are two forms of pregnancy-induced hypertension: preeclampsia, the nonconvulsive form, and eclampsia, the convulsive form.
2 Discuss the cause of pregnancy-induced hypertension.	The cause of pregnancy-induced hypertension is unknown, but it appears to be related to several conditions: —Inadequate prenatal care, especially poor nutrition —The woman's age and number of pregnancies (women over age 30 or under age 20, as well as those in their first pregnancies, seem more prone)

—Multiple pregnancies
—Preexisting diabetes mellitus or hypertension
—Hydramnios (excess of amniotic fluid)
—Hydatidiform mole (an intrauterine neoplastic mass that mimics pregnancy).

| **3** Discuss the signs and symptoms associated with pregnancy-induced hypertension. | The signs and symptoms associated with pregnancy-induced hypertension are as follows:
—Mild preeclampsia produces hypertension; proteinuria (protein in the urine); generalized edema (swelling) of the hands, face, and feet; and sudden weight gain of more than 3 lb (1.4 kg) a week during the second trimester or 1 lb (0.5 kg) a week during the third trimester.
—Severe preeclampsia is marked by increased hypertension and protein in the urine, eventually leading to oliguria (absence of urine).
—Symptoms that may indicate worsening preeclampsia include blurred vision, epigastric pain or heartburn, irritability, emotional tension, and severe frontal headache.
—In eclampsia, all the clinical manifestations of preeclampsia are magnified and are associated with convulsions and possibly coma.
—Possible complications of persistent convulsions include stroke due to cerebral hemorrhage, blindness, abruptio placentae (separation of the placenta from the inner uterine wall), premature labor, stillbirth, kidney failure, and liver damage. |
| **4** Explain how the diagnosis of pregnancy-induced hypertension is made. | The diagnosis of pregnancy-induced hypertension is made as follows:
—In mild preeclampsia, higher-than-normal blood pressure and protein in the urine are found.
—In severe preeclampsia, higher-than-normal blood pressure readings (during bed rest), increased amounts of protein in the urine, decreased urine output, and increased deep tendon reflexes are found.
—Eclampsia is strongly suggested by typical clinical features (especially convulsions) combined with typical findings for severe preeclampsia. In addition, ophthalmoscopic examination may reveal vascular changes in the eyes.
—Tests are usually performed to evaluate the condition of the fetus. A nonstress test (see the "Antepartal Nonstress Test" teaching plan in this chapter), an oxytocin challenge test (see the "Oxytocin Challenge Test" teaching plan in this chapter), and a urine estriol test (see the "Estriol Measurement Test" teaching plan in this chapter) may be performed. |

5 Describe the treatment for pregnancy-induced hypertension.	The treatment for pregnancy-induced hypertension is designed to halt the disorder's progress, especially the signs of eclampsia, and ensure the survival of the baby. —If the patient is near term, her physician might want to induce labor. —Other therapy may include sedatives, complete bed rest, and a high-protein, low-sodium, low-carbohydrate diet, with increased fluid intake. (See *Managing Pregnancy-Induced Hypertension at Home*, pp. 298-299.) —If the patient's blood pressure fails to respond to bed rest and sedation, magnesium sulfate may be administered to produce generalized sedation, promote diuresis (increased fluid excretion through her kidneys), reduce her blood pressure, and prevent convulsions. —If all the preceding measures fail to improve her condition or if her baby's life is in danger (determined by nonstress and stress tests), a cesarean or induced delivery may be necessary.
6 Describe the medication regimen.	A drug commonly used for this disorder is magnesium sulfate. For specific medication instructions, see Chapter 10, Drug Therapy.
7 Explain the importance of routine medical follow-up.	The patient is strongly encouraged to follow her medical regimen and keep all her medical appointments. Pregnancy-induced hypertension can be detrimental to her health and the life and health of her baby. Early detection and careful observation of her condition may prevent serious complications.

HYDATIDIFORM MOLE

Patient objectives	*Teaching plan content*
1 Define hydatidiform mole.	Hydatidiform mole is an uncommon developmental malfunction of the placenta in which a mass of grapelike tissue forms within the uterus.
2 Discuss the cause of hydatidiform mole.	The cause of hydatidiform mole is unknown, but loss of fetal circulation and death of the embryo seem to precede formation of the mole. Hydatidiform mole occurs most commonly in women over age 45, in Oriental women, and in women whose ovulatory cycles have been stimulated by clomiphene.
3 Discuss the signs and symptoms associated with hydatidiform mole.	The signs and symptoms associated with hydatidiform mole are as follows: —The early stages of a pregnancy in which a hydatidi-

form mole develops seem normal, except that the uterus grows more rapidly than usual.
—The patient may also experience excessive nausea and vomiting. (See the "Hyperemesis Gravidarum" teaching plan in this chapter.)
—The first obvious sign of trouble may be vaginal bleeding (ranging from spotting to hemorrhage) and lower abdominal cramps; these symptoms mimic spontaneous abortion. The blood may contain grapelike vesicles and may be bright red or brownish (prune-juice color).
—Signs of preeclampsia may be present. (See the "Pregnancy-Induced Hypertension" teaching plan in this chapter.)
—The patient may also experience uterine discomfort from overstretching.

4 Explain how the diagnosis of hydatidiform mole is made.	Diagnosis of hydatidiform mole is based on the following subjective and objective findings: —Persistent bleeding and an abnormally enlarged uterus —Passage and identification of hydatid vesicles (grapelike structures) —A pregnancy test that shows very high levels of human chorionic gonadotropin (HCG) —Absence of fetal heart rate and inability to identify fetal parts on palpation of the abdomen —Evidence of preeclampsia developing earlier than usual in the pregnancy (see the "Pregnancy-Induced Hypertension" teaching plan in this chapter) —Pelvic ultrasound that confirms the absence of a fetus —Possible decreased hemoglobin and hematocrit (red blood cell count) due to bleeding —Possible increased white blood cell count due to infection.
5 Describe the treatment of hydatidiform mole.	Hydatidiform mole necessitates uterine evacuation via dilatation and curettage (see the "Dilatation and Curettage" teaching plan in this chapter). If this is ineffective, an abdominal hysterectomy (see the "Hysterectomy" teaching plan in this chapter) or suction curettage (see the "Dilatation and Vacuum Extraction" teaching plan in this chapter) may have to be performed. The patient's postoperative care and length of hospitalization will depend on her condition and on any complications that may arise.

6 **Explain the importance of routine medical follow-up.**	Because of the possibility of choriocarcinoma after hydatidiform mole, follow-up care is essential. Such care includes monitoring HCG levels until they return to normal and taking chest X-rays to check for lung involvement. Most physicians advise postponing another pregnancy for at least 1 year after HCG levels return to normal and regular ovulation and menstrual cycles are reestablished.

PLACENTA PREVIA

Patient objectives	*Teaching plan content*
1 **Define placenta previa.**	Placenta previa is characterized by the abnormal implantation of the placenta over or in proximity to the internal os (opening) of the cervix. The placenta may cover all (total, complete, or central), part (partial or incomplete), or a fraction (marginal or low-lying) of the internal cervical os. The degree of placenta previa depends largely on the extent of cervical dilation at the time of examination because the dilating cervix gradually uncovers the placenta.
2 **Discuss the cause of placenta previa.**	In placenta previa, the lower segment of the uterus fails to receive as much nourishment as the fundus (upper portion). The placenta tends to spread out, seeking the blood supply it needs, and becomes larger and thinner than normal. Hemorrhage occurs as the internal cervical os effaces and dilates, tearing the uterine vessels. Although the specific cause of placenta previa is unknown, factors that may affect the site of the placenta's attachment to the uterine wall include the following: —Early or late fertilization —Receptivity and adequacy of the uterine lining —Multiple pregnancy (the placenta requires a larger surface for attachment) —Previous uterine surgery —Previous multiple pregnancies —Advanced maternal age.
3 **Discuss the signs and symptoms of placenta previa.**	Placenta previa usually produces painless third trimester bleeding (often the first complaint). Various fetal malpresentations occur because the placenta's location interferes with proper descent of the fetal head. (The fetus remains active, however, with good heart tones.)

4 **Explain how the diagnosis of placenta previa is made.**

Findings that may support the diagnosis of placenta previa include position of the fetal presenting part in the pelvis and decreased blood cell count due to blood loss. Radiologic testing (soft-tissue X-rays) may be used to locate the placenta, but it has limited value. Definitive diagnosis of placenta previa requires one of the following special measures:
—Pelvic ultrasound scanning for placental position (see the "Pelvic Ultrasonography" teaching plan in this chapter)
—Pelvic examination, performed immediately before delivery, to confirm diagnosis. (This examination is done in the delivery room, with equipment available in case of hemorrhage.)

5 **Describe the treatment of placenta previa.**

The goals of treatment of placenta previa are to assess, control, and replace the amount of blood lost; to deliver a viable infant; and to prevent coagulation disorders.
—Immediate therapy includes the following:
• Starting an I.V. line using a large-bore catheter
• Drawing blood for hemoglobin and hematocrit levels as well as typing and cross matching
• Initiating external electronic fetal monitoring
• Monitoring maternal blood pressure, pulse rate, and respirations
• Assessing the amount of vaginal bleeding.
—If the fetus is premature, treatment consists of careful observation, following determination of the degree of placenta previa and necessary fluid and blood replacement. If clinical evaluation confirms complete placenta previa, the patient is usually hospitalized because of the increased risk of hemorrhage.
• As soon as the fetus is sufficiently mature, or in case of intervening severe hemorrhage, immediate cesarean delivery may be necessary.
• Vaginal delivery is sometimes chosen to provide tamponade (stoppage of the blood flow by pressure) by compressing the detached placenta against the implantation site during labor. Because of the possibility of fetal blood loss through the placenta, a pediatric team is usually on hand during such deliveries to immediately assess and treat neonatal problems.

6 **Explain the importance of routine medical follow-up.**

Medical follow-up will vary, depending on the patient's course of treatment.
—Cesarean delivery will necessitate staple or suture removal within a 1- to 2-week period, along with a postoperative checkup by her physician.
—Vaginal delivery will necessitate a 4- to 6-week postpartum checkup by her physician.

—In either case, the physician will want to assess her for low hemoglobin and hematocrit levels and, depending on the viability of the infant and its survival, for her psychological condition.
—The physician will also want to counsel her about birth control and future pregnancies.

ABRUPTIO PLACENTAE (Placental abruption)

Patient objectives	Teaching plan content
1 Define abruptio placentae.	Abruptio placentae is the premature separation of the placenta from the uterine wall. This usually occurs after the 20th week of gestation and produces heavy bleeding.
2 Discuss the cause of abruptio placentae.	The cause of abruptio placentae is unknown, but the following are predisposing factors: —Trauma, such as a direct blow to the uterus —Possible placental site bleeding from a needle puncture during amniocentesis —Chronic hypertension —Eclampsia (see the "Pregnancy-Induced Hypertension" teaching plan in this chapter) —Pressure on the vena cava (the large vessel that brings blood back to the heart from systemic circulation) from an enlarged uterus —Five or more previous pregnancies —Maternal age over 30 —Excessive intrauterine pressure due to hydramnios (excess of amniotic fluid) or multiple pregnancy.
3 Discuss the effects of abruptio placentae.	Abruptio placentae produces a wide range of clinical effects, depending on the extent of placental separation and the amount of blood lost from maternal circulation. —Mild abruptio placentae (marginal separation) develops gradually, and fetal heart tones remain strong and regular. It causes the following: • Mild-to-moderate bleeding (with dark red blood or none seen at all) • Vague lower abdominal discomfort • Mild-to-moderate abdominal tenderness • Uterine irritability. —Moderate abruptio placentae (about 50% placental separation) may develop gradually or abruptly. Labor usually starts within 2 hours and often proceeds rapidly. The following signs and symptoms occur: • Continuous abdominal pain • Moderate dark red vaginal bleeding

- A very tender uterus that remains firm between contractions
- Barely audible or irregular and slow fetal heart tones
- Possibly, signs of shock (dizziness, fainting, disorientation, chills and possibly shivering, and rapid heartbeat).

—Severe abruptio placentae (nearly 70% placental separation) usually develops abruptly and causes the following:

- Agonizing, unremitting uterine pain (often described as tearing or knifelike)
- A boardlike, tender uterus
- Moderate dark red vaginal bleeding
- Rapidly progressive shock
- Absence of fetal heart tones.

---

4 Identify the possible complications of abruptio placentae.

In addition to hemorrhage and shock, complications of abruptio placentae may include the following:

—Kidney failure

—Disseminated intravascular coagulation (DIC), a disorder that accelerates clotting, causing the occlusion of small blood vessels, depletion of circulating clotting factors and platelets, and elevation of fibrinogen in circulation, all of which can exacerbate or provoke severe hemorrhage

—Maternal or fetal death.

---

5 Explain how the diagnosis of abruptio placentae is made.

Diagnostic measures for abruptio placentae include the following:

—Observation of clinical features, such as bleeding, pain, uterine contractions and irritability, and other presenting signs and symptoms

—Pelvic examination, usually done in the delivery room, with equipment ready to handle delivery or complications

—Pelvic ultrasonography to rule out placenta previa (see the "Pelvic Ultrasonography" and "Placenta Previa" teaching plans in this chapter)

—Periodic blood tests to monitor the progression of the abruption and to detect the development of DIC.

---

6 Describe the treatment of abruptio placentae.

The goals of treatment of abruptio placentae are to assess, control, and restore the amount of blood lost; to deliver a viable infant; and to prevent coagulation disorders.

—Immediate treatment measures for the patient with abruptio placentae include the following:

- Starting an I.V. infusion with appropriate fluids to help combat fluid loss

• Initiating blood tests to determine blood components lost during bleeding and typing and cross matching in case blood transfusions have to be administered
• External fetal monitoring
• Monitoring the patient's pulse rate, blood pressure, and respirations
• Assessing the amount of vaginal bleeding.
—After determination of the severity of her condition and after appropriate fluid and blood replacement, prompt cesarean delivery will be performed if the fetus is alive but in distress.
—If the fetus is not in distress, the patient will be monitored continuously. Delivery is usually performed at the earliest sign of fetal distress.
—If the tone of the uterus cannot be restored to a point where it will contract to stop the bleeding, a hysterectomy may be performed.

7 Explain the importance of routine medical follow-up.	Severe abruptio placentae and its resultant hemorrhage may cause future problems that the physician must assess. If the patient begins lactating at the proper time, the physician will know her pituitary gland has not been seriously damaged. He will want to determine if her menses have returned to normal and counsel her on birth control and future plans for pregnancy. Also, he will want to test her thyroid and adrenal gland function 4 to 6 months after the episode.

PREMATURE RUPTURE OF MEMBRANES (P.R.O.M.)

Patient objectives	*Teaching plan content*
1 Define PROM.	PROM is a spontaneous break or tear in the fetal membranous sac before the onset of regular contractions (a premature break in the bag of waters).
2 Discuss the cause of PROM.	Although the cause of PROM is unknown, malpresentation of the fetus and a contracted pelvis (variation in the shape or diameter of the pelvic inlet) commonly accompany PROM. There are also predisposing factors, which include the following: —Poor maternal nutrition and hygiene —Lack of proper prenatal care —Incompetent cervix (cervical opening does not remain closed) —Increased intrauterine tension resulting from multiple pregnancy or hydramnios (excess of amniotic fluid) —Defects in the membrane's tensile strength.

3 **Discuss the signs and symptoms of PROM.**	Typically, PROM causes blood-tinged amniotic fluid containing vernix particles to gush or leak from the vagina. If the patient's membranes have been ruptured for more than 24 hours, there is a risk of infection for both her and the fetus. With infection, she would exhibit a fever over 100.4° F. (38° C.) and a foul-smelling vaginal discharge. On examination, the fetal heart rate would be very high.
4 **Explain how the diagnosis of PROM is made.**	When the patient's fetal membranes rupture, she may experience a gush of warm fluid or a slow trickle, suggesting urinary incontinence. A physical examination will show amniotic fluid in her vagina. —Tests will be performed on a sample of this fluid to determine the presence of infectious organisms and assess fetal maturity. —Abdominal palpation (Leopold's maneuvers) will assess fetal presentation and size. Physical examination will also determine the possibility of a multiple pregnancy. —The following data will be used to determine gestational age: • Dates of last menstrual period and quickening • Initial detection of fetal heart rate with amplification, measurement of uterine fundus height above her symphysis pubis, and pelvic ultrasound measurements of the fetal skull (biparietal diameter) • Lecithin-sphingomyelin (L/S) ratio. (L/S ratio greater than 2.0 indicates pulmonary maturity of the fetus.)
5 **Describe the treatment of PROM.**	Treatment of PROM depends on fetal age and the risk of infection. —A term pregnancy usually requires induction of labor with oxytocin or, when induction fails, cesarean delivery if spontaneous labor and delivery are not achieved within a relatively short time (usually within 24 hours after membranes rupture). —If gross uterine infection is present, the physician may perform a hysterectomy. —A preterm pregnancy of less than 28 weeks also necessitates induction of labor, since fetal mortality is almost certain and carrying the fetus in a ruptured amniotic sac exposes the mother to infection. —With a preterm pregnancy of 28 to 35 weeks, treatment includes hospitalization and observation for signs of infection (increased maternal white blood cell count or fever and very fast fetal heart rate) while awaiting fetal maturation. Antibiotics will be given both prophy-

lactically and curatively by the I.V. route while she is hospitalized.

6 Explain the importance of routine medical follow-up.	Considerations for preterm and postpartum follow-up are as follows: —If the preterm patient is sent home on antibiotics and bed rest, she must keep all her medical appointments and take her temperature twice daily. If her temperature rises above 100.4° F. (38° C.), she should notify her physician immediately. —If the patient had an induced or cesarean delivery, her physician will want to see her in his office after discharge from the hospital for a postpartum check. He will also want to follow her progress to make sure no infection is present. At that time, the physician will also counsel her on birth control measures and future pregnancy plans.

PRETERM LABOR

Patient objectives	Teaching plan content
1 Define preterm labor.	Preterm labor is the onset of rhythmic uterine contractions after 28 weeks but before 37 weeks of pregnancy. Preterm labor could also be interpreted as premature contractions after fetal viability but before fetal maturity.
2 Discuss the cause of preterm labor.	There are many possible causes of preterm labor. —Fetal stimulation may trigger labor. Genetically imprinted information tells the fetus that nutrition is inadequate and that a change in environment is required for well-being; this provokes the onset of labor. —Decreased placental production of progesterone (thought to be the hormone that maintains pregnancy) triggers labor. —Labor may begin because the myometrium (the inner lining of the uterus) becomes too sensitive to oxytocin, the hormone that normally induces uterine contractions. —A maternal genetic defect may shorten gestation and precipitate premature labor. —Maternal cardiovascular disease may result in insufficient blood flow to the uterus and placenta, causing problems with fetal oxygenation and triggering labor. In addition, preterm labor may be caused by the following: —Premature rupture of membranes (see the "Premature Rupture of Membranes" teaching plan in this chapter)

—Preeclampsia (see the "Pregnancy-Induced Hypertension" teaching plan in this chapter)
—Chronic hypertension (maternal high blood pressure)
—Hydramnios (see the "Hydramnios and Oligohydramnios" teaching plan in this chapter)
—Multiple pregnancy
—Placenta previa (see the "Placenta Previa" teaching plan in this chapter)
—Abruptio placentae (see the "Abruptio Placentae" teaching plan in this chapter)
—Incompetent cervix (the cervix dilates before the end of pregnancy, releasing the products of conception)
—Abdominal surgery
—Trauma
—Structural malformations of the uterus
—Infections
—Fetal death.

---

3 Identify the signs and symptoms of preterm labor.

Like labor at term, preterm labor produces the following signs and symptoms:
—Rhythmic uterine contractions
—Cervical dilation and effacement
—Possible rupture of the membranes
—Expulsion of the cervical mucous plug
—Bloody discharge.

---

4 Explain how the diagnosis of preterm labor is made.

Preterm labor is confirmed by the patient's prenatal history, physical examination, presenting signs and symptoms, and possibly, pelvic ultrasonography showing the position of the fetus in relation to the pelvis. A vaginal examination will show progressive cervical effacement and dilation.

---

5 Describe the treatment of preterm labor.

Treatment is designed to suppress preterm labor when tests show immature fetal lung development, cervical dilation of 2″ (5 cm), and absence of any other problems that may affect the continuation of the pregnancy. This treatment consists of bed rest and, when necessary, drug therapy.

---

6 Describe the medication regimen.

Some drugs commonly used for this disorder are ritodrine and terbutaline. For specific medication instructions, see Chapter 10, Drug Therapy.

---

7 Explain the importance of routine medical follow-up.

Routine medical follow-up is important for the following reasons:
—Prevention of preterm labor requires good prenatal care, adequate nutrition, and proper rest. Insertion of a

purse-string suture to reinforce an incompetent cervix at 14 to 18 weeks' gestation may prevent preterm labor in women with a history of this problem.

—If the patient in preterm labor is to be managed at home, she must comply with all her physician's instructions, including all visits with him to check on her progress.

—If a preterm infant is delivered, the patient will need to visit the physician for postdelivery assessment.

—Because the delivery of a preterm infant can cause guilt and anxiety for a woman and her family, the patient needs psychological support at this time. She should talk with delivery nurses, postpartum nurses, physicians, or nursery personnel after her discharge to cope with depression or problems that normally occur after preterm delivery.

HYDRAMNIOS AND OLIGOHYDRAMNIOS

Patient objectives	Teaching plan content
1 Define hydramnios.	Hydramnios (also called polyhydramnios) is a disorder of pregnancy in which the patient accumulates more than 2,000 ml of amniotic fluid in her uterus.
2 Define oligohydramnios.	Oligohydramnios is a rare disorder of pregnancy in which the patient exhibits 300 ml or less of amniotic fluid.
3 Explain the two types of hydramnios.	There are two types of hydramnios: chronic and acute. —In the chronic type, the fluid volume increases gradually throughout the gestational period. —In the acute type, the fluid volume increases rapidly over a period of a few days.
4 Discuss the causes of hydramnios and oligohydramnios.	The exact causes are unknown; however, both disorders tend to develop in certain circumstances. —Hydramnios often occurs in the presence of major congenital anomalies (malformations) that affect fetal swallowing and in neurologic disorders that expose the meninges (coverings of the brain) of the fetus. Hydramnios can also occur along with maternal diabetes, Rh sensitization, and multiple pregnancy. —Oligohydramnios can be found in cases of postmaturity with intrauterine growth retardation (a condition in which the fetus is smaller than gestational dates signify because of placental insufficiency) and in cases of fetal renal and urinary malfunction.

5 Explain how the diagnosis of hydramnios or oligohydramnios is made.

The diagnosis is made as follows:
—Hydramnios may be suspected when the height of the patient's uterus increases disproportionately to fetal gestational age. Pelvic ultrasonography will reveal large spaces between the fetus and the uterine wall.
—If oligohydramnios is suspected, pelvic ultrasonography will show smaller than normal spaces between the fetus and the uterine wall.

6 Discuss the effects of hydramnios and oligohydramnios.

There are both maternal and fetal effects of hydramnios and oligohydramnios.
—In hydramnios, the maternal effects may include shortness of breath and edema of the lower extremities. There is also a possibility of pain associated with the increased stretching of the uterus.
—Fetal effects of hydramnios include premature delivery, malpresentations, malformations, and possibly prolapsed umbilical cord when the membranes (bag of waters) rupture.
—Maternal effects of oligohydramnios may include dysfunctional, preterm labor or protracted labor (labor arrests at some point and fails to progress any further).
—Fetal effects of oligohydramnios may include umbilical cord compression, resulting in fetal hypoxia. Skeletal malformations may also be found.

7 Describe the treatment for hydramnios.

If the patient has accumulated a large amount of fluid, causing pain and shortness of breath, her physician may hospitalize her to remove some of the excess. This procedure can be done vaginally or through amniocentesis (see the "Amniocentesis" teaching plan in this chapter). (At present, there is no treatment for oligohydramnios.)

Explaining treatments

POSTPARTUM FUNDAL CHECKS

Patient objectives

Teaching plan content

1 State the purpose of postpartum fundal checks.

Postpartum fundal checks allow the physician to follow the progress of involution (the gradual decrease in size and descent of the uterus into prepregnancy position).

2 Describe the procedure used in a postpartum fundal check.	A postpartum fundal check is performed as follows: —The patient will be placed on her back, with her head down. If this position is too uncomfortable, her head may be slightly elevated. —Her abdomen and perineum will be exposed, in privacy. —One of the examiner's hands will be placed on the lower portion of the uterus to provide stability. —The other hand will be placed on her abdomen, and the fundus of her uterus will be gently palpated. At this time, the height of the fundus will be measured in fingerbreadths from the umbilicus, and the firmness of the uterus will be evaluated. —If her uterus is soft or boggy, the examiner will gently massage her fundus. —During evaluation of firmness and massage of the uterus, her perineum will be observed for bleeding and clot expulsion.
3 Discuss patient guidelines for postpartum fundal checks.	Patient guidelines include the following: —Unless the patient's physician orders otherwise, fundal checks will be performed as follows: • Every 10 to 15 minutes for 60 to 90 minutes in the recovery room • Every 30 minutes for the next 2 hours • Every hour for the next 3 hours • Every 4 hours for the rest of the first postpartum day • Every 24 hours, once a day, until discharge. —The patient's urinary bladder will have to be empty for a proper fundal check; a full bladder causes distention, which impairs contraction by pushing the uterus up and to the side. —If she is unable to urinate, her physician may order catheterization (passing a tube through her urethra into her bladder, to empty it of urine). —A patient who has had a cesarean delivery may receive pain medication beforehand to minimize her discomfort. —If massage does not help stimulate contraction of the uterus, synthetic oxytocics may be administered. Breast-feeding releases natural oxytocics that help to maintain or stimulate contractions.

EPISIOTOMY

Patient objectives	*Teaching plan content*
1 Define episiotomy.	An episiotomy is a surgical incision made during the vaginal delivery of an infant. The incision extends downward from the vaginal orifice.

2 State the purpose of an episiotomy.	An episiotomy is done to minimize perineal stretching and tearing and to decrease trauma to the fetal head during the birth process.
3 Describe the procedure used in an episiotomy.	An episiotomy may be performed just before delivery. —When the presenting part of the fetus is visible in the vaginal opening, the physician may give the mother a local anesthetic or a light general anesthetic and will make either a mediolateral incision (off to the side) or a midline incision (straight down the perineum toward the rectum). —After delivery of the baby and the placenta, the incision will be sutured (sewn up) by the physician.
4 Discuss patient guidelines for an episiotomy.	Patient guidelines include the following: —For the first 8 hours, ice packs will be used to decrease pain and swelling. —After the first 8 hours, hot sitz baths are recommended to increase circulation of blood to the area, thereby helping the healing process. (See *Giving Yourself a Sitz Bath,* pp. 300-301.) —Analgesic sprays and oral analgesics will be available if the patient needs pain relief. —Due to the trauma to the perineum during birth, a hematoma (collection of blood in the tissues) may form near the episiotomy, causing pain and discomfort. A nurse will inspect the perineum frequently to watch the progress of healing. —Because of the location of the episiotomy, cleanliness after emptying the bladder or bowel is extremely important to prevent infection. (See the "Postpartum Perineal Care" teaching plan in this chapter.)

POSTPARTUM PERINEAL CARE

Patient objectives	*Teaching plan content*
1 State the purpose of postpartum perineal care.	Postpartum perineal care promotes comfort and healing and prevents infection.
2 Describe the procedure for postpartum perineal care.	After elimination, the patient assesses the lochia (blood and debris eliminated from the uterus after delivery), cleanses and dries her perineum, and applies a clean perineal pad. —Perineal cleansing may be performed with a hand-held peri-bottle or a water-jet irrigation system. —After elimination and while still on the commode,

the patient rinses the perineum for at least 2 minutes, from front to back.
—She pats the area dry with either toilet tissue or cotton wipes, from front to back.
—She applies a fresh perineal pad and stands before flushing the commode, to avoid being sprayed with contaminated water.

3 Discuss the types of lochia.	Evaluation of lochia is important in assessing uterine involution and the healing of the placental site. The patient will experience three types of lochia after giving birth. —Lochia rubra, named for its dark red color, occurs for the first 2 to 3 days. —Lochia serosa is pink and not as dense in consistency as lochia rubra. It lasts from the 3rd to the 10th day. —Lochia alba is a creamy or yellowish color and may persist for an additional week or two.

RhoGAM ADMINISTRATION

Patient objectives	*Teaching plan content*
1 Define RhoGAM.	RhoGAM is a concentrated solution of gamma globulin containing $Rh_o(D)$ antibodies.
2 Discuss the purpose of RhoGAM administration.	RhoGAM administration prevents the Rh-negative mother from producing antibodies in response to an Rh-positive infant.
3 Discuss the administration of RhoGAM.	RhoGAM is administered I.M. at two possible times during the period of pregnancy and delivery. —At 28 weeks' gestation, RhoGAM is administered prophylactically to all Rh-negative patients. This is done to prevent maternal sensitization to the fetus due to small areas of bleeding at the site of the placenta. —RhoGAM is also given 72 hours after an Rh-negative mother delivers an Rh-positive infant or has an abortion or ectopic pregnancy. This is to prevent future problems with pregnancies involving Rh-positive fetuses.

SITZ BATH

Patient objectives	*Teaching plan content*
1 Define sitz bath.	A sitz bath is the immersion of the pelvic area in tepid or hot water.

2 State the purpose of a sitz bath.

A sitz bath relieves discomfort, especially after episiotomy and childbirth. The bath promotes wound healing by cleansing the perineum and anus, increasing circulation, and reducing inflammation. It also helps relax perineal muscles.

3 Describe the procedure for a sitz bath.

The procedure for a sitz bath involves the following:
—First, the patient should urinate to empty her bladder.
—Water placed in the bathtub or sitz tub should register approximately 110° to 115° F. (43.3° to 46.1° C.) on a bath thermometer and should rise to the proper fill line.
—Either she will sit in the water for the prescribed time (15 to 20 minutes), or a constant stream of warm water will flow over the wound site for that amount of time.
—She will then blot her perineum dry, from front to back.
—She will apply antiseptic or anesthetic creams or sprays as needed and put on a new perineal pad. (See *Giving Yourself a Sitz Bath,* pp. 300-301.)
—The warmth and the position may make the patient light-headed or faint. This is normal. A nurse will check on her frequently and the call light should be handy for her to use.

DILATATION AND CURETTAGE (D&C)

Patient objectives	*Teaching plan content*
1 State the purpose of a D&C.	A D&C removes the endometrial lining of the uterus to empty the uterine cavity after an incomplete abortion.
2 Describe the procedure used in a D&C.	The surgical procedure for a D&C is as follows: —After the patient has received a general anesthetic, she will be placed in the lithotomy position, with her feet in stirrups. —Her cervix will be slowly dilated by increasingly larger cervical sounds (round-tipped rods used to dilate the cervix). —The endometrial lining of her uterus will then be scraped away with a curette (a teaspoonlike instrument).
3 Describe the preoperative procedures for a D&C.	In addition to routine preoperative procedures (see Appendix B, *Preoperative and Postoperative Teaching*), the patient can expect the following for a D&C:

—An anesthesiologist or anesthetist will visit the patient the day before surgery (or, in an emergency, right before surgery) to discuss what type of anesthetic she will be given. Either a general or spinal anesthetic will be used. In either case, the patient will not wake up or feel any pain during the procedure.

—The surgeon will visit, either the day before surgery or right before surgery, to explain the procedure. At that time, the operative permit will be signed. The patient should not sign the permit until all her questions about the risks of surgery have been answered by her physician.

—The patient will receive a sleeping pill the night before surgery to help her relax and sleep. She will also receive a sedative just before going to the operating room to help her relax (in an emergency, a sedative will be given right before surgery). This sedative will be given by I.M. injection.

—She is not to eat or drink after midnight or on the morning of surgery.

—The morning of surgery (or right before surgery, in an emergency), a nurse will start an I.V. line, so that medications and blood (if needed) can be administered during the operation.

---

4 Explain what to expect postoperatively.

Postoperatively, the patient can expect the following:
—She will wake up in the recovery room. A nurse will check her often, and she will be wearing a sanitary pad to catch any vaginal discharge or blood.

—When she is awake enough to respond to her name and her pulse, blood pressure, and breathing are stable, she will be taken back to her room. Pain medication will be available if she needs it.

—As soon as the patient is awake and able to keep clear liquids down, her I.V. line will be discontinued.

—That night she will be expected to walk in her room and urinate in the bathroom.

—She will be discharged in the morning, if all goes well.

—Pain medication will be provided for cramps.

—She will experience bleeding for a few days, similar to her menses.

—She will have to limit activities for a week or two, then may resume her normal activities.

---

5 Explain the importance of routine medical follow-up.

—In postoperative follow-up appointments, the physician will check the patient for infection or other complications and will discuss future pregnancies and birth control.

DILATATION AND VACUUM EXTRACTION (D&E) (Suction curettage)

Patient objectives	Teaching plan content
1 Define D&E.	A D&E is the dilation of the cervix and aspiration of the endometrium, including the products of conception, using a suction pump or vacuum container.
2 State the purpose of a D&E.	A D&E evacuates the uterine contents; it is used as an abortion technique up to the 12th week of gestation.
3 Describe the procedure used in a D&E.	A D&E may be done on an outpatient basis or with an overnight hospital stay. Preoperative preparation is the same as for a D&C. (See the "Dilatation and Curettage" teaching plan in this chapter.) —In some hospitals, the patient may be asked to come the day before surgery to have a Laminaria inserted into her cervix. This is a tent made of sterilized seaweed. In the cervix, it absorbs moisture and allows for gentle dilation of the cervix. If this is not done, then cervical dilation will be carried out during the procedure, as in a D&C. —In the operating room, a suction tip will be introduced into the partially dilated cervix and a suction pump or vacuum container will gently evacuate the contents of the uterus.
4 Explain what to expect postoperatively.	Postoperatively, the patient can expect the following: —She will be asked to remain in bed for a few hours. —At that time her vital signs will be taken and perineal care will be administered, along with an oxytocin medication (to contract her uterus and control bleeding). A prophylactic antibiotic may also be given. —She may be allowed to leave the hospital 4 to 6 hours after the procedure. —Mild cramping is normal, and acetaminophen may be taken. —She can expect to have bleeding similar to her menstrual flow for the first week and possible spotting for 2 weeks. —She should not douche, use tampons, or have sexual intercourse before returning for her follow-up visit.
5 Discuss guidelines for follow-up care.	The patient should watch for signs of infection, such as fever over 100.4° F. (38° C.) and malodorous secretions on her sanitary pads. She should call the physician immediately if bleeding seems excessive (more than two

pads saturated in 1 hour, with or without the passage of clots). In a 2- to 3-week follow-up visit, her physician will check on her healing and discuss contraception and future pregnancies.

SALINE OR PROSTAGLANDIN INDUCTION

Patient objectives	Teaching plan content
1 Define saline or prostaglandin induction.	An injection of saline solution (salt water) or prostaglandins (hormonelike substances) is administered during the second trimester of pregnancy to induce labor. Prostaglandins may also be given by vaginal suppository.
2 State the purpose of saline or prostaglandin induction.	Saline or prostaglandin induction ends a pregnancy that is 16 to 24 weeks long.
3 Describe the general procedure for saline or prostaglandin induction.	The patient can expect the following general procedure: —For saline induction, she will be admitted to the labor floor and asked to urinate and change into a hospital gown. A small amount of saline solution will be injected into her uterus after the removal of some amniotic fluid by means of amniocentesis. (See the "Amniocentesis" teaching plan in this chapter.) Within 12 to 36 hours, labor will probably begin. Labor is sometimes augmented with oxytocins. Delivery of the products of conception is usually carried out in the labor room. —For prostaglandin induction, she will be admitted to the labor floor and asked to urinate and change into a hospital gown. Prostaglandins will be administered, either by means of amniocentesis or by vaginal suppository. Uterine contractions usually begin ½ to 1 hour after prostaglandin administration, and delivery of the products of conception is usually carried out in the labor room. Generally, no oxytocin is necessary.
4 Discuss patient guidelines for postoperative care.	Douching and sexual intercourse should be discontinued until after the patient's postabortion checkup with her physician. She should expect spotting for at least 2 weeks after the abortion and a menstrual flow for 2 to 8 weeks following the procedure. She should also watch for a fever of over 100° F. (37.8° C.), which might signal infection. If this happens, she should notify her physician immediately.

HYSTERECTOMY

Patient objectives	Teaching plan content
1 Define hysterectomy.	A hysterectomy is the surgical removal of a diseased, ruptured, or cancerous uterus (or uterus, fallopian tubes, ovaries, cervix, and/or vagina).
2 Describe the surgical procedure used in a hysterectomy.	The surgical procedure for a hysterectomy is as follows: —After the patient has been put to sleep, a vaginal or an abdominal incision will be made. If a vaginal procedure is used, the incision is made above and around the cervix. There are two types of abdominal incisions: • The Pfannenstiel (bikini) incision extends transversely across the lower abdomen. Because it leaves a less noticeable scar, this incision is often chosen for cosmetic reasons. However, it may cause more postoperative discomfort than the vertical incision. • The vertical incision extends along the patient's midline from upper to lower abdomen. This incision takes longer to heal and may be weaker after healing. —Depending on the patient's condition, one of the following types of hysterectomy will be performed: • Subtotal, or partial, which is removal of only the uterus • Total, which is removal of the uterus and cervix • Panhysterectomy, or total abdominal hysterectomy with bilateral salpingo-oophorectomy, which is removal of the uterus, ovaries, and fallopian tubes (must be done abdominally) • Wertheim's operation, which is removal of the uterus, cervix, fallopian tubes, and ovaries, as well as a partial vaginectomy and pelvic lymph node dissection (must be done abdominally).
3 Describe the preoperative procedures for a hysterectomy.	In addition to routine preoperative procedures (see Appendix B, *Preoperative and Postoperative Teaching*), the patient can expect the following: —An anesthesiologist or anesthetist will visit her the day before surgery to discuss what type of anesthetic she will be given. Hysterectomies are usually done under a general anesthetic; however, if the patient has a breathing problem, a spinal anesthetic may be used. She will not awaken during surgery, and if a spinal anesthetic is used, she will not feel any pain. —The surgeon will also visit the day before surgery to explain the hysterectomy procedure to be used and the risks involved. The patient should ask questions if she

does not understand something and should write down her questions so she does not forget them. She will be asked to sign the operative permit at that time, giving her consent for the procedure. She should not sign the permit until all her questions have been answered and she understands everything that will happen.

—She will be shaved from her nipple line down to and including her perineum and rectum. This is to prevent any infection in the incision from bacteria in the hair.

—She may have to use a medicated douche to rid her vagina of any discharge or secretions that might harbor bacteria.

—She may also need to have an enema to clear her lower bowel. This is to decompress the bowel and flatten it out, thus lessening the risk of trauma during the operation.

—She will receive a sleeping pill the night before surgery to help her relax and sleep. She will receive one or two I.M. injections to sedate her before going to the operating room.

—After midnight, she should have no food or fluids by mouth. This is to prevent her from vomiting during surgery.

—The morning of the operation, a nurse will start an I.V. line. This is done routinely to administer medications or blood during the operation. The I.V. line will also provide nourishment to her until she can take solid foods again.

—The morning of surgery an indwelling (Foley) catheter will be placed in her urinary bladder. This is to keep the bladder empty, so she does not have to worry about getting up to go to the bathroom postoperatively and so the bladder will not be traumatized with any instruments during surgery.

---

4 Explain what to expect postoperatively.

Postoperatively, the patient can expect the following:

—She will wake up in the recovery room, where a nurse will check her frequently until she is awake enough to go back to her room.

—She will have a large bandage on her abdomen (if she had an abdominal incision) and will be wearing a sanitary pad for any bleeding or drainage from her vagina.

—She will have sutures or staples on her incision.

—Medication for pain will be available.

—When she is almost fully awake and her pulse, breathing, and blood pressure are stable, she will be taken back to her room.

—She will probably sleep most of the first day and she

may experience nausea from the anesthetic.

—Once her urinary catheter and I.V. line have been removed and she can keep her food down and walk in the hall, the physician will write her discharge. This is usually 4 to 6 days postoperatively.

—The sutures or staples may be removed before she is discharged.

—Any medications she will be taking at home will be reviewed, including name, dosage, adverse effects, and precautions.

5 **Discuss patient guidelines for postoperative care.**	The patient should follow any dietary restrictions or instructions that the physician has given her.

—Her physician may provide other specific instructions. Light activity will be allowed at first, with increasing exercises and amounts of activity as time progresses. (See *After a Hysterectomy: How to Care for Yourself*, pp. 302-304.)

—The incision must be kept clean and dry. She can expect itching and discomfort as it heals, but she should call the physician if her incision becomes red or very tender, starts draining, or opens.

—She should also call the physician if she develops a fever, nausea, malaise, or other signs of systemic infection.

—If her ovaries were removed, she should know the signs and symptoms of menopause. Once the discharge from the operation has stopped, she will no longer have her menses.

—A hysterectomy will probably affect her emotionally as well as physically. She should know that the surgery will not affect her sexuality, only her ability to have children.

—The physician will want to check her healing and check for any signs of complications in a follow-up visit.

Patient-Teaching Aid

MANAGING PREGNANCY-INDUCED HYPERTENSION AT HOME

Dear Patient:

You have pregnancy-induced hypertension (PIH), also called preeclampsia. Since your condition is mild, you can manage it at home if you follow the instructions below. Keep in mind, however, that mild PIH can quickly become severe. So follow this home care plan carefully. Keep regular appointments with your physician and call him if you have any concerns or questions.

Immediately notify your physician if you experience severe headaches, dizziness, spots before your eyes, blurred vision, stomach pain, nausea, or vomiting; if you begin urinating only small amounts; or if the baby becomes less active than usual.

Check with your physician before traveling any distance from home.

Physician's phone # _____

Nurse's phone # _____

Activities

Limit your household activities, such as laundry, housecleaning, and grocery shopping. Sit whenever possible, for example, while you are folding laundry or ironing. Rest in bed at least 1 hour daily. Be sure to lie on your left side while resting.

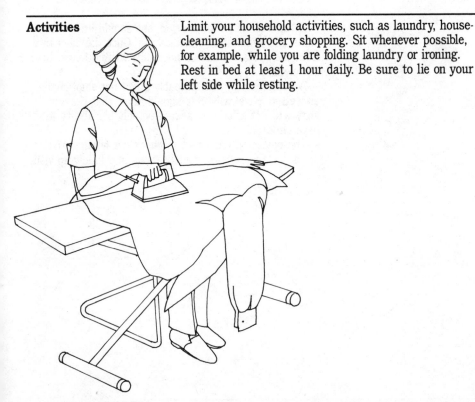

MANAGING PREGNANCY-INDUCED HYPERTENSION AT HOME—*continued*

Diet

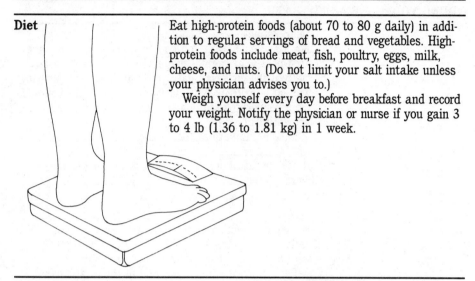

Eat high-protein foods (about 70 to 80 g daily) in addition to regular servings of bread and vegetables. High-protein foods include meat, fish, poultry, eggs, milk, cheese, and nuts. (Do not limit your salt intake unless your physician advises you to.)

Weigh yourself every day before breakfast and record your weight. Notify the physician or nurse if you gain 3 to 4 lb (1.36 to 1.81 kg) in 1 week.

Urine testing

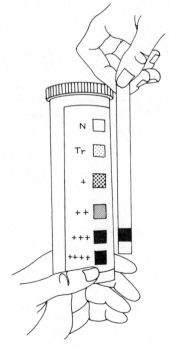

Test your urine for protein twice a day (a.m. and p.m.), using the test strips that were given you. Be sure to perform the test in a well-lighted room so you can clearly see the color changes on the strip.

Before starting the test, wash your hands thoroughly with soap and water. Then wash your genital area with soap and water, rinse it, and dry it completely with a towel.

Collect a midstream urine specimen in a clean container, and dip the test strip into the specimen. Compare the color changes on the strip with the table of values on your test strip bottle. Notify your physician or nurse immediately if your test results are 3+ or 4+.

IMPORTANT: Avoid drinking a lot of water before the test. Water dilutes your urine and may produce false-low results.

Patient-Teaching Aid

GIVING YOURSELF A SITZ BATH

Dear Patient:

For a few days after you go home, your perineum (the area near your vagina) may feel uncomfortable, especially if the physician gave you stitches after your baby was born or if you have hemorrhoids. To make yourself more comfortable, take warm-water sitz baths, as shown in this aid.

Take a sitz bath at these times: _____

If the physician orders, add this medication to the warm water: _____

1

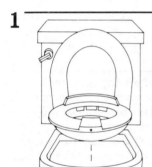

For your convenience, we have provided you with a sitz bath kit. It contains a plastic pan and a plastic bag with attached tubing. Here is how to use it:

First, raise the toilet seat and fit the plastic pan onto the toilet bowl. Position the pan so its drainage holes are along the back of the bowl, as shown here. If you have placed the pan correctly, you will see a single slot in front.

2

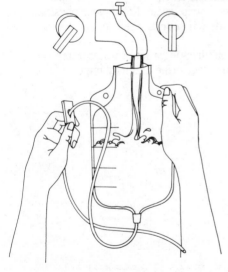

Next, close the clamp on the bag's tubing. Fill the bag with warm water and medication (if ordered).

GIVING YOURSELF A SITZ BATH—*continued*

3

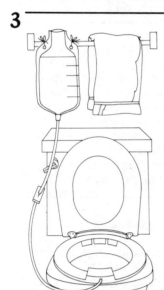

Snap the free end of the tubing into the slot at the front of the pan. Then, hang the bag on the doorknob or towel bar. Make sure the bag is higher than the toilet.

4

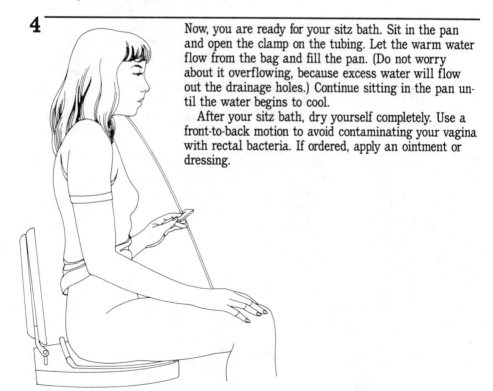

Now, you are ready for your sitz bath. Sit in the pan and open the clamp on the tubing. Let the warm water flow from the bag and fill the pan. (Do not worry about it overflowing, because excess water will flow out the drainage holes.) Continue sitting in the pan until the water begins to cool.

After your sitz bath, dry yourself completely. Use a front-to-back motion to avoid contaminating your vagina with rectal bacteria. If ordered, apply an ointment or dressing.

Patient-Teaching Aid

AFTER A HYSTERECTOMY: HOW TO CARE FOR YOURSELF

Dear Patient:

Because you have just had a hysterectomy, you will want to take special precautions to speed your recovery. Take care not to overexert yourself until your incision heals completely. The nurse has filled in the physician's specific instructions on the following list. Read it carefully. If you have any questions, talk to your nurse. Then, when you go home, make a special effort to follow these guidelines:

• Restrict your activities. For example, avoid heavy lifting and cleaning, as well as vigorous sports, for 6 to 8 weeks. Also wait at least _____ weeks before driving a car.

• Avoid sexual activity and douching for _____ weeks after surgery.

• Take a shower _____ days after surgery. Before taking a tub bath, get your physician's OK.

• Call your physician if you have heavy bleeding, abnormal cramps, hot flashes, or changes in your bowel habits.

Now here are some exercises to help strengthen your abdomen. You can begin this exercise program _____ days after surgery. Add a new exercise each day. Repeat each exercise four times, twice a day, in the morning and in the evening. Continue this program for _____ weeks, or as ordered by your physician.

IMPORTANT: If any of these exercises is painful, stop it immediately. If the pain persists, notify the physician.

1

Sit at the edge of your bed or chair. Take a slow, deep breath. Breathe in through your nose, and concentrate on fully expanding your chest. Breathe out through your mouth and concentrate on drawing in your abdominal muscles.

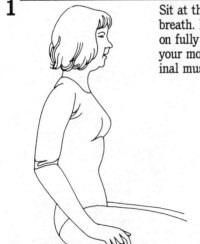
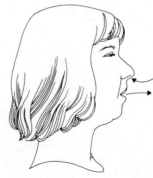

AFTER A HYSTERECTOMY: HOW TO CARE FOR YOURSELF—*continued*

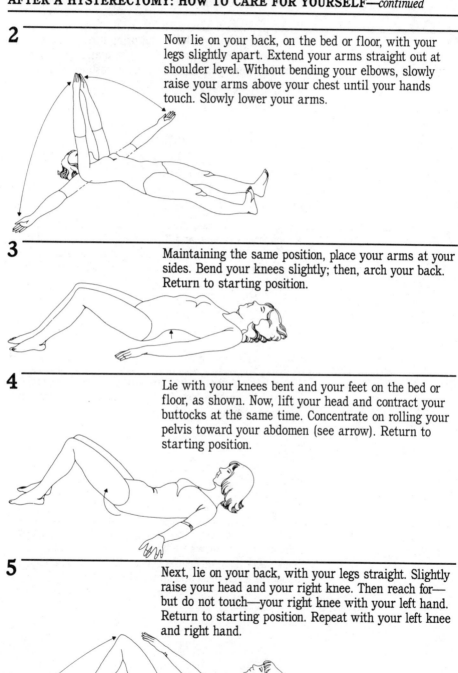

2

Now lie on your back, on the bed or floor, with your legs slightly apart. Extend your arms straight out at shoulder level. Without bending your elbows, slowly raise your arms above your chest until your hands touch. Slowly lower your arms.

3

Maintaining the same position, place your arms at your sides. Bend your knees slightly; then, arch your back. Return to starting position.

4

Lie with your knees bent and your feet on the bed or floor, as shown. Now, lift your head and contract your buttocks at the same time. Concentrate on rolling your pelvis toward your abdomen (see arrow). Return to starting position.

5

Next, lie on your back, with your legs straight. Slightly raise your head and your right knee. Then reach for—but do not touch—your right knee with your left hand. Return to starting position. Repeat with your left knee and right hand.

AFTER A HYSTERECTOMY: HOW TO CARE FOR YOURSELF—*continued*

6

Now, bend your right knee and bring it toward your chest, as close as possible. Straighten and lower your right leg, until your right foot again rests on the bed or floor. Repeat with your left leg.

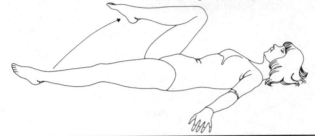

7

Keeping your knees and hips straight and toes pointed upward, raise your right leg as high as possible. Return to starting position, and repeat with your left leg.

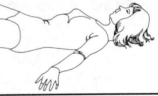

8

Keeping your knees and hips straight and toes pointed upward, raise *both* legs as high as possible. Return to starting position.

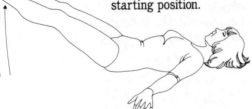

9

For this exercise, kneel on the bed or floor and support your weight on your elbows and knees, as shown. Hump your back upward as you contract your buttocks and pull in your abdomen. Then relax and breathe deeply.

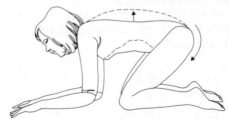

AIDS and Its Complications

 Patient-learner data base*

Areas of potential knowledge deficit
Groups at risk for contracting acquired
    immunodeficiency syndrome (AIDS)
—Sexually active homosexual and bisexual men
—Present or past abusers of intravenous drugs
—Persons with hemophilia
—Heterosexual sex partners of someone with AIDS or
    at risk for AIDS
—Persons having had transfusions of blood or blood
    products
—Infants who may have contracted AIDS before,
    during, or after birth.
Specific level of knowledge about AIDS
—Definition of AIDS
—Cause of AIDS
—Signs and symptoms associated with AIDS
—Treatment of AIDS
—Prevention of AIDS
—Home care
History or presence of AIDS-related diseases
—*Candida albicans* infection
—Cytomegalovirus infection
—*Cryptosporidium* enterocolitis
—Herpes simplex
—Herpes zoster
—Histoplasmosis
—Kaposi's sarcoma
—*Mycobacterium avium intracellulare* infection
—*Pneumocystis carinii* pneumonia
—Progressive multifocal leukoencephalopathy
—Toxoplasmosis

*A general assessment should be done for all patients. For general assessment guidelines, see Chapter 1, Principles of Patient Teaching.

Explaining diagnostic tests

H.I.V. ANTIBODY TEST

Patient objectives	*Teaching plan content*
1 Describe the human immunodeficiency virus (HIV) antibody test.	The HIV antibody test detects the presence of antibodies to the virus responsible for AIDS. If infected with HIV, the body naturally produces antibodies to that virus. The physician or laboratory technician will obtain a blood sample from the patient to use in the test.
2 Discuss the implications of the presence of antibodies to HIV.	The presence of antibodies to HIV in the blood (a positive result) indicates previous exposure to the virus. Most people with antibodies to HIV are infected with active virus and, therefore, may be contagious and capable of transmitting the virus. A positive result does not mean that the patient has or will get AIDS-related complex (ARC) or AIDS.
3 Discuss the implications of the absence of antibodies to HIV.	The absence of antibodies to HIV in the blood is a negative result. This does not mean the patient does not have or will not develop ARC or AIDS. It indicates any of the following: —The patient has not been infected with the virus. —The patient has had contact with the virus but has not become infected and has not produced antibodies. —The patient has been infected with the virus but has not yet produced antibodies.

BRONCHOSCOPY

Patient objectives	*Teaching plan content*
1 Define bronchoscopy.	Bronchoscopy is the visual examination of the larynx, trachea, and bronchi using a bronchoscope, which is a flexible tube with a light at its tip. (An illustration can be used to demonstrate anatomic structures.) (See *Patient's Guide to Bronchoscopy,* pp. 328-329.)
2 State the purpose of bronchoscopy as it relates to AIDS.	Bronchoscopy may be done to visually examine the tracheobronchial tree for abnormalities and to assist in laboratory diagnosis of infections through sputum samples and biopsies obtained during the procedure. Find-

ings may include *Pneumocystis carinii* pneumonia, cytomegalovirus or *Mycobacterium avium intracellulare* infection, and histoplasmosis.

3 **Discuss patient guidelines for bronchoscopy.**	Before bronchoscopy, the patient can expect the following: —He should not eat or drink for 8 to 12 hours before the procedure. —He should remove jewelry and constricting garments before the procedure. Dentures and eyeglasses will need to be removed immediately before the procedure. —After the purpose, preparation, expectations, and potential complications of the procedure have been explained by a physician, the patient will sign a consent form. —Arterial blood gas analysis may be done before the procedure. —The patient should perform good oral hygiene the evening before and the morning of the procedure so fewer bacteria will be present in his mouth. —Chest X-rays should be done within 24 hours of the procedure, if ordered. —The patient will receive atropine (to decrease secretions) and morphine sulfate and diazepam (to decrease apprehension) before the procedure.
4 **Describe the procedure used in bronchoscopy.**	During bronchoscopy, the patient can expect the following: —His mouth, throat, and tongue will be topically anesthetized to decrease gagging and discomfort during insertion of the bronchoscope. (A general anesthetic may be used.) He should relax and breathe around the tube or through his nose. —Communication will need to be by hand signals since the patient will not be able to talk while the bronchoscope is in place. —The procedure will be done with the patient on his back with his neck hyperextended. A pillow may be placed under the neck to achieve hyperextension. —The physician may wear gloves, a mask, and a gown. These are standard precautions when handling potentially infected material or when splattering might occur.
5 **Describe the procedure for bronchoalveolar lavage.**	Through the channel of the bronchoscope, small amounts of normal saline solution are instilled and immediately aspirated. The fluid is analyzed for cells, foreign substances, and indicators of inflammation or immune changes.

6 **Describe postbronchoscopy care.**	Postbronchoscopy procedures include the following: —The nurse will monitor the patient's vital signs frequently. —Until the gag reflex returns, the conscious patient will be in a semi-Fowler position to prevent aspiration. The unconscious patient will be on his side with his head elevated to prevent aspiration. —No food or drink will be allowed until the gag reflex returns. The gag reflex will be tested by touching or tickling the back of the throat with a cotton-tipped applicator or tongue blade. —Copious amounts of sputum may result from trauma caused by the passing of the bronchoscope into the lungs. Adequate hydration will help make respiratory secretions easier to expectorate. —Difficult breathing or excessive bleeding should be reported immediately to the physician. —Blood-tinged sputum may be expected for 24 to 48 hours. —An ice collar may relieve a sore throat. After the return of the gag reflex, saline solution gargles or throat lozenges may relieve the sore throat. —The patient should avoid smoking, coughing, and talking immediately after the procedure to decrease throat irritation. Any hoarseness or change in voice is common and only temporary. —The patient should not drive for 12 hours because of potential drowsiness from the sedative.

UPPER GASTROINTESTINAL ENDOSCOPY

Patient objectives	*Teaching plan content*
1 **Define upper gastrointestinal endoscopy.**	Upper gastrointestinal (GI) endoscopy is the visual examination of the pharynx, esophagus, stomach, and small intestine using an endoscope, which is a flexible tube with a light at its tip. (An illustration can be used to demonstrate anatomic structures.)
2 **State the purpose of upper GI endoscopy as it relates to AIDS.**	This procedure identifies abnormalities of the upper GI tract. Findings may include cytomegalovirus, Kaposi's sarcoma, esophagitis, or esophageal candidiasis.
3 **Discuss patient guidelines for upper GI endoscopy.**	Before endoscopy, the patient can expect the following: —He should not eat or drink for at least 6 hours before the procedure. The absence of food or liquid permits better visualization and prevents aspiration. —He should remove jewelry and constricting garments

before the procedure. Dentures and eyeglasses need to be removed immediately before the procedure.
—After the purpose, preparation, expectations, and potential complications of the procedure have been explained by a physician, the patient will sign a consent form.
—An I.V. line or a heparin lock may be started for medication administration.

---

4 Describe the procedure used in upper GI endoscopy.

During endoscopy, the patient can expect the following:
—Topical anesthesia of the posterior pharynx (with gargle or spray) will be necessary. The anesthetic may cause the mouth and throat to feel swollen.
—Swallowing may be difficult as the anesthetic begins to take effect; saliva may drain from the mouth into an emesis basin. If necessary, a suction machine will be used to remove saliva.
—The jaw will be supported by a mouthpiece during the procedure; however, this will not obstruct breathing.
—The patient will be positioned on his left side. He will remain conscious throughout the procedure, although he may be drowsy.
—The lights in the room will be dimmed to allow better visualization of the GI tract.
—The physician may wear gloves, a gown, and a mask. These are standard precautions when handling potentially infected materials or when splattering may occur.
—Once the gag reflex has disappeared, the physician will insert the endoscope into the mouth and toward the back of the throat. The patient will then be asked to swallow repeatedly, and the tube will gently slide into the stomach.
—It is not uncommon to feel pressure in the stomach due to the presence of the tube. A feeling of fullness may result from air used to inflate the stomach. Inflating the stomach allows greater visualization of the stomach folds.

---

5 Describe postendoscopy care.

Postendoscopy procedures include the following:
—The nurse will frequently monitor the patient's vital signs immediately after the test.
—Until the gag reflex returns, the patient will be kept in a semi-Fowler position to prevent aspiration.
—No food or drink will be allowed until the gag reflex returns, within 2 to 4 hours. Fluids and a light meal will then be permissible. The gag reflex will be tested by touching or tickling the back of the throat with a cotton-tipped applicator or tongue blade.

—Burping and a sore throat that lasts for several days
may occur. Warm saline solution gargles and throat
lozenges may ease the discomfort.
—The physician should be notified immediately if the
patient experiences persistent swallowing difficulty,
pain, fever, black stools, or vomiting of blood.

COMPUTED TOMOGRAPHY (C.T.) SCAN OF THE BRAIN

Patient objectives	Teaching plan content
1 **Define computed tomography (CT).**	CT is an X-ray technique that visualizes specific layers of tissue, usually in cross section, so that abnormalities can be precisely located. It detects small differences in tissue density that conventional X-rays do not. An iodine contrast material may be given intravenously to enhance tissue density. When a CT scan of the brain is performed, a head scanner is used to provide images of only the brain, not the whole body. (See *Patient's Guide to Computed Tomography [CT, or CAT] Scan*, pp. 330-331.)
2 **State the purpose of a CT scan of the brain as it relates to AIDS.**	A CT scan of the brain is performed to determine the cause of a change in neurologic status or to detect lesions that may suggest an infectious process or a lymphoma. A CT scan also may help diagnose toxoplasmosis and progressive multifocal leukoencephalopathy, two conditions found in persons with AIDS.
3 **Discuss patient guidelines for a CT scan of the brain.**	Before a CT scan of the brain, the patient can expect the following: —He should remove jewelry or other pieces of metal from the head or neck region. —He will be asked about any previous allergic reactions to contrast material or dye. These may be indications for not receiving contrast material intravenously. —An I.V. line or a heparin lock may be started for administration of a sedative or contrast material. —The CT scan itself does not cause discomfort, but the patient may find it difficult to lie still for 30 minutes. Sedation may be given for anxiety or restlessness.
4 **Describe what will happen during a CT scan of the brain.**	During a CT scan of the brain, the patient can expect the following: —He must lie quietly on his back for 30 minutes with his head resting in a stationary box. Although his head is enclosed, his face is not covered.

—The scanner will produce a fanlike beam of radiation through the brain. A movable frame will rotate around the head, making clacking sounds, and a computer will calculate the amount of radiation absorbed and construct a picture.

—When this series of X-rays is complete, contrast material is injected, if ordered, and another series of scans is taken.

—A two-way intercom allows communication between the patient and the X-ray personnel.

5 Describe post–CT scan care.	Post–CT scan procedures include the following: —If contrast material has been administered, the patient should increase fluid intake for 24 hours. —If a sedative has been administered, he must not drive until the effects of the medication have worn off. —No other special care measures are needed.

SPUTUM CULTURE

Patient objectives	*Teaching plan content*
1 State the purpose of a sputum culture as it relates to AIDS.	The purpose of a sputum culture is to detect the cause of respiratory infection in the AIDS patient. The test is a laboratory procedure to identify infectious organisms present in sputum (the mucus-containing material from the lungs). Infections diagnosed in persons with AIDS may include *Mycobacterium tuberculosis* and *Pneumocystis carinii* pneumonia.
2 Describe the steps in sputum specimen collection.	Sputum specimen collection involves the following: —The patient will be given a sterile container. He must not touch the inside of the container. —The specimen is best collected on first arising because the sputum is more concentrated. In addition, sputum is more plentiful because secretions may have pooled during sleep. —The patient should rinse his mouth with plain water before sputum collection so the specimen is not contaminated with saliva and mouth bacteria. He should not use toothpaste or antiseptic solution before collecting the specimen since this will decrease the viability of organisms. —To obtain sputum rather than saliva, the patient should take several deep breaths, cough from deep down in his chest, and expectorate the mucus directly into the container. (The lid is then secured tightly.) A specimen that is only from the upper respiratory passages will not be adequate for laboratory examination.

—When tuberculosis is suspected, collections are needed at three different times (three mornings in a row).
—The specimen will be submitted to the laboratory as soon as possible after collection.
—Sputum specimens should be obtained before antibiotic therapy is started to ensure more accurate results.

STOOL CULTURE

Patient objectives	Teaching plan content
1 State the purpose of a stool culture as it relates to AIDS.	The purpose of a stool culture is to detect the cause of gastrointestinal infection in the AIDS patient. The test is a laboratory procedure to identify bacteria, viruses, and protozoa. Normally, many varieties of bacteria as well as some harmless parasites can be found in the stool. Due to an immunodeficiency, however, AIDS patients frequently develop infections from such organisms, which are not problematic in a person with an intact immune system. The organisms include, but are not limited to, *Cryptosporidium*, *Campylobacter*, *Salmonella*, *Shigella*, *Giardia*, and *Strongyloides*.
2 Describe the steps in stool specimen collection.	The steps in collecting a stool specimen are as follows: —The patient will be given a disposable stool container. If someone is assisting the patient, he or she should wear gloves. —The patient may defecate into a clean bedpan or directly into a stool cup. He should not combine stool with urine, as the latter may kill some organisms. Diarrheic stool can also be cultured; only a small amount (2 tbs) is needed. —The specimen should include any fecal material that contains blood or mucus or is otherwise unusual in appearance. —If the patient defecates into a bedpan, a tongue blade can be used to transfer the stool to the stool container. —The lid must be secure on the container. —The container is placed in a zip-locked plastic bag. —Hands should be washed thoroughly on completing the procedure. —Fresh stool specimens are obtained on three different days. —Stools should be collected before the start of antibiotic therapy to ensure more accurate results.

Explaining AIDS and related disorders

ACQUIRED IMMUNODEFICIENCY SYNDROME (A.I.D.S.)

Patient objectives	Teaching plan content
1 Define acquired immunodeficiency syndrome (AIDS).	AIDS is characterized by a defect in the immune system. The syndrome is characterized by opportunistic infections and/or neoplasms occurring in a person with no known cause for diminished resistance to those diseases.
2 Define opportunistic infection.	The body normally harbors many bacteria, protozoa, viruses, and fungi. When the immune system no longer is completely intact, these normally occurring organisms take the opportunity to cause damage and thus are known as opportunistic infections. Opportunistic infections that occur in many persons with AIDS include, but are not limited to, *Pneumocystis carinii* pneumonia (PCP), mucocutaneous herpes simplex, and candidal esophagitis.
3 Describe the signs and symptoms of AIDS.	There is wide variation in the clinical course before an initial diagnosis of AIDS. —Some patients have a history (weeks or months) of nonspecific weakness, malaise, fever, diarrhea, or weight loss. —Other patients have no constitutional symptoms until lesions develop from Kaposi's sarcoma or until shortness of breath results from PCP. —Shortness of breath and other changes in respiratory status may be due to PCP or, less commonly, cytomegalovirus (CMV) or *Mycobacterium avium intracellulare.* —Uncontrollable copious, watery diarrhea may be due to such organisms as *Cryptosporidium* or *Giardia.* —Neurologic changes may range from acute meningitis (*Cryptococcus*) to progressive dementia (progressive multifocal leukoencephalopathy). —Vision loss may result from CMV. —Extensive genital or perirectal ulcerations or mouth inflammation may be caused by reactivated herpes simplex.

—Purple lesions on the skin or mucous membranes or in the gastrointestinal tract may be caused by Kaposi's sarcoma.

4 Describe AIDS-related complex (ARC).

The term *AIDS-related complex (ARC)* was developed to describe persons who manifest signs and symptoms suggestive of AIDS and who are HIV antibody–positive but have no opportunistic infections or neoplasms. Persons with ARC may exhibit mild to severe symptoms of fatigue, fever, weight loss, night sweats, persistent diarrhea, and lymphadenopathy.

5 Discuss how the diagnosis of AIDS is made.

The diagnosis of AIDS depends on clinical signs and symptoms and the presence of opportunistic infections and/or neoplasms rather than on laboratory criteria. The HIV antibody test may aid the diagnosis in the absence of clearly identified opportunistic infections.

6 Explain the cause and transmission of AIDS.

The cause of AIDS is a virus called the human immunodeficiency virus (HIV). HIV is spread by contact with sexual secretions (semen, vaginal secretions), direct inoculation of infectious material such as blood or blood products, or perinatal transmission from mother to fetus. There is no scientific evidence to support the transmission of the virus through casual contact with persons who have AIDS.

7 Identify the six groups at increased risk for contracting AIDS.

Currently, there are six groups at risk for contracting AIDS:
—sexually active homosexual and bisexual men
—present or past abusers of intravenous drugs
—persons with hemophilia
—persons having had transfusions of blood or blood products
—heterosexual sex partners of someone with AIDS or at risk for AIDS
—infants who may have contracted AIDS before or during birth or as a result of postpartum breast-feeding.

8 Explain ongoing research in the area of AIDS treatment.

Currently, no cure exists for AIDS. However, researchers continue to explore methods to arrest the growth of HIV or to restore lost immune function.
—Although bone marrow transplantation has failed to improve immune function, I.V. infusion of interleukin-2 and interferon has shown limited effectiveness.
—The experimental antiviral drug azidothymidine (AZT) has shown promise in impeding progress of HIV and is being made more widely available to AIDS patients.

AIDS and Its Complications   315

—Other drug treatment for AIDS varies, depending on the AIDS-related disorder present. Although many of the causative infectious organisms are responsive to drugs, infection tends to recur when treatment is discontinued. For specific medication instructions, see Chapter 10, Drug Therapy.
—The development of a vaccine to help combat AIDS is now under investigation by researchers. It will be many years before such a vaccine is available for general use.

9 Discuss measures to prevent the spread of AIDS.

Measures to prevent the spread of AIDS include the following:
—Practice protective sex or safer sex, or avoid vaginal or anal intercourse with infected individuals.
  • Wear a rubber condom during vaginal or anal intercourse.
  • Sexual practices in which no semen, vaginal fluid, or blood is exchanged is considered safer.
  • Know your sexual partner and his or her habits.
  • Do not have sex with prostitutes.
—Blood transmission can be avoided if needles and syringes are not shared.
  • Use of recreational drugs should be avoided. These can do serious harm to the patient with AIDS. Opiates, alcohol, and marijuana, which can act as immunosuppressants, may increase the patient's vulnerability to infection. Moreover, research suggests that, although inhaled nitrates do not play a role in the development of AIDS itself, they may increase the risk of Kaposi's sarcoma in homosexual men afflicted with AIDS.
—Mothers who are HIV-positive should avoid pregnancy.
  • Mother-to-infant transmission can occur during pregnancy, or after pregnancy when breast-feeding.
—Individuals who test positive for HIV should not donate blood, body organs or tissues, or sperm.
—Individuals who test positive for HIV should follow infection-control guidelines. (See *AIDS and Community Living*, pp. 334-335.)

10 Explain infection-control measures for home care of the AIDS patient.

Infection-control precautions include the following:
—The patient/caregiver should wash his hands after contact with body fluids, such as blood, urine, stool, and drainage from wounds.
—Clean, disposable (not sterile) gloves should be available in the home to assist with care when body fluids will be contacted.

—Gowns may be worn if drainage is expected to soil clothes. Wearing of gowns is to protect clothing, not to prevent the spread of infectious organisms.

—Masks are not necessary unless *Mycobacterium tuberculosis* is suspected and has not been treated with antibiotics. The patient should wear a mask until therapy has been completed to protect others from infectious pulmonary secretions.

—Soiled linens or clothing can be cleaned in the washing machine with hot water, detergent, and 1 cup of bleach. (Detergent and bleach should be added to water before clothes or linens to prevent fading from the bleach.)

—Soiled tabletops, toilets, showers, or floors can be cleaned by washing spills with hot, soapy water, then disinfecting with a solution of one part bleach to nine parts water.

—Separate eating or cooking utensils are unnecessary for the person with AIDS. Eating utensils should be washed in hot, soapy water after each use.

—Toothbrushes and razors should not be shared since bleeding may occur during their use.

—If needles are used in the care of the person with AIDS, an impermeable disposal unit should be kept in the home.

—Disposal of all disposable items should be handled as follows:

• Gloves, soiled underpads or dressings, or other items that may contain body fluids of the person with AIDS should be placed in a heavy-duty plastic bag and secured firmly at the top to prevent spillage.

• Needles should be placed in impermeable plastic containers.

• These containers and heavy-duty plastic bags can then be disposed of in accordance with local regulations for disposal of solid wastes. (In most communities, these items can be disposed of through normal city trash pickup.)

(See *Preventing the Spread of AIDS*, p. 336.)

11 Explain how to adapt the home environment for the AIDS patient.

The following methods can be used to improve comfort and safety:

—Furniture should be arranged so that the patient can walk safely. The patient may move more freely if he can rest on chairs or against walls.

—Area rugs can be hazardous and may cause falls. They should be removed as the patient becomes weaker and more prone to falls.

—A walker or a wheelchair may allow the patient increased independence to move about in the house.

—A shower chair or a bathtub rail may allow the person increased independence in personal care activities.

A nonskid bath mat may also be helpful.

—A bedside commode may assist the patient who has diarrhea or is unable to walk to the bathroom unassisted.

—A bedside table and a telephone may allow the bedridden patient independence in some activities of daily living and therefore afford him a greater sense of control.

—A clock and a bedside calendar with space for noting appointments can help minimize confusion.

—To ensure a safe environment, 24-hour supervision is needed as the patient's mental status deteriorates.

—As the patient becomes weaker, a physical therapist should be consulted regarding energy conservation. (See *How to Conserve Your Energy,* p. 333, and *Adapting the Home Environment to the AIDS Patient,* p. 337.)

---

12 **Discuss the value of community resources.**

A variety of community resources (see Appendix A, *Educational Resources*) is available specifically for persons with AIDS and for their families or other caregivers. These resources provide educational and financial information and psychological support and networking.

---

13 **Describe the services provided by various members of the health care team.**

Patients with AIDS may have special physical and psychological needs. Various health care team members working together provide the following services.

The hospital and/or home health care nurse monitors the patient's condition, provides care, and coordinates the plan of care. Social workers make legal and financial arrangements, provide psychological support, and make funeral plans when needed. The homemaker/home health aide provides assistance with activities of daily living, personal care, and light housework. Physical therapists assist with rehabilitation or strengthening exercises, as appropriate. Volunteers help with respite and with emotional and spiritual support. All team members work closely with the physician.

CANDIDA ALBICANS INFECTION

Patient objectives	*Teaching plan content*

1 **Define *Candida albicans* infection and explain how it relates to AIDS.**

Candida albicans is a fungus that causes one of the most common opportunistic infections associated with AIDS. *C. albicans* is commonly present in the mucous membranes of the mouth, throat, esophagus, or rectum. Candidal infection of the mouth or esophagus (candidiasis) may be the initial manifestation of AIDS. It is an uncommon infection in healthy individuals who have not received prior antibiotic, hormonal, or immunosuppressive therapy.

2 Explain how *C. albicans* infection is diagnosed.	*C. albicans* infection is diagnosed as follows: —Clinical diagnosis is made on the basis of characteristic signs and symptoms. —If laboratory testing is done, the diagnosis is made through microscopic examination of tissue from the oral or rectal lesion.
3 Identify two common signs and symptoms of oral and esophageal candidiasis.	The two most common signs and symptoms of oral and esophageal candidiasis are the presence of white, cottage cheese–like patches in the mouth and of dysphagia (swallowing difficulty).
4 Identify three common symptoms of candidal proctitis.	The three most common symptoms of candidal proctitis are rectal pain, pruritus, and discharge.
5 Describe the medication regimen.	The medications used for *C. albicans* infection are as follows: —For oral candidiasis, clotrimazole troches and nystatin oral suspension are used. —For esophageal candidiasis, ketoconazole is administered. —For candidal proctitis, clotrimazole cream is applied to the affected area. —Treatment generally will continue for the entire course of the illness because of the underlying immunodeficiency. For specific medication instructions, see Chapter 10, Drug Therapy.
6 Describe other measures to help control symptoms related to *C. albicans* infection.	The following measures help control symptoms related to candidal infection: —For oral lesions, rinse the mouth frequently with dilute mouthwash, and brush the teeth with a soft toothbrush twice a day. —For rectal lesions, cleanse the anus gently with warm water after each bowel movement, and pat it dry with a soft towel. Sitz baths and analgesics may relieve associated discomfort.

CYTOMEGALOVIRUS (C.M.V.) INFECTION

Patient objectives	*Teaching plan content*
1 Define cytomegalovirus (CMV) infection and explain how it relates to AIDS.	CMV, one of the herpesviruses, often will cause no apparent illness in healthy individuals but may result in serious, widespread infection in AIDS patients. The most common sites for CMV infection include the lungs,

adrenal glands, eyes, central nervous system, gastrointestinal tract, male genitourinary tract, and blood.

2 **Explain how CMV infection is diagnosed.**

A blood titer for CMV is one method of diagnosing CMV infection. Tissue biopsy is another method.

3 **Identify the signs and symptoms of CMV infection.**

Unexplained fever, malaise, gastrointestinal ulcers, swollen lymph nodes, enlarged liver and spleen, and blurred vision are common signs and symptoms that may be related to CMV infection. Vision changes leading to blindness are not uncommon.

4 **Describe the medication regimen.**

There is no effective therapy for CMV infection at this time. DHPG, an experimental drug, may help to slow the virus, particularly when eye infection is identified. For specific medication instructions, see Chapter 10, Drug Therapy.

5 **Describe comfort and safety measures for vision impairment caused by CMV infection.**

The following comfort and safety measures are used for vision impairment due to CMV infection:
—Occupational therapy may help reorient the patient to his home, and rearranging furnishings may allow for an increased level of independence.
—The patient should contact local organizations for the blind for such resources as talking books, large-print newspapers, and radios for the blind.
—If the patient is unable to safely manage a stove or an oven, he may use an attendant for meal preparation or a home meal program.

CRYPTOSPORIDIUM ENTEROCOLITIS

Patient objectives

Teaching plan content

1 **Define *Cryptosporidium* enterocolitis and explain how it relates to AIDS.**

Cryptosporidium enterocolitis is an intestinal infection caused by a protozoan (one-celled animal). The disease may be untreatable and very distressing in the person with AIDS. The causal organism is found primarily in the small bowel and rarely in other organs.

2 **Explain how *Cryptosporidium* enterocolitis is diagnosed.**

Diagnosis is established by examination of stool specimens (see "Explaining Diagnostic Tests" in this chapter) or by examination of biopsy specimens of small-bowel or large-bowel mucosa.

3 Identify two major symptoms of the disease.	The two major symptoms of *Cryptosporidium* enterocolitis are cramping abdominal pain and chronic, profuse, watery diarrhea.
4 Describe the medication regimen.	Therapy for *Cryptosporidium* enterocolitis has been largely ineffective. Spiramycin, an antibiotic with anti-*Toxoplasma* activity, has been helpful in some cases of severe diarrhea. For specific medication instructions, see Chapter 10, Drug Therapy.
5 Describe other measures to control or manage diarrhea caused by *Cryptosporidium* enterocolitis.	The following measures may be used to help control or manage diarrhea: —Discontinue foods that may aggravate diarrhea. —For mild diarrhea, take kaolin and pectin mixtures after each bowel movement. —For severe diarrhea, as ordered, take either diphenoxylate hydrochloride with atropine, or loperamide. (For specific medication instructions, see Chapter 10, Drug Therapy.) —Consider using incontinence pads, such as Attends, Depends, or Chux, and a bedside commode.

HERPES SIMPLEX

Patient objectives	*Teaching plan content*
1 Define herpes simplex and explain how it relates to AIDS.	Herpes simplex is a chronic infection caused by a herpes simplex virus. It is marked by groups of small blisters—often on the borders of the lips or the nares, or on the anus or genitals. Lesions may also be found on the esophageal and tracheobronchial mucosa in AIDS. Herpes simplex is often a reactivation of an earlier herpes infection. Open lesions are highly contagious: gloves should be worn and hand-washing techniques used by the patient and his caregivers.
2 Explain how herpes simplex is diagnosed.	The diagnosis of herpes simplex is made as follows: —Clinical diagnosis is made by the presence of characteristic lesions. —Laboratory diagnosis is made by culturing the virus from active lesions. Viral growth can be recognized in 1 to 4 days.
3 Identify the common signs and symptoms of herpes simplex.	The most common signs and symptoms of herpes simplex virus are red, blisterlike lesions occuring in oral, anal, and genital areas. The patient generally will complain of pain, bleeding, or discharge.

4 Describe the medication regimen.	Acyclovir ointment is used topically to adequately cover all lesions. The drug is given orally in capsule form. Treatment may have to continue indefinitely to prevent recurrence. For specific medication instructions, see Chapter 10, Drug Therapy.
5 Describe other measures to help control symptoms related to rectal lesions.	The following measures help control symptoms related to rectal lesions: —After each bowel movement, the anus should be cleansed gently with warm water and patted dry with a soft towel. —Toilet paper may scratch blisters and should not be used. —Sitz baths and analgesics may relieve associated discomfort.

HERPES ZOSTER

Patient objectives	*Teaching plan content*
1 Define herpes zoster and explain how it relates to AIDS.	Herpes zoster, also known as shingles, is an acute infection caused by the chicken pox virus. It is characterized by small clusters of painful, reddened papules (small, circumscribed, superficial skin elevations) that follow the route of inflamed nerves. It may be disseminated. Herpes zoster may develop in AIDS because the immune system is impaired, allowing opportunistic infections to occur.
2 Explain how herpes zoster is diagnosed.	A clinical diagnosis based on signs and symptoms is usually sufficient. Laboratory diagnosis can be made by scraping the blister and examining the specimen under the microscope.
3 Identify the common signs and symptoms of herpes zoster.	Small clusters of painful, reddened papules are the most common signs and symptoms of herpes zoster.
4 Describe the medication regimen.	Herpes zoster is most often treated with acyclovir capsules until healed. Treatment may have to continue indefinitely to prevent recurrence. Intravenous acyclovir has been effective in treating disseminated herpes zoster lesions in some patients. Medications may be used to relieve pain associated with herpes zoster infection. For specific medication instructions, see Chapter 10, Drug Therapy.

KAPOSI'S SARCOMA (K.S.)

Patient objectives	*Teaching plan content*
1 Define Kaposi's sarcoma (KS) and describe how it relates to AIDS.	KS is a neoplasm characterized by purple or blue patches, plaques, or nodular skin lesions that spread widely in the AIDS patient. The most common sites for these lesions include the skin, oral mucosa, lymph nodes, GI tract, lungs, and visceral organs.
2 Explain how KS is diagnosed.	The following diagnostic measures are used for KS: —Clinical diagnosis is made by the presence of characteristic skin lesions. —Internal examination by GI endoscopic procedures may reveal lesions in the upper and lower GI tract. —Laboratory diagnosis is made by skin biopsy.
3 Identify the signs and symptoms of KS.	Signs and symptoms of KS may vary, depending on the location of the lesions. Lesions may be present externally, on the surface of the skin; and internally, in organs or systems of the body. These lesions seldom drain or bleed. —When lesions are present on the skin surface, the most common signs of KS include purple or blue patches, plaques, or nodular skin lesions. —When lesions are present internally, location of the lesions may determine signs and symptoms: • Lesions of the GI tract are associated with diarrhea, nausea, loss of appetite, and weight loss. • Lesions of the lungs are associated with congestion and difficulty breathing. • Lesions of the lymphatic system are associated with severe extremity and facial swelling and pain secondary to swelling.
4 Identify treatments used for KS.	The following treatments are used for KS: —Skin lesions may be successfully removed by surgical incision with no further treatment indicated. —Tumors that require further treatment are generally responsive to local irradiation. —Chemotherapeutic agents are also used. These include doxorubicin, vinblastine, bleomycin, etoposide (VP-16), interferon, and interleukin-2. For specific medication instructions, see Chapter 10, Drug Therapy. —Many experimental protocols are being tested in the treatment of KS in AIDS. The physician should be asked about availability and more information.

5 Describe other measures to help control or manage symptoms related to KS lesions.	The following measures may help control or manage symptoms related to KS lesions: —For swelling of the extremities, elevate the affected extremities, and use support stockings if possible. —For facial swelling, apply cool, moist towels, and elevate the head of the bed. —Swelling associated with KS will not usually be relieved by diuretics; it is related to local lymphatic blockage and not to systemic involvement. —For diarrhea, discontinue foods that may aggravate the condition. • For mild diarrhea, take kaolin and pectin mixtures after each bowel movement. • For severe diarrhea, take either diphenoxylate hydrochloride with atropine, or loperamide. (For specific medication instructions, see Chapter 10, Drug Therapy.) • Use incontinence pads, such as Attends, Depends, or Chux, and a bedside commode. —Routine doses of acetaminophen, aspirin, or ibuprofen may be taken to relieve fever. Since fevers may be persistent, a round-the-clock regimen of medication should be initiated. Conventional methods, such as sponge baths, may also be implemented for the relief of elevated temperatures. —Weight loss and fatigue may be difficult to control. Emotional support and energy conservation activities should be utilized.

MYCOBACTERIUM AVIUM-INTRACELLULARE (M.A.I.) INFECTION

Patient objectives	Teaching plan content
1 Define *Mycobacterium avium-intracellulare (MAI)* infection and explain how it relates to AIDS.	MAI infection is caused by bacteria commonly found in the environment. The bacteria rarely cause infection in the healthy individual. However, because of the immunodeficiency in AIDS, the bacteria may spread throughout the patient's blood, lymph nodes, bone marrow, liver, lungs, and gastrointestinal tract.
2 Explain how MAI infection is diagnosed.	Diagnosis is generally made by the presence of the bacteria in body fluid or tissue cultures. Blood culture results may be available within 5 to 10 days, although tissue biopsy results may take 2 to 3 weeks. MAI may be confused with *Mycobacterium tuberculosis*, since the

two organisms are similar and difficult to distinguish. Special stains are used to help distinguish these infections in laboratory examination of the cultures.

3 Describe four common signs and symptoms of MAI infection.	The four most common signs and symptoms of MAI infection are fever, diarrhea, weight loss, and debilitation. These signs and symptoms are often masked by or confused with those of other opportunistic infections.
4 Describe the medication regimen.	The following regimen is used in the treatment of MAI infection: —Treatment involves a multidrug regimen, including isoniazid, ethambutol, and rifampin. Ansamycin and clofazimine are experimental drugs that may be added to this regimen. (This regimen has shown poor results, however.) For specific medication instructions, see Chapter 10, Drug Therapy. —Besides ansamycin and clofazimine, other experimental protocols to treat MAI infection may be available. The physician should be asked about this.
5 Describe other measures to help control symptoms of MAI infection.	See the "Kaposi's Sarcoma" teaching plan in this chapter for comfort measures related to diarrhea, fever, and weight loss.

PNEUMOCYSTIS CARINII PNEUMONIA (P.C.P.)

Patient objectives	*Teaching plan content*
1 Describe *Pneumocystis carinii* pneumonia and explain how it relates to AIDS.	PCP is a protozoan infection found in the air sacs of the lungs. It is the most common lung infection found in persons with AIDS. PCP is an otherwise uncommon infection in healthy individuals who have not received prior antibiotic, hormonal, or immunosuppressive therapy.
2 Explain how PCP is diagnosed.	The following diagnostic measures are used for PCP: —Clinical diagnosis may be made by the presence of common signs and symptoms. (Clinical diagnosis is often made, and treatment implemented, without further diagnostic procedures.) —Laboratory diagnosis is made by examination of sputum or tissue samples. Tissue samples may be obtained during bronchoscopy. (See "Explaining Diagnostic Tests" in this chapter.)

—X-rays and gallium scans may also be used to assess pulmonary status.
—Arterial blood gases may be analyzed. These may be normal in the patient with AIDS despite the presence of PCP. However, hypoxemia may occur.

3 **Identify three common signs and symptoms of PCP.**	The three most common signs and symptoms of PCP are fever, shortness of breath, and a dry, nonproductive cough.
4 **Describe the medication regimen.**	PCP is treated with co-trimoxazole (sulfamethoxazole-trimethoprim) or pentamidine isethionate. For specific medication instructions, see Chapter 10, Drug Therapy. —Because of immune system impairment, many persons with AIDS experience adverse effects from co-trimoxazole, such as rash, fevers, and chills. If such reactions occur, pentamidine therapy should be considered. —Pyrimethamine with sulfadoxine also is being used as prophylactic treatment in AIDS.
5 **Describe other measures to help control symptoms related to PCP.**	The following measures help control symptoms: —The patient should take routine doses of acetaminophen, aspirin, or ibuprofen to relieve fever. —The patient should use energy conservation techniques. (See *How to Conserve Your Energy,* p. 333.) —He should use oxygen therapy continuously or as needed. An oxygen concentrator may be more cost-effective for long-term home intervention. —He should take oral morphine solution as ordered to reduce respiratory rate and anxiety.* For specific medication instructions, see Chapter 10, Drug Therapy.

*Since dosages of certain drugs may be substantially different in hospice care, *Oral Morphine in Advanced Cancer* (Twycross, Robert, and Lack, Sylvia. Beaconsfield, England: Beaconsfield Publishers Ltd., 1984.) may be a useful reference.

PROGRESSIVE MULTIFOCAL LEUKOENCEPHALOPATHY (P.M.L.)

Patient objectives	*Teaching plan content*
1 **Define progressive multifocal leukoencephalopathy as it relates to AIDS.**	PML is a central nervous system disorder caused by a papovavirus that causes gradual brain degeneration. Before AIDS, PML was an uncommon infection that was occasionally seen in patients with other immunodeficiency-related diseases.

2 Explain how PML is diagnosed.	The following diagnostic measures are used for PML: —Clinical diagnosis may be made by the presence of characteristic neurologic signs and symptoms. —CT scans may show hypodensity of white-matter lesions. —Definitive diagnosis may be made by brain biopsy, although this procedure is done infrequently to confirm diagnosis of PML.
3 Identify common symptoms of PML.	Progressive dementia, memory loss, confusion, and weakness are the most common symptoms of PML. Other neurologic complications, such as seizures, may occur.
4 Describe measures to help manage symptoms in PML.	No treatments are currently available for PML, but the following measures help manage symptoms: —A large clock in the room and a bedside calendar with appointments noted can help minimize confusion. —As the disease progresses, a physical therapist should be consulted for energy conservation exercises. —To ensure a safe environment, 24-hour supervision is needed as the patient's mental status deteriorates.

TOXOPLASMOSIS

Patient objectives	*Teaching plan content*
1 Define toxoplasmosis as it relates to AIDS.	Toxoplasmosis, caused by a protozoan, results in acute or chronic brain infection in persons with AIDS. Toxoplasmosis generally occurs as a secondary opportunistic infection and less frequently as a primary infection. Before AIDS, toxoplasmosis caused illness in other immunocompromised patients. In these patients, the organism caused other problems, such as swollen lymph nodes, and disease spread to the muscles and internal organs.
2 Explain how toxoplasmosis is diagnosed.	The following diagnostic measures are used for toxoplasmosis: —Clinical diagnosis is made by the presence of characteristic neurologic deficits. —CT scans are frequently used to identify the presence of brain lesions, although these are nonspecific tests. —Lumbar puncture (spinal tap) is a nonspecific test for toxoplasmosis.

—Definitive diagnosis is made by brain biopsy and the observation of *Toxoplasma* organisms. However, this procedure is seldom performed.

3 **Identify common signs and symptoms of toxoplasmosis in AIDS.**	Localized neurologic defects, such as seizures, memory loss, confusion, weakness, and lethargy, are common signs and symptoms of toxoplasmosis.
4 **Describe the medication regimen.**	Pyrimethamine and sulfadiazine is the most common regimen used for toxoplasmosis. For specific medication instructions, see Chapter 10, Drug Therapy.
5 **Describe other measures to help manage symptoms of toxoplasmosis.**	See the "Progressive Multifocal Leukoencephalopathy" teaching plan in this chapter for comfort measures related to dementia.

Patient-Teaching Aid

PATIENT'S GUIDE TO BRONCHOSCOPY

Dear Patient:
Your physician has ordered a special procedure called bronchoscopy for you. This guide will help answer many of the questions you may have concerning this procedure.

What is bronchoscopy?

Bronchoscopy is the direct visualization of the trachea and tracheobronchial tree (large airways). It is performed using a bronchoscope, a special flexible tube with a light source.

Why is bronchoscopy done?

Bronchoscopy is done for diagnostic purposes to visualize obstructions that have been seen on an X-ray, to help determine the cause of such respiratory symptoms as shortness of breath, and to obtain tissue or mucus specimens for examination. It may also be done to locate and treat bleeding in the tracheobronchial tree or to remove foreign bodies, mucous plugs, or excessive secretions from the airways.

How is bronchoscopy done?

Bronchoscopy is usually performed in a special laboratory or in the X-ray department; the room will be darkened. You will be placed in a supine position (flat on your back) on a bed or table, although you may be asked to sit upright in a chair. After a local anesthetic is sprayed into your mouth, the physician will begin inserting the bronchoscope into the airway; he will flush small amounts of anesthetic through the tube deeper into the airway to suppress coughing. You may feel slightly short of breath, but you will not suffocate; oxygen will be given through the bronchoscope. The physician then will examine the airways closely and obtain any needed specimens. The bronchoscope will be removed, and you will be returned to your room. The procedure usually takes 45 to 60 minutes.

PATIENT'S GUIDE TO BRONCHOSCOPY—*continued*

What is my role before, during, and after bronchoscopy?

Before bronchoscopy:
- Do not eat or drink for 6 hours before the test.
- You may receive a sedative intravenously to help you relax.

During bronchoscopy:
- Try to remain relaxed, and keep your arms at your sides.
- Breathe through your nose during the procedure.

After bronchoscopy:
- Lie on your side or with your head up until the gag reflex returns (usually in about 2 hours).
- Do not try to eat or drink until the gag reflex returns.
- When the gag reflex returns, you may gargle or use lozenges to ease the sore throat and hoarseness that can be expected.
- Report bloody mucus, shortness of breath, wheezing, or chest pain immediately to the physician or nurse.
- You may receive the test results in 1 day.

Patient-Teaching Aid

PATIENT'S GUIDE TO COMPUTED TOMOGRAPHY (C.T., OR C.A.T.) SCAN

Dear Patient:

Your physician has ordered a test called a CT scan for you. This is a safe and accurate test that provides more detailed pictures of soft tissues than conventional X-rays do. This guide will help answer many of the questions you may have concerning this procedure.

What is a CT scan?

A CT scan is a specialized X-ray that provides cross-sectional images of various layers of body tissue. A CT scan will show minute differences in the density of the tissue or area being studied, thereby allowing faster, more accurate diagnosis.

Why is a CT scan done?

A CT scan can be done on any part of the body to detect and identify structural abnormalities, edema (swelling), or lesions.

How is a CT scan done?

A CT scan is done in the X-ray department.
• You will be positioned on an X-ray table, and a strap will be placed across the part of your body that will be scanned, to restrict any movement. The table then will slide into the circular opening of the scanner.
• You will not be able to see the technician performing the test, but he will be able to hear and see you from an adjacent room.
• If a contrast medium is ordered, you will receive it intravenously over a period of about 5 minutes. This permits enhanced visualization of the area being studied.
• The X-rays will then be taken—you will hear noises from the scanner and may notice the machine revolving around you.
• You will then be returned to your room or be permitted to go home.
• The test takes about 30 to 60 minutes.

PATIENT'S GUIDE TO COMPUTED TOMOGRAPHY (C.T., OR C.A.T.) SCAN—
continued

What is my role before, during, and after a CT scan?

There is no special preparation necessary for a CT scan.
- You may wear a hospital gown or comfortable clothing.
- If the physician has told you that a contrast medium will be used, do not eat or drink for 4 hours before the test.
- During the CT scan, remain as still as possible.
- If you receive a contrast medium, report any discomfort, breathing difficulty, or itching immediately to the technician.
- After the CT scan, you may resume your normal activities and diet; however, increase your fluid intake the rest of the day to help expel the contrast medium.

Patient-Teaching Aid

DENTAL CARE FOR THE A.I.D.S. PATIENT

Dear Patient:

Dental care, or oral hygiene, means keeping the whole mouth—the teeth or dentures, tongue, roof of the mouth, and gums—clean and healthy. The keys to good oral hygiene are regular dental checkups, good nutrition, and frequent brushing. As a patient with AIDS, it is important that you see your dentist to avoid possible problems. Keep in mind that your dentist or dental hygienist will use certain procedures—such as the wearing of gloves—to prevent contracting or transmitting infection.

Why is mouth care so important?

• Mouth care prevents tooth decay and bad breath.
• It prevents mouth infections that can spread to other parts of the body.
• It stimulates the gums to help prevent gum disease.
• It makes the mouth feel clean and fresh, which can boost the appetite and improve nutrition by making eating more enjoyable.

Here are the basics of good mouth care.

• Brush after every meal, if not more often.
• Use a soft toothbrush with toothpaste or tooth powder. Brush the surface of each tooth with 8 to 10 strokes, moving from the gums to the tooth crowns. Use short vibrating strokes where the gum meets the tooth. If your dentist permits, an electric toothbrush may be used.
• Brush the tongue and the roof of your mouth to help remove thickened saliva that can collect there.
• If mouth problems exist, causing sensitivity, a damp face cloth may be used to clean the teeth and gums.
• Rinse with cool water to remove the toothpaste foam and loosened food particles. For a final rinse, use warm tap water flavored with lemon juice.

Remember—it is most important that you avoid getting infections. See your dentist early in the course of your illness. Give him the name of the physician who is treating you for AIDS so that they may share information regarding any problems you may be having, medications you are taking, or treatments you are receiving.

Patient-Teaching Aid

HOW TO CONSERVE YOUR ENERGY

To help maintain a sense of well-being, save your strength by learning to conserve your energy. The following guidelines will help you to accomplish this.

- Sit down while performing routine daily activities.
- Shop at home using the telephone, mail order, and delivery services to avoid making trips to stores, the library, or the dry cleaner.
- Avoid rushing by planning carefully. Spread your activities out during the day. Prioritize your chores and eliminate or postpone the less urgent ones.
- Take time out to rest between activities. Sit or lie down as soon as you feel tired to avoid overexertion.
- Avoid working with your arms raised, which can tire you more quickly. Work with objects at waist level instead.
- Have all necessary materials close at hand before you begin a task.
- Use electrical equipment whenever possible. Preparing meals with electric kitchen appliances can help you save your strength.
- Wear clothing that is easy to put on and take off. Zippers and Velcro strips are simpler to fasten than buttons.
- Eat frequent, small meals instead of three large ones if chewing tires you.
- Be careful not to overexert yourself when you walk. Remember to move slowly, and take a moment to rest if you get tired.
- If you live in a two-story home, consider moving your bedroom to the first floor so you won't have to climb the stairs so often.
- Ask family, friends, and community service organizations for help when you need it.
- Ask your physical therapist to recommend further energy-saving methods specific to your personal needs.

Patient-Teaching Aid

A.I.D.S. AND COMMUNITY LIVING

Dear Patient:
Even though you have been diagnosed with AIDS, your physician feels you are well enough to care for yourself at home. You can safely live with healthy individuals and other persons with AIDS if the following common-sense hygienic measures are followed to protect you and your housemates. For answers to any questions or concerns, contact your physician or AIDS information center.

1 Maintain a state of personal cleanliness.

- Bathe regularly.
- Wash your hands after using bathroom facilities or after contact with your own body fluids, such as semen, mucus, or blood.
- Wash your hands before preparing food.
- When you cough, cover your mouth with tissues or handkerchiefs; dispose of or launder them properly.
- Flush body wastes down the toilet.

2 Do not share body secretions, especially blood or semen.

- Practice safer sex using condoms, avoiding exchange of body fluids, and exercising extreme care in the choice of a sexual partner.

3 Kitchen and bathroom facilities may be shared. Use normal sanitary practices to prevent growth of fungi and bacteria that may cause illness to AIDS patients.

- Clean kitchen counters with scouring powder to remove food particles.
- *Never* use the same sponge to clean the kitchen and the bathroom. Dirty-looking sponges *should not* be used to wash dishes or kitchen countertops.
- Clean the inside of the refrigerator with soap and water to control molds.
- Mop the kitchen floor at least once a week; clean spills as they occur.
- Mop the bathroom floor at least once a week, and clean up spills immediately. Bleach at 1:9 strength (one part bleach to nine parts water) can be used to disinfect the floor, shower, and sink. Full-strength bleach poured into the bowl will disinfect the toilet.
- Immediately clean up any spills of body fluids— blood, urine, stool, vomitus, and so on—and disinfect the surface with 1:9 bleach solution.
- *DO NOT* use sponges used to clean body fluid spills to wash dishes or to clean food preparation areas.

A.I.D.S. AND COMMUNITY LIVING—*continued*

- *DO NOT* pour mop water down a sink where food is prepared.
- Disinfect sponges and mops by soaking in 1:9 bleach solution for 5 minutes (longer may disintegrate the sponge).

---

4 Eating utensils may be shared with others, provided they are properly washed.

- Separate eating utensils are not necessary.
- While eating, do not share utensils.
- Eating utensils should be washed in hot, soapy water after each use.

---

5 Take precautions with the food you eat.

- Do not eat raw organically grown food (composted with human or animal feces) or unpeeled fruits. Organic lettuce is not safe.
- Do not use unpasteurized milk and milk products; these are associated with *Salmonella* infections. *Salmonella* infections are not well tolerated by people with AIDS.
- You may cook for others, as long as you wash your hands before starting and do not lick your fingers or taste from the mixing spoon while cooking.

---

6 Take precautions with equipment.

- Do not share towels or washcloths without first laundering them.
- Do not share toothbrushes, razors, enema equipment, or sexual devices.

---

7 Take precautions with trash disposal.

- Line trash cans with plastic bags.
- Place soiled disposable items (such as underpads) in the plastic liner.
- When full, trash bags should be tightly secured at top, then disposed of in the normal trash pickup.
- Do not overfill bags, as this is a cause of breakage.

---

8 Take precautions with pets.

- Wear gloves when cleaning bird cages (to prevent psittacosis) and cat litter boxes (to prevent toxoplasmosis).
- Tropical fish tanks may contain organisms in the *Mycobacterium* family, which are not well tolerated by AIDS patients. Get someone else to clean your tank.

Adapted with permission from *Infection Precautions for People with AIDS Living in the Community.* Lusby, G., and Schietinger, H. San Francisco: San Francisco General Hospital Medical Special Care Unit and San Francisco Bay Area Association for Practitioners of Infection Control AIDS Resource Group, 1984.

Patient-Teaching Aid

PREVENTING THE SPREAD OF A.I.D.S.

Dear Patient:

Measures to prevent the spread of AIDS include the following:

• Practice protective sex or safer sex, or avoid vaginal or anal intercourse with infected individuals.
—Wear a rubber condom during vaginal or anal intercourse.
—Sexual practices in which no semen, vaginal fluid, or blood is exchanged are considered safer.
—Know your sexual partner and his or her habits.
—Do not have sex with prostitutes.

• Blood transmission can be avoided if needles and syringes are not shared.
—Use of recreational drugs should be avoided. These can do serious harm to the patient with AIDS. Opiates, alcohol, and marijuana, which can act as immunosuppressants, may increase the patient's vulnerability to infection. Moreover, research suggests that, although inhaled nitrates do not play a role in the development of AIDS itself, they may increase the risk of Kaposi's sarcoma in homosexual men afflicted with AIDS.

• Women who are HIV-positive should avoid pregnancy.
—Mother-to-infant transmission can occur during pregnancy or after pregnancy when breast-feeding.

• Individuals who test positive for HIV should not donate blood, body organs or tissues, or sperm and should follow infection-control guidelines. (See *AIDS and Community Living*, pp. 334-335.)

Patient-Teaching Aid

ADAPTING THE HOME ENVIRONMENT TO THE A.I.D.S. PATIENT

Dear Caregiver:
The following methods can be used to improve the comfort and safety of the home:

- Furniture should be arranged so that the patient can walk safely. The patient may move more freely if he can rest on chairs or against walls.
- Area rugs can be hazardous and may cause falls. They should be removed as the patient becomes weaker and more prone to falls. At this point, a physical therapist should be consulted regarding energy conservation.

- A walker or a wheelchair may allow the patient increased independence to move about in the house.
- A shower chair or a bathtub rail may allow the person increased independence in personal care activities.
- A nonskid bath mat may also be helpful.

- A bedside commode may assist the patient who has diarrhea or is unable to walk to the bathroom unassisted.
- A bedside table and a telephone may allow the bedridden patient independence in some activities of daily living and therefore afford him a greater sense of control.
- A clock and a bedside calendar with space for noting appointments can help minimize confusion.

- To ensure a safe environment, 24-hour supervision is needed as the patient's mental status deteriorates.

Patient-Teaching Aid

HOME CARE INFECTION CONTROL

Dear Patient/Caregiver:

Because AIDS impairs the body's ability to fight infection, prevention of infection is extremely important. However, if you do come down with an infection, always remember that early recognition and treatment are equally important. They can prevent worsening of your condition and improve the quality of your life. The following guidelines will help you control infection:

• Wash your hands after contact with body fluids, such as blood, urine, stool, and drainage from wounds.
• Clean, disposable (not sterile) gloves should be available in the home to assist with care when body fluids will be contacted.

• Gowns may be worn if drainage is expected to soil clothes. Wearing of gowns is to protect clothing, not to prevent the spread of infectious organisms.
• Masks are not necessary unless *Mycobacterium tuberculosis* is suspected and has not been treated with antibiotics. The patient should wear a mask until therapy has been completed to protect others from infectious pulmonary secretions.
• Soiled linens or clothing can be cleaned in the washing machine with hot water, detergent, and 1 cup of bleach. (Detergent and bleach should be added to water before clothes or linens to prevent fading from the bleach.)
• Soiled tabletops, toilets, showers, or floors can be cleaned by washing spills with hot, soapy water, then disinfecting with a solution of one part bleach to nine parts water.
• Separate eating or cooking utensils are unnecessary for the person with AIDS. Eating utensils should be washed in hot, soapy water after each use.
• Toothbrushes and razors should not be shared since bleeding may occur during their use.
• If needles are used in the care of the person with AIDS, an impermeable disposal unit should be kept in the home.

HOME CARE INFECTION CONTROL—*continued*

• Disposal of all disposable items should be handled as follows:

—Gloves, soiled underpads or dressings, or other items that may contain body fluids of the person with AIDS should be placed in a heavy-duty plastic bag and secured firmly at the top to prevent spillage.

—Needles should be placed in impermeable plastic containers.

—These containers and heavy-duty plastic bags can then be disposed of in accordance with local regulations for disposal of solid wastes. (In most communities, these items can be disposed of through normal city trash pickup.)

Drug Therapy

Patient-learner data base*

Areas of potential knowledge deficit
Risk factors (for noncompliance with medication regimen)
—Fear of addiction
—Misconceptions about medication
—Unpleasant side effects
—Multiple drug regimen
—Presence of administration difficulty
—Presence of financial difficulty
—Previous medication teaching inadequate/ineffective
Name of medication
Dosage prescribed
Ordered frequency of administration
Medication action
Side effects of medication
Administration guidelines

Explaining medications

ACETAMINOPHEN (Datril Extra-Strength, Liquiprin, Tempra, Tylenol)

Patient objectives	Teaching plan content
1 State the name of the medication, the dose prescribed, and the ordered frequency of administration.	This information should be obtained from the patient's physician.

*A general assessment should be done for all patients. For general assessment guidelines, see Chapter 1, Principles of Patient Teaching.

2 Explain the use of acetaminophen.	Acetaminophen is used to treat pain because of its ability to block the generation of pain impulses. Acetaminophen relieves fever by increasing blood flow through the skin, producing sweating and heat loss.
3 Identify potential side effects of acetaminophen.	Acetaminophen has the following side effects: Hepatic: severe hepatotoxicity with large doses Skin: rash, urticaria (hives)
4 Discuss guidelines to follow while taking acetaminophen.	The patient should follow these guidelines while taking acetaminophen: —Take only as directed by the physician. —High doses or chronic use can cause liver damage—do not abuse the drug. —Avoid drinking alcohol while using this drug.

ACETIC ACID (OTIC) (Domeboro Otic, VōSol Otic)

Patient objectives	*Teaching plan content*
1 State the name of the medication, the dose prescribed, and the ordered frequency of administration.	This information should be obtained from the patient's physician.
2 Explain the use of acetic acid.	Acetic acid is used to treat external ear canal infection and as a prophylactic for swimmer's ear because of its ability to inhibit or destroy bacteria present in the ear canal.
3 Identify potential side effects of acetic acid.	Acetic acid has the following side effects: Ear: irritation or itching Skin: urticaria (hives) Other: overgrowth of nonsusceptible organisms
4 Discuss guidelines to follow while using acetic acid.	The patient should follow these guidelines while using acetic acid: —Use only as directed by the physician. —Notify the physician of persistent ear drainage.

ACYCLOVIR (Zovirax)

Patient objectives	*Teaching plan content*
1 State the name of the medication, the dose prescribed, and the ordered frequency of administration.	This information should be obtained from the patient's physician.
2 Explain the use of acyclovir.	Acyclovir is used to treat herpes simplex virus because of its ability to inhibit viral multiplication.
3 Identify potential side effects of acyclovir.	Acyclovir has the following side effects: CNS: headache, lethargy, tremors, confusion, hallucinations, agitation, seizures, coma CV: hypotension (low blood pressure) GI: nausea GU: hematuria (blood in urine) Local: inflammation and phlebitis at injection site Skin: rash, itching
4 Discuss guidelines to follow while taking acyclovir.	The patient should follow these guidelines while taking acyclovir: —Report any unusual adverse effects to the nurse or physician. —Take plenty of fluids during treatment.

ALLOPURINOL (Lopurin, Zyloprim)

Patient objectives	*Teaching plan content*
1 State the name of the medication, the dose prescribed, and the ordered frequency of administration.	This information should be obtained from the patient's physician.
2 Explain the use of allopurinol.	Allopurinol is used to treat gout and to prevent acute gouty attacks by lowering blood and urine uric acid levels in primary gout.
3 Identify potential side effects of allopurinol.	Allopurinol has the following side effects: Blood: agranulocytosis (decrease in number of granulocytes), anemia, aplastic anemia CNS: drowsiness EENT: cataracts, retinopathy

GI: nausea, vomiting, diarrhea, abdominal pain
Hepatic: altered liver function studies, hepatitis
Skin: rash—usually maculopapular (raised), exfoliative (peeling), urticarial (itchy hives), and purpuric lesions; erythema multiforme; severe furunculosis of nose; toxic epidermal necrolysis

4 Discuss guidelines to follow while taking allopurinol.	The patient should follow these guidelines while taking allopurinol: —Take only as directed. Do not adjust the dose or discontinue the drug without the physician's approval. —Discontinue the drug at the first sign of skin rash, and report it immediately to the physician. —Drink plenty of liquids while taking allopurinol. —Minimize GI adverse effects by administering with meals or immediately after. —This drug may cause drowsiness; do not drive a car or perform tasks requiring mental alertness until CNS response to drug is known. —Daily urinary output of at least 2 liters is desirable.

AMITRIPTYLINE (Amitid, Amitril, Elavil, Endep, Enovil)

Patient objectives	*Teaching plan content*
1 State the name of the medication, the dose prescribed, and the ordered frequency of administration.	This information should be obtained from the patient's physician.
2 Explain the use of amitriptyline.	Amitriptyline is used to treat depression because of its ability to increase the amount of norepinephrine or serotonin (or both) in the central nervous system.
3 Identify potential side effects of amitriptyline.	Amitriptyline has the following side effects: CNS: drowsiness, dizziness, excitation, tremors, weakness, confusion, headache, nervousness CV: orthostatic hypotension (light-headedness on rising), tachycardia, EKG changes, hypertension EENT: blurred vision, tinnitus (ringing in the ears), mydriasis GI: dry mouth, constipation, nausea, vomiting, anorexia, paralytic ileus GU: urinary retention

Skin: rash, urticaria (hives)
Other: sweating, allergy
After abrupt withdrawal of long-term therapy: nausea,
headache, malaise (general feeling of tiredness). These
symptoms do not indicate addiction.

4 **Discuss guidelines to follow while taking amitriptyline.**	The patient should follow these guidelines while taking amitriptyline: —Take only as directed. Do not adjust the dose or discontinue the drug without the physician's approval. —Do not drink alcohol without the physician's permission. —Increase fluids to alleviate constipation. Inquire about a stool softener, if needed. —Avoid activities that require alertness and good psychomotor coordination until CNS response to drug is determined. —Relieve dry mouth with sugarless hard candy or gum. —Do not take any other drugs (prescription or over-the-counter) without first consulting the physician.

AMPHOTERICIN B (Fungizone)

Patient objectives	*Teaching plan content*
1 **State the name of the medication, the dose prescribed, and the ordered frequency of administration.**	This information should be obtained from the patient's physician.
2 **Explain the use of amphotericin B.**	Amphotericin B is used to treat systemic fungal infections such as *Cryptococcus* because of its ability to bind to the fungal cell membrane and alter it, allowing cell contents to leak out and ultimately destroying the fungal cell.
3 **Identify potential side effects of amphotericin B.**	Amphotericin B has the following side effects: Blood: normochromic anemia (anemia characterized by hemoglobin in the normal range), normocytic anemia (anemia characterized by a decrease in hemoglobin and red cell volume) CNS: headache, peripheral neuropathy; with intrathecal administration (injection into the spinal cord)—peripheral nerve pain, paresthesias (altered sensations) GI: anorexia, weight loss, nausea, vomiting, dyspepsia (indigestion), diarrhea, epigastric cramps

GU: abnormal renal function with hypokalemia (abnormally low serum potassium level), azotemia (excess of urea in the blood), renal tubular acidosis; with large doses—permanent renal impairment, anuria (lack of urine formation), oliguria (scanty urine formation)
Local: burning, stinging, irritation, tissue damage with extravasation, thrombophlebitis, pain at injection site
Other: arthralgia (pain in the joints), myalgia (muscle pain), muscle weakness secondary to hypokalemia, fever, chills, malaise, generalized pain

4 **Discuss guidelines to follow while receiving amphotericin B.**	The patient should follow these guidelines while receiving amphotericin B: —Report any change in urine appearance or amount to the nurse or physician. —Keep topical ointment away from clothing; staining may occur. —Report any unusual adverse effects to the nurse or physician.

AMPICILLIN (Amcill, Omnipen, Polycillin)

Patient objectives	*Teaching plan content*
1 **State the name of the medication, the dose prescribed, and the ordered frequency of administration.**	This information should be obtained from the patient's physician.
2 **Explain the use of ampicillin.**	Ampicillin is used to treat systemic infections, acute and chronic urinary tract infections, meningitis, and uncomplicated gonorrhea because of its bactericidal action against microorganisms.
3 **Identify potential side effects of ampicillin.**	Ampicillin has the following side effects: Blood: anemia, thrombocytopenia, thrombocytopenic purpura, eosinophilia, leukopenia GI: nausea, vomiting, diarrhea, glossitis, stomatitis Local: pain at injection site, vein irritation, thrombophlebitis Other: hypersensitivity (rash, urticaria, anaphylaxis), overgrowth of nonsusceptible organisms
4 **Discuss guidelines to follow while taking ampicillin.**	The patient should follow these guidelines while taking ampicillin: —Take the medication exactly as prescribed, even after

you feel better. The entire quantity prescribed should be taken.
—Call the physician if rash, fever, or chills develop. (A rash is the most common allergic reaction.)
—Take the medication 1 to 2 hours before meals or 2 to 3 hours after.
—Never use leftover ampicillin for a new illness or share ampicillin with family and friends.

ANSAMYCIN (L.M. 427)

Patient objectives	Teaching plan content
1 State the name of the medication, the dose prescribed, and the ordered frequency of administration.	This information should be obtained from the patient's physician.
2 Explain the use of ansamycin.	Ansamycin is an investigational drug used to treat tuberculosis and *Mycobacterium avium intracellulare.*
3 Identify potential side effects of ansamycin.	Ansamycin has the following side effects: CNS: possible seizures GI: nausea, vomiting, diarrhea, abdominal pain Blood: possible bone marrow dysfunction
4 Discuss guidelines to follow while taking ansamycin.	The patient should follow these guidelines while taking ansamycin: —Take only as directed. Do not adjust the dose or discontinue the drug without the physician's approval. —Report any unusual adverse effects to the nurse or physician.

ARTIFICIAL TEARS (Adsorbotear, Hypotears, Isopto Alkaline, Isopto Plain, Isopto Tears, Lacril, Lacrisert, Liquifilm Forte, Liquifilm Tears, Lyteers, Neo-Tears, Tearisol, Tears Naturale, Tears Plus, Ultra Tears)

Patient objectives	Teaching plan content
1 State the name of the medication, the dose prescribed, and the ordered frequency of administration.	This information should be obtained from the patient's physician.

2 Explain the use of artificial tears.	Artificial tears are used to treat insufficient tear production.
3 Identify potential side effects of artificial tears.	Artificial tears have the following side effects: Eye: discomfort, burning, pain on instillation, blurred vision (especially with Lacrisert), crust formation on eyelids and eyelashes from products with high viscosity, such as Adsorbotear, Isopto Tears, and Tearisol
4 Discuss guidelines to follow while using artificial tears.	The patient should follow these guidelines while using artificial tears: —Do not touch the tip of the container to the eye, surrounding tissue, or any other surface. —Do not share medication. —Insert Lacrisert rod with the special applicator that is included in the package.

ASCORBIC ACID (VITAMIN C) (Ascorbicap, Cecon, Cemill, Cenolate, Cetane, Cevalin, Cevi-Bid, Ce-Vi-Sol, Cevita, C-Long, Solucap C, Vita-C)

Patient objectives	*Teaching plan content*
1 State the name of the medication, the dose prescribed, and the ordered frequency of administration.	This information should be obtained from the patient's physician.
2 Explain the use of ascorbic acid.	Ascorbic acid is used for wound healing, chronic disease states, and prevention of vitamin C deficiency due to poor nutrition. Ascorbic acid is essential for the proper synthesis and metabolism of body protein.
3 Identify potential side effects of ascorbic acid.	Ascorbic acid has the following side effects: CNS: faintness or dizziness with fast I.V. administration GI: diarrhea, epigastric burning GU: acidic urine, oxaluria (excessive amounts of oxalate in the urine), renal calculi (kidney stones) Skin: discomfort at injection site
4 Discuss guidelines to follow while taking ascorbic acid.	The patient should follow these guidelines while taking ascorbic acid: —Take only as directed. Do not adjust the dose or discontinue the drug without the physician's approval. —Ascorbic acid can be found in chewable wafers and tablets, or in regular pill form.

ASPIRIN (A.S.A., Ecotrin, Empirin)

Patient objectives	Teaching plan content
1 State the name of the medication, the dose prescribed, and the ordered frequency of administration.	This information should be obtained from the patient's physician.
2 Explain the use of aspirin.	Aspirin is used to treat mild pain and arthritis pain and inflammation because of its ability to block the generation of pain impulses and to inhibit prostaglandin synthesis.
3 Identify potential side effects of aspirin.	Aspirin has the following side effects: Blood: prolonged bleeding time EENT: tinnitus (ringing in the ears), hearing loss (first signs of toxicity) GI: nausea, vomiting, GI distress, occult bleeding Hepatic: abnormal liver function studies, hepatitis Skin: rash, bruising Other: hypersensitivity manifested by anaphylaxis (severe allergic response) and/or asthma
4 Discuss guidelines to follow while taking aspirin.	The patient should follow these guidelines while taking aspirin: —Take only as directed. Do not adjust the dose or discontinue the drug without the physician's approval. —Do not use with large doses of antacids. —Do not use with cimetidine unless ordered to do so by a physician. —Do not take with oral anticoagulants or steroids unless under a physician's care. —Take with food, milk, an antacid, or a large glass of water to reduce GI adverse effects. —Avoid drinking alcohol while using this drug.

ATROPINE INJECTION

Patient objectives	Teaching plan content
1 State the name of the medication, the dose prescribed, and the ordered frequency of administration.	This information should be obtained from the patient's physician.

2 Explain the use of atropine.	Atropine is used preoperatively to reduce the secretions in the nasopharynx and the mouth, which prevents aspiration and its consequences.
3 Identify potential side effects of atropine.	Atropine has the following side effects: With usual doses of 0.4 to 0.6 mg, there are few adverse effects other than dry mouth. However, individual tolerance varies greatly. CNS: disorientation, restlessness, irritability, incoherence, hallucinations, headache CV: palpitations, tachycardia, paradoxical bradycardia (variable, slow heart rate) with doses less than 0.4 mg EENT: dilated pupils, blurred vision, photophobia, increased intraocular pressure, eye pain, dysphagia GI: constipation, mouth dryness, nausea, vomiting GU: urinary hesitancy or retention Skin: flushing, dryness Other: bronchial plugging, fever Above adverse effects may be due to pending atropine toxicity and are dose-related.
4 Discuss guidelines to follow with administration of atropine.	The patient should follow these guidelines while receiving atropine: —Alert the nurse to any unusual adverse effects. —Empty your bladder before receiving atropine; the drug may cause urinary retention and hesitancy. —Remain in bed after administration of atropine.

ATROPINE (OPHTHALMIC) (Atropisol, Isopto Atropine)

Patient objectives	*Teaching plan content*
1 State the name of the medication, the dose prescribed, and the ordered frequency of administration.	This information should be obtained from the patient's physician.
2 Explain the use of atropine (ophthalmic).	Atropine (ophthalmic) is used for acute iris inflammation and cycloplegic refraction (paralysis of the ciliary muscle of the eye) because of its ability to dilate the pupil of the eye.
3 Identify potential side effects of atropine (ophthalmic).	Atropine (ophthalmic) has the following side effects: Eye: increased intraocular pressure, ocular congestion in long-term use, conjunctivitis, contact dermatitis,

edema, blurred vision, eye dryness, photophobia
Systemic: flushing, dry skin and mouth, fever, tachycardia, abdominal distention in infants, ataxia, irritability, confusion, somnolence (sleepiness)

4 Discuss guidelines to follow while using atropine (ophthalmic).	The patient should follow these guidelines while using atropine (ophthalmic): —Wear dark glasses to ease the discomfort of photophobia. —Atropine (ophthalmic) is not for internal use. Treat drops and ointment as poison. Physostigmine is an antidote for poisoning. Signs of poisoning are disorientation and confusion. —Do not touch the dropper or the tip of the tube to the eye or surrounding tissue. —Do not operate machinery or drive a car until the temporary visual impairment caused by this drug wears off. —Wash your hands before and after administration. —Apply light finger pressure on lacrimal (tear) sac for 1 minute following instillation. This minimizes systemic absorption.

BACILLE CALMETTE-GUÉRIN (B.C.G.) VACCINE

Patient objectives	*Teaching plan content*
1 State the name of the medication, the dose prescribed, and the ordered frequency of administration.	This information should be obtained from the patient's physician.
2 Explain the use of BCG vaccine.	BCG vaccine is used for cancer immunotherapy because of its ability to initiate formation of specific antibodies by stimulating the host's antigen-antibody mechanism, providing active, acquired immunity, and its ability to destroy tumor cells.
3 Identify potential side effects of BCG vaccine.	BCG vaccine has the following side effects: Local: lymphangitis, lymph node and skin abscess, ulceration at injection site (2 to 3 weeks after injection), lupuslike reaction Other: urticaria (hives) of trunk and limbs, anaphylaxis (severe allergic reaction)

4 Discuss guidelines to follow while receiving the BCG vaccine.	The patient should follow these guidelines while receiving the BCG vaccine: —Give a detailed history of any allergies and reactions to immunizations to your nurse or physician before receiving the BCG vaccine.

BENZOCAINE (Dermoplast)

Patient objectives	*Teaching plan content*
1 State the name of the medication, the dose prescribed, and the ordered frequency of administration.	This information should be obtained from the patient's physician.
2 Explain the use of benzocaine.	Benzocaine is used as a local anesthetic for episiotomy stitches and hemorrhoids after childbirth because of its ability to inhibit or dull pain.
3 Identify potential side effects of benzocaine.	Benzocaine has the following side effects: Local: sensitivity, rash
4 Discuss guidelines to follow while using benzocaine.	The patient should follow these guidelines while using benzocaine: —Use only as directed by the physician. —Discontinue use if rash or irritation develops. —If spray preparation is used, hold can 6″ to 12″ (15 to 30 cm) from the affected area, and spray liberally. Avoid inhalation. —If using rectally, cleanse and thoroughly dry the rectal area before applying.

BENZTROPINE (Cogentin)

Patient objectives	*Teaching plan content*
1 State the name of the medication, the dose prescribed, and the ordered frequency of administration.	This information should be obtained from the patient's physician.
2 Explain the use of benztropine.	Benztropine is used to treat problems of muscle tonicity associated with acute dystonic reaction and parkinsonism because of its ability to inhibit the effects of acetylcholine (a neurotransmitter).

3 Identify potential side effects of benztropine.	Benztropine has the following side effects: CNS: disorientation, restlessness, irritability, incoherence, hallucinations, headache, sedation, depression, muscular weakness CV: palpitations, tachycardia, paradoxical bradycardia (variable, slow heartbeat) EENT: dilated pupils, blurred vision, photophobia, difficulty swallowing GI: constipation, mouth dryness, nausea, vomiting, epigastric distress GU: urinary hesitancy or retention Some adverse effects may be due to pending atropine-like toxicity and are dose-related.
4 Discuss guidelines to follow while taking benztropine.	The patient should follow these guidelines while taking benztropine: —Take only as directed. Do not adjust the dose or discontinue the drug without the physician's approval. —Inform physician if taking amantadine. —Avoid activities that require alertness until CNS response to this drug is determined. —Watch for intermittent constipation, abdominal distention, and abdominal pain; these may signal onset of paralytic ileus. —Relieve dry mouth with cool drinks, ice chips, or sugarless gum or hard candy. —To help prevent gastric irritation, take after meals.

BIPERIDEN (Akineton)

Patient objectives	*Teaching plan content*
1 State the name of the medication, the dose prescribed, and the ordered frequency of administration.	This information should be obtained from the patient's physician.
2 Explain the use of biperiden.	Biperiden is used to treat problems of muscle tonicity associated with parkinsonism and extrapyramidal disorders because of its ability to inhibit the effects of acetylcholine (a neurotransmitter).
3 Identify potential side effects of biperiden.	Biperiden has the following side effects: CNS: disorientation, euphoria, restlessness, irritability, incoherence, dizziness, increased tremors CV: transient postural hypotension

EENT: blurred vision
GI: constipation, mouth dryness, nausea, vomiting, epigastric distress
GU: urinary hesitancy or retention
Adverse effects are dose-related and may resemble those of atropine toxicity.

4 **Discuss guidelines to follow while taking biperiden.**	The patient should follow these guidelines while taking biperiden: —Take only as directed. Do not adjust the dose or discontinue the drug without the physician's approval. —Take oral doses with or after meals to decrease GI adverse effects. —Avoid activities that require alertness until CNS response to this drug is determined. —Relieve dry mouth with cool drinks, ice chips, or sugarless gum or hard candy.

BLEOMYCIN (Blenoxane)

Patient objectives	*Teaching plan content*
1 **State the name of the medication, the dose prescribed, and the ordered frequency of administration.**	This information should be obtained from the patient's physician.
2 **Explain the use of bleomycin.**	Bleomycin is used to treat Kaposi's sarcoma because of its ability to inhibit DNA synthesis of cancer cells.
3 **Identify potential side effects of bleomycin.**	Bleomycin has the following side effects: CNS: headache GI: anorexia, nausea, vomiting, diarrhea Skin: tenderness, rash, darkening of palms of hands and soles of feet Other: reversible alopecia, fever, chills, weight loss, pneumonia or fibrosis of lungs
4 **Discuss guidelines to follow while taking bleomycin.**	The patient should follow these guidelines while taking bleomycin: —Do not use adhesive dressings on skin. —Report all unusual adverse effects to the nurse or physician. —Treat bleomycin-induced fever with antipyretics, as ordered.

BORIC ACID (OPHTHALMIC) (Blinx, Collyrium Eye Lotion)

Patient objectives	Teaching plan content
1 State the name of the medication, the dose prescribed, and the ordered frequency of administration.	This information should be obtained from the patient's physician.
2 Explain the use of boric acid (ophthalmic).	Boric acid (ophthalmic) is used to soothe and cleanse the eye after ocular procedures and in conjunction with contact lenses.
3 Identify potential side effects of boric acid (ophthalmic).	Boric acid (ophthalmic) has the following side effects: Boric acid is toxic if absorbed through abraded (scraped) skin areas, granulating (healing) wounds, or ingestion.
4 Discuss guidelines to follow while using boric acid (ophthalmic).	The patient should follow these guidelines while using boric acid (ophthalmic): —Do not apply to abraded cornea or skin. —Always wash your hands before and after instilling solution or ointment. —Do not share with another person.

BORIC ACID (OTIC) (Ear-Dry, Swim-Ear, Swim 'n Clear)

Patient objectives	Teaching plan content
1 State the name of the medication, the dose prescribed, and the ordered frequency of administration.	This information should be obtained from the patient's physician.
2 Explain the use of boric acid (otic).	Boric acid (otic) is used to treat external ear canal infection because of its ability to inhibit or destroy bacteria present in the ear canal.
3 Identify potential side effects of boric acid (otic).	Boric acid (otic) has the following side effects: Ear: itching or irritation Skin: urticaria (hives) Other: overgrowth of nonsusceptible organisms

4 Discuss guidelines to follow while using boric acid (otic).	The patient should follow these guidelines while using boric acid (otic): —If a cotton earplug is used, always moisten it with medication. —Avoid touching the ear with the dropper. —Watch for signs of superinfection (continual pain, inflammation, fever).

BROMPTON'S COCKTAIL (A mixture containing varying amounts of the following ingredients: morphine or methadone, cocaine or amphetamine, syrup or honey, alcohol [90% to 98%] or gin, chloroform water)

Patient objectives	*Teaching plan content*
1 State the name of the medication, the dose prescribed, and the ordered frequency of administration.	This information should be obtained from the patient's physician.
2 Explain the use of Brompton's cocktail.	Brompton's cocktail is used to treat severe chronic pain of terminal illness because of its ability to relieve moderate-to-severe pain by altering both the perception of and emotional response to pain.
3 Identify potential side effects of Brompton's cocktail.	Brompton's cocktail has the following side effects: CNS: sedation, somnolence (sleepiness), clouded sensorium, euphoria, convulsions with large doses CV: hypotension (low blood pressure), bradycardia GI: nausea, vomiting, constipation, ileus GU: urinary retention Other: respiratory depression, physical dependence
4 Discuss guidelines to follow while taking Brompton's cocktail.	The patient should follow these guidelines while taking Brompton's cocktail: —Take only as directed. Do not adjust the dose or discontinue the drug without the physician's approval. —Do not drink alcoholic beverages or take other drugs (especially CNS depressants) without first consulting the physician. —If cocaine is one of the ingredients in the cocktail, swish the mixture in the mouth to aid absorption. —Store the mixture in the refrigerator.

CHLORAL HYDRATE

Patient objectives	*Teaching plan content*
1 State the name of the medication, the dose prescribed, and the ordered frequency of administration.	This information should be obtained from the patient's physician.
2 Explain the use of chloral hydrate.	Chloral hydrate is used for sedation and to treat insomnia.
3 Identify potential side effects of chloral hydrate.	Chloral hydrate has the following side effects: Blood: eosinophilia CNS: hangover, drowsiness, nightmares, dizziness, ataxia (loss of coordination) GI: nausea, vomiting, diarrhea, flatulence Skin: hypersensitivity reactions
4 Discuss guidelines to follow while taking chloral hydrate.	The patient should follow these guidelines while taking chloral hydrate: —Take only as directed. Do not adjust the dose without the physician's approval. —Do not drink alcoholic beverages or take other drugs (such as CNS depressants or narcotic analgesics). —Dilute or administer with liquid to minimize unpleasant taste and stomach irritation. Take after meals. —Store in a dark container. —Store suppositories in the refrigerator.

CHLORAMBUCIL (Leukeran)

Patient objectives	*Teaching plan content*
1 State the name of the medication, the dose prescribed, and the ordered frequency of administration.	This information should be obtained from the patient's physician.
2 Explain the use of chlorambucil.	Chlorambucil is used to treat chronic lymphocytic leukemia, lymphosarcoma, giant follicular lymphoma, Hodgkin's disease, ovarian carcinoma, and mycosis fungoides because of its ability to cause an imbalance of growth that leads to the death of certain cells.

3 Identify potential side effects of chlorambucil.	Chlorambucil has the following side effects: Blood: leukopenia (reduction in leukocytes), delayed up to 3 weeks, lasting up to 10 days after last dose; thrombocytopenia (decrease in platelets); anemia; myelosuppression (depression of bone marrow), usually moderate, gradual, and rapidly reversible GI: nausea, vomiting Metabolic: hyperuricemia (increased amount of serum uric acid) Skin: exfoliative dermatitis (inflammation of the skin, causing peeling of layers of skin), rashes Other: allergic febrile reactions
4 Discuss guidelines to follow while taking chlorambucil.	The patient should follow these guidelines while taking chlorambucil: —Screen urine for stones. —Watch closely for signs of bleeding when using anticoagulants.

CHLORAMPHENICOL (OTIC) (Chloromycetin Otic)

Patient objectives	*Teaching plan content*
1 State the name of the medication, the dose prescribed, and the ordered frequency of administration.	This information should be obtained from the patient's physician.
2 Explain the use of chloramphenicol (otic).	Chloramphenicol (otic) is used to treat external ear canal infection because of its ability to inhibit and destroy bacteria present in the ear canal.
3 Identify potential side effects of chloramphenicol (otic).	Chloramphenicol (otic) has the following side effects: Ear: itching or burning Local: pruritus (itching), burning, urticaria (hives), vesicular or maculopapular dermatitis Systemic: sore throat, angioedema Other: overgrowth of nonsusceptible organisms
4 Discuss guidelines to follow while using chloramphenicol (otic).	The patient should follow these guidelines while using chloramphenicol (otic): —Avoid prolonged use. —Avoid touching the ear with the dropper.

—Notify the physician of signs of superinfection (continued pain, inflammation, fever), persistent drainage, or sore throat (early sign of toxicity).

CHLORDIAZEPOXIDE (A-poxide, Libritabs, Librium, Sereen, SK-Lygen)

Patient objectives	Teaching plan content
1 State the name of the medication, the dose prescribed, and the ordered frequency of administration.	This information should be obtained from the patient's physician.
2 Explain the use of chlordiazepoxide.	Chlordiazepoxide is used to treat anxiety, tension, and withdrawal symptoms of acute alcoholism because of its ability to depress the central nervous system, which results in sedation and relaxation.
3 Identify potential side effects of chlordiazepoxide.	Chlordiazepoxide has the following side effects: CNS: drowsiness, lethargy, hangover, fainting CV: transient hypotension GI: nausea, vomiting, abdominal discomfort Local: pain at injection site
4 Discuss guidelines to follow while taking chlordiazepoxide.	The patient should follow these guidelines while taking chlordiazepoxide: —Take only as directed. Do not adjust the dose or discontinue the drug without the physician's approval. —Avoid activities that require alertness and good psychomotor coordination until the response to the drug is determined. —Do not combine with alcohol or other depressants. —Do not share medication with others.

CHLORPROMAZINE (Ormazine, Promapar, Promaz, Sonazine, Thorazine)

Patient objectives	Teaching plan content
1 State the name of the medication, the dose prescribed, and the ordered frequency of administration.	This information should be obtained from the patient's physician.

2 Explain the use of chlorpromazine.	Chlorpromazine is used to treat mild alcohol withdrawal, nausea and vomiting, and psychosis.

3 Identify potential side effects of chlorpromazine.	Chlorpromazine has the following side effects: Blood: transient leukopenia (reduction in the number of leukocytes), agranulocytosis (decrease in granulocytes) CNS: extrapyramidal reactions (tremors, choppy gait, problems with coordination—moderate incidence), sedation (high incidence), pseudoparkinsonism, EEG changes, dizziness CV: orthostatic hypotension (light-headedness on rising), tachycardia, EKG changes EENT: ocular changes, blurred vision GI: dry mouth, constipation GU: urinary retention, dark urine, menstrual irregularities, gynecomastia, inhibited ejaculation Hepatic: jaundice, abnormal liver function tests Skin: mild photosensitivity, dermal allergic reactions, exfoliative dermatitis (inflammation of the skin in which skin peels in layers) Local: pain on I.M. injection, sterile abscesses Other: weight gain, increased appetite After abrupt withdrawal of long-term therapy: gastritis, nausea, vomiting, dizziness, tremors, feeling of warmth or cold, sweating, tachycardia, headache, insomnia

4 Discuss guidelines to follow while taking chlorpromazine.	The patient should follow these guidelines while taking chlorpromazine: —Take only as directed. Do not adjust the dose or discontinue the drug without the physician's approval. —Do not take antacids, antidepressants and antiparkinsonism agents, barbiturates, lithium, or alcohol without consulting the physician. —Hold dose and notify the physician if you develop jaundice, symptoms of blood dyscrasias (fever, sore throat, infection, cellulitis, weakness), or extrapyramidal reactions (such as restlessness, muscular weakness, numbness, spasms, rigidity, or tremors). This is especially important if you are a pregnant woman or if you are giving this medication to a child. —Use sunscreening agents and protective clothing to avoid photosensitivity reactions. —Avoid activities that require alertness or good psychomotor coordination until CNS response to the drug is determined.

—Protect liquid concentrate from light. Dilute with fruit juice, milk, or semisolid food just before administration.
—Relieve dry mouth with sugarless gum or sour hard candy or by rinsing with mouthwash.

CISPLATIN (CIS-PLATINUM) (Platinol)

Patient objectives	Teaching plan content
1 State the name of the medication, the dose prescribed, and the ordered frequency of administration.	This information should be obtained from the patient's physician.
2 Explain the use of cisplatin.	Cisplatin is used to treat advanced bladder cancer, as an adjunctive therapy in metastatic testicular cancer, and as an adjunctive therapy in metastatic ovarian cancer because of its ability to cause an imbalance of growth that leads to the death of certain cells.
3 Identify potential side effects of cisplatin.	Cisplatin has the following side effects: Blood: reversible myelosuppression (depression of bone marrow) in 25% to 30% of patients, leukopenia (decrease in leukocytes), thrombocytopenia (decrease in platelets), anemia CNS: peripheral neuritis, loss of taste, seizures EENT: tinnitus (ringing in the ears), hearing loss GI: nausea, vomiting, beginning 1 to 4 hours after dose and lasting 24 hours; diarrhea GU: more prolonged and severe renal toxicity with repeated courses of therapy Other: anaphylactic reaction (severe allergic reaction)
4 Discuss guidelines to follow while taking cisplatin.	The patient should follow these guidelines while taking cisplatin: —Inform the physician if you are taking antibiotics. —Report tinnitus immediately to prevent permanent hearing loss. —Take antiemetics, as ordered, 24 hours before therapy with cisplatin.

CLOFAZIMINE (Lamprene)

Patient objectives	*Teaching plan content*
1 State the name of the medication, the dose prescribed, and the ordered frequency of administration.	This information should be obtained from the patient's physician.
2 Explain the use of clofazimine.	Clofazimine is a new, investigational drug used to treat tuberculosis and *Mycobacterium avium intracellulare*.
3 Identify potential side effects of clofazimine.	Clofazimine has the following side effects: Eye: ocular pigmentation GI: nausea, vomiting, abdominal pain, diarrhea Skin: discoloration and pigmentation; dry, scaly skin
4 Discuss guidelines to follow while taking clofazimine.	The patient should follow these guidelines while taking clofazimine: —Take only as directed. Do not adjust the dose or discontinue the drug without the physician's approval. —Report any unusual adverse effects to the physician or nurse.

CLORAZEPATE (Tranxene)

Patient objectives	*Teaching plan content*
1 State the name of the medication, the dose prescribed, and the ordered frequency of administration.	This information should be obtained from the patient's physician.
2 Explain the use of clorazepate.	Clorazepate is used to treat acute alcohol withdrawal and anxiety because of its ability to depress the central nervous system, resulting in sedative, relaxant, and anticonvulsant effects.
3 Identify potential side effects of clorazepate.	Clorazepate has the following side effects: CNS: drowsiness, lethargy, hangover, fainting CV: transient hypotension GI: nausea, vomiting, abdominal discomfort

4 Discuss guidelines to follow while taking clorazepate.	The patient should follow these guidelines while taking clorazepate: —Take only as directed. Do not adjust the dose or discontinue the drug without the physician's approval. —Do not combine with alcohol or other depressants. —Avoid activities requiring alertness and psychomotor coordination until response to the drug is determined. —Relieve dry mouth with sugarless chewing gum or hard candy.

CLOTRIMAZOLE (Canesten, Lotrimin, Mycelex)

Patient objectives	*Teaching plan content*
1 State the name of the medication, the dose prescribed, and the ordered frequency of administration.	This information should be obtained from the patient's physician.
2 Explain the use of clotrimazole.	Clotrimazole is used to treat superficial fungal infections, such as candidiasis.
3 Identify potential side effects of clotrimazole.	Clotrimazole has the following side effects: GU: with vaginal use—mild vaginal burning, irritation Hepatic: elevated SGOT levels (from lozenges) Skin: blistering, erythema, edema, pruritus, burning, stinging, peeling, urticaria, skin fissures, general irritation
4 Discuss guidelines to follow while using clotrimazole.	The patient should follow these guidelines while using clotrimazole: —Watch for and report irritation or sensitivity. If either occurs, discontinue use. —Do not use occlusive dressings.

CODEINE

Patient objectives	*Teaching plan content*
1 State the name of the medication, the dose prescribed, and the ordered frequency of administration.	This information should be obtained from the patient's physician.

2 Explain the use of codeine.	Codeine is used to treat mild-to-moderate pain because of its ability to alter both the perception of and emotional response to pain.
3 Identify potential side effects of codeine.	Codeine has the following side effects: CNS: sedation, clouded sensorium, euphoria, convulsions with large doses CV: hypotension (low blood pressure), bradycardia GI: nausea, vomiting, constipation, ileus GU: urinary retention Other: respiratory depression, physical dependence
4 Discuss guidelines to follow while taking codeine.	The patient should follow these guidelines while taking codeine: —Take only as directed. Do not adjust the dose or discontinue the drug without the physician's approval. —Do not take with alcoholic beverages or other depressant drugs without the physician's permission. —Avoid activities that require alertness. —Codeine may cause constipation; eat more fruits and vegetables, or check with the physician about a laxative. —Take before pain is intense for full analgesic effect.

COLCHICINE (Colchicine)

Patient objectives	*Teaching plan content*
1 State the name of the medication, the dose prescribed, and the ordered frequency of administration.	This information should be obtained from the patient's physician.
2 Explain the use of colchicine.	Colchicine is used to treat gout and gouty arthritis by inhibiting migration of granulocytes (one of many types of white blood cells) to an area of inflammation. It decreases lactic acid production and interrupts the cycle of urate crystal deposition and inflammatory response.
3 Identify potential side effects of colchicine.	Colchicine has the following side effects: Blood: aplastic anemia and agranulocytosis (decrease in granulocytes) with prolonged use, nonthrombocytopenic purpura (bruising without a loss of platelets)

CNS: peripheral neuritis
GI: nausea, vomiting, abdominal pain, diarrhea
Local: severe local irritation if extravasation occurs
when given I.V.
Skin: urticaria (hives), dermatitis
Other: alopecia (loss of hair)

4 **Discuss guidelines to follow while taking colchicine.**	The patient should follow these guidelines while taking colchicine: —Take only as directed. Do not adjust the dose or discontinue the drug without the physician's approval. —Be alert for signs of overdosage: weakness, anorexia, nausea, vomiting, or diarrhea. —Take with meals to reduce GI adverse effects. —Be aware that laboratory studies, including complete blood count, should be repeated periodically. —Monitor intake and output carefully. —Store in a tightly closed, light-resistant container.

CORYNEBACTERIUM PARVUM

Patient objectives	*Teaching plan content*
1 **State the name of the medication, the dose prescribed, and the ordered frequency of administration.**	This information should be obtained from the patient's physician.
2 **Explain the use of *Corynebacterium parvum*.**	*Corynebacterium parvum* is a species of bacteria used as an adjunctive cancer chemotherapy because of its ability to stimulate the body's immune system to fight malignant cells.
3 **Identify potential side effects of *Corynebacterium parvum*.**	*Corynebacterium parvum* has the following side effects: CNS: hyperesthesia, transient hemiparesis GI: abdominal pain, nausea, vomiting Metabolic: fever Respiratory: dyspnea Other: hypotension, shaking, chills, malaise
4 **Discuss guidelines to follow while taking *Corynebacterium parvum*.**	The patient should follow these guidelines while taking *Corynebacterium parvum*: —Report any unusual adverse effects to the nurse or physician. —Remain on bed rest to conserve energy.

—Come to a sitting position slowly before arising, to minimize hypotension.

CO-TRIMOXAZOLE (SULFAMETHOXAZOLE-TRIMETHOPRIM) (Bactrim, Bactrim DS, Cotrim, Cotrim DS, Septra, Septra DS)

Patient objectives	*Teaching plan content*
1 State the name of the medication, the dose prescribed, and the ordered frequency of administration.	This information should be obtained from the patient's physician.
2 Explain the use of co-trimoxazole.	Co-trimoxazole is used to treat *Pneumocystis carinii* pneumonia because of its ability to inhibit bacterial cell proliferation.
3 Identify potential side effects of co-trimoxazole.	Co-trimoxazole has the following side effects: Blood: agranulocytosis (decreased number of granulocytes), thrombocytopenia (decreased number of platelets), leukopenia (reduction in the number of leukocytes), hemolytic anemia CNS: headache, mental depression, convulsions, hallucinations GI: nausea, vomiting, diarrhea, abdominal pain, anorexia, stomatitis (inflammation of the mucous membranes of the mouth) GU: toxic nephrosis with oliguria (scanty urine) and anuria (lack of urine production), crystalluria (excretion of crystals in the urine), hematuria (blood in urine) Hepatic: jaundice Skin: photosensitivity, urticaria (hives), pruritus (itching) Other: hypersensitivity, serum sickness, drug fever, anaphylaxis (severe allergic reaction)
4 Discuss guidelines to follow while taking co-trimoxazole.	The patient should follow these guidelines while taking co-trimoxazole. —Take only as directed. Do not adjust the dose or discontinue the drug without the physician's approval. —Promptly report skin rash, sore throat, fever, or mouth sores. —May take by oral suspension if tablets are too large to swallow.

CYCLOPHOSPHAMIDE (Cytoxan, Neosar)

Patient objectives	Teaching plan content
1 State the name of the medication, the dose prescribed, and the ordered frequency of administration.	This information should be obtained from the patient's physician.
2 Explain the use of cyclophosphamide.	Cyclophosphamide is used to treat breast, colon, head, neck, lung, ovarian, and prostatic cancer; Hodgkin's disease; chronic lymphocytic leukemia; chronic myelocytic leukemia; acute lymphoblastic leukemia; neuroblastoma; retinoblastoma; non-Hodgkin's lymphomas; multiple myeloma; mycosis fungoides; and sarcomas because of its ability to cause an imbalance of growth that leads to the death of certain cells.
3 Identify potential side effects of cyclophosphamide.	Cyclophosphamide has the following side effects: Blood: leukopenia (decrease in leukocytes), thrombocytopenia (decrease in platelets), anemia CV: cardiotoxicity (with very high doses and in combination with doxorubicin) GI: anorexia; nausea and vomiting beginning within 6 hours, lasting 4 hours; stomatitis (inflammation of the mouth); mucositis (inflammation of mucous membranes) GU: gonadal suppression (may be irreversible), hemorrhagic cystitis, bladder fibrosis, sterility, nephrotoxicity Metabolic: hyperuricemia (increased levels of serum uric acid), syndrome of inappropriate antidiuretic hormone secretion (with high doses) Other: reversible alopecia (loss of hair) in 50% of patients, especially with high doses; secondary malignancies, pulmonary fibrosis (fibrotic growths in the lungs) with high doses
4 Discuss guidelines to follow while taking cyclophosphamide.	The patient should follow these guidelines while taking cyclophosphamide: —Both males and females should practice contraception while taking this drug and for 4 months after; this drug can cause fetal abnormalities. —Alopecia is likely to occur but is reversible. —Watch closely for signs of bleeding when using anticoagulants. —Take an antiemetic, as ordered, before administration of this drug.

CYCLOSERINE (Seromycin)

Patient objectives	Teaching plan content
1 State the name of the medication, the dose prescribed, and the ordered frequency of administration.	This information should be obtained from the patient's physician.
2 Explain the use of cycloserine.	Cycloserine is used to treat tuberculosis because of its ability to inhibit bacterial wall synthesis.
3 Identify potential side effects of cycloserine.	Cycloserine has the following side effects: CNS: drowsiness, headache, tremors, vertigo, confusion, loss of memory, possible suicidal tendencies and other psychotic symptoms, nervousness, hallucinations, depression, hyperirritability, paresthesias (numbness and tingling), weakness, hyperreflexia (increased response of reflexes) Other: hypersensitivity (allergic dermatitis)
4 Discuss guidelines to follow while taking cycloserine.	The patient should follow these guidelines while taking cycloserine: —Take only as directed. Do not adjust the dose or discontinue the drug without the physician's approval. —Inform the physician if taking isoniazid.

DANAZOL (Danocrine)

Patient objectives	Teaching plan content
1 State the name of the medication, the dose prescribed, and the ordered frequency of administration.	This information should be obtained from the patient's physician.
2 Explain the use of danazol.	Danazol is an investigational drug used for patients with low platelet counts because of its ability to enhance the manufacture of red blood cells.
3 Identify potential side effects of danazol.	Danazol has the following side effects: Androgenic: acne, edema, weight gain, hirsutism, hoarseness, clitoral enlargement, decrease in breast size, changes in libido, male-pattern baldness, oiliness of skin or hair

CNS: dizziness, headache, sleep disorders, fatigue, tremor, irritability, excitation, lethargy, mental depression, chills, paresthesias (numbness and tingling)
CV: elevated blood pressure
GI: gastric irritation, nausea, vomiting, diarrhea, constipation, appetite changes
GU: hematuria
Hepatic: reversible jaundice
Hypoestrogenic: flushing; sweating; vaginitis, including itching, dryness, burning, and vaginal bleeding; nervousness; emotional lability
Other: muscle cramps or spasms, decreased testicular size

4 Discuss guidelines to follow while taking danazol.	The patient should follow these guidelines while taking danazol: —Take only as directed. Do not adjust the dose or discontinue the drug without the physician's approval. —Eat a diet high in calories and protein unless contraindicated. —Report any unusual adverse effects to the nurse or physician.

DEMECARIUM BROMIDE (Humorsol)

Patient objectives	*Teaching plan content*
1 State the name of the medication, the dose prescribed, and the ordered frequency of administration.	This information should be obtained from the patient's physician.
2 Explain the use of demecarium bromide.	Demecarium bromide is used to treat glaucoma and postiridectomy patients because of its ability to cause pupillary constriction and accommodation spasm.
3 Identify potential side effects of demecarium bromide.	Demecarium bromide has the following side effects: CNS: headache CV: hypotension, bradycardia Eye: iris cysts (reversible with discontinuation), lens opacity, ciliary spasm, blurred vision, eye or brow pain, photosensitivity, eyelid twitching, conjunctival and intraocular hyperemia (an excess of blood accumulation), ocular pain, photophobia, acute attack of narrow-angle glaucoma

GI: nausea, vomiting, abdominal pain, diarrhea, excessive salivation
GU: frequent urination
Skin: contact dermatitis
Other: flushing, bronchial constriction

4 Discuss guidelines to follow while using demecarium bromide.	The patient should follow these guidelines while using demecarium bromide: —Use only as directed and prescribed. —Stop drug and report immediately if excessive salivation, diaphoresis, urinary incontinence, diarrhea, or muscle weakness occurs. —Use this drug at bedtime, since it blurs vision. —Do not touch the tip of the dropper to the eye or surrounding tissue. —Apply light finger pressure on lacrimal (tear) sac for 1 minute following instillation to minimize systemic absorption. —If solution contacts skin, wash promptly with large amounts of water. —Wash hands immediately before and after administration. —Maintain close and constant medical supervision. —Store in a tightly closed container.

DESIPRAMINE (Norpramin, Pertofrane)

Patient objectives	*Teaching plan content*
1 State the name of the medication, the dose prescribed, and the ordered frequency of administration.	This information should be obtained from the patient's physician.
2 Explain the use of desipramine.	Desipramine is used to treat depression because of its effect on the central nervous system.
3 Identify potential side effects of desipramine.	Desipramine has the following side effects: CNS: drowsiness, dizziness, excitation, tremors, weakness, confusion, headache, nervousness CV: orthostatic hypotension (light-headedness on rising), tachycardia, EKG changes, hypertension EENT: blurred vision, tinnitus (ringing in the ears), mydriasis GI: dry mouth, constipation, nausea, vomiting, anorexia, paralytic ileus

GU: urinary retention
Skin: rash, urticaria (hives)
Other: sweating, allergy
After abrupt withdrawal of long-term therapy: nausea, headache, malaise. (These symptoms do not indicate addiction.)

---

4 Discuss guidelines to follow while taking desipramine.

The patient should follow these guidelines while taking desipramine:
—Take only as directed. Do not adjust the dose or discontinue the drug without the physician's approval.
—Get up slowly to minimize orthostatic hypotension.
—Increase fluids to lessen constipation. Inquire about a stool softener, if needed.
—Avoid activities that require alertness and good psychomotor coordination until response to drug is determined.
—Relieve dry mouth with sugarless hard candy or gum.
—Do not drink alcoholic beverages or take any other drugs (prescription or over-the-counter) without first consulting the physician.

DEXAMETHASONE (Decadron)

Patient objectives	*Teaching plan content*
1 State the name of the medication, the dose prescribed, and the ordered frequency of administration.	This information should be obtained from the patient's physician.
2 Explain the use of dexamethasone.	Dexamethasone is used to treat inflammation because of its ability to accelerate protein breakdown.
3 Identify potential side effects of dexamethasone.	Dexamethasone has the following side effects: CNS: euphoria, insomnia, psychotic behavior CV: congestive heart failure, hypertension, edema EENT: cataracts, glaucoma GI: peptic ulcer, gastrointestinal irritation, increased appetite Local: atrophy at I.M. injection site Metabolic: possible hypokalemia (decrease in serum potassium level), hyperglycemia (increase in serum glucose level), and carbohydrate intolerance; growth suppression in children

Skin: delayed wound healing, acne, various skin eruptions

Other: muscle weakness, pancreatitis, hirsutism, susceptibility to infections. Acute adrenal insufficiency may follow increased stress (infection, surgery, trauma) or abrupt withdrawal after long-term therapy.

Withdrawal symptoms: rebound inflammation, fatigue, weakness, arthralgia, fever, dizziness, lethargy, depression, fainting, orthostatic hypotension, dyspnea, anorexia, hypoglycemia. *Sudden withdrawal may be fatal.*

4 **Discuss guidelines to follow while taking dexamethasone.**	The patient should follow these guidelines while taking dexamethasone: —Take only as directed. Do not adjust the dose or discontinue the drug without the physician's approval. —Do not take with barbiturates, phenytoin, rifampin, indomethacin, or aspirin, unless prescribed by a physician. —Watch for petechiae (pinpoint, nonraised, perfectly round purplish red spots caused by slight bleeding under the skin) and easy bruising. —Take oral dose with food whenever possible.

DEXAMETHASONE (NASAL) (Decadron Phosphate, Decadron Phosphate Respihaler, Decadron Phosphate Turbinaire)

Patient objectives	*Teaching plan content*
1 **State the name of the medication, the dose prescribed, and the ordered frequency of administration.**	This information should be obtained from the patient's physician.
2 **Explain the use of dexamethasone (nasal).**	Dexamethasone (nasal) is used to treat allergic or inflammatory conditions and nasal polyps (protruding growths within the nose).
3 **Identify potential side effects of dexamethasone (nasal).**	Dexamethasone (nasal) has the following side effects: EENT: nasal irritation, dryness, rebound nasal congestion Other: hypersensitivity, systemic adverse effects with prolonged use (pituitary-adrenal suppression, sodium retention, congestive heart failure, hypertension, hypokalemia [decreased serum potassium level], headaches, convulsions, peptic ulcer, ecchymoses [bruises], petechiae [pinpoint, round purplish spots caused by bleeding under the skin], masking of secondary infection)

| **4** Discuss guidelines to follow while using dexamethasone (nasal). | The patient should follow these guidelines while using dexamethasone (nasal):
—Irritation or sensitivity may require stopping the drug.
—Gradually reduce dose, as ordered by physician, as nasal condition improves.
—Mothers should not breast-feed, as systemic absorption can occur.
—Only one person should use the nasal spray.
—Do not break, incinerate, or store in extreme heat; contents are under pressure. |

DEXAMETHASONE (OTIC) (Decadron)

Patient objectives	*Teaching plan content*
1 State the name of the medication, the dose prescribed, and the ordered frequency of administration.	This information should be obtained from the patient's physician.
2 Explain the use of dexamethasone (otic).	Dexamethasone (otic) is used to treat inflammation of the external ear canal because of its ability to control inflammation, edema, and pruritus (itching).
3 Identify potential side effects of dexamethasone (otic).	Dexamethasone (otic) has the following side effects: Systemic: adrenal suppression with long-term use Other: masking or exacerbation (flare-up) of underlying infection
4 Discuss guidelines to follow while using dexamethasone (otic).	The patient should follow these guidelines while using dexamethasone (otic): —Avoid touching the ear with the dropper. —Take medication only as directed.

D.H.P.G.

Patient objectives	*Teaching plan content*
1 State the name of the medication, the dose prescribed, and the ordered frequency of administration.	This information should be obtained from the patient's physician.

2 Explain the use of DHPG.	DHPG is a drug used investigationally to treat cyto-megalovirus infections in immunologically depressed patients.
3 Identify potential side effects of DHPG.	DHPG has the following side effects: Blood: granulocytopenia (decrease in the amount of granulocytes)
4 Discuss guidelines to follow while taking DHPG.	The patient should follow these guidelines while taking DHPG: —Cooperate with the medical team as to dosage, route, and times of administration. Since this is an experimental drug, permission will have to be given by you for its use. —Report any unusual side effects to the physician or nurse.

DIAZEPAM (Valium)

Patient objectives	*Teaching plan content*
1 State the name of the medication, the dose prescribed, and the ordered frequency of administration.	This information should be obtained from the patient's physician.
2 Explain the use of diazepam.	Diazepam is used to treat tension, anxiety, and muscle spasms because of its ability to depress the central nervous system, resulting in sedative, skeletal muscle relaxant, and anticonvulsive effects.
3 Identify potential side effects of diazepam.	Diazepam has the following side effects: CNS: drowsiness, lethargy, hangover, fainting CV: transient hypotension GI: nausea, vomiting, abdominal discomfort Local: desquamation (peeling), pain, phlebitis at injection site
4 Discuss guidelines to follow while taking diazepam.	The patient should follow these guidelines while taking diazepam: —Take only as directed. Do not adjust the dose or discontinue the drug without the physician's approval. —Do not take with cimetidine unless monitored by a physician.

—Avoid activities that require alertness and good psychomotor coordination until CNS response to drug is determined.
—Do not combine with alcohol or other depressant drugs without first consulting the physician.
—Do not give medication to others.

DIPHENHYDRAMINE (Allerdryl, Benadryl, Benahist, Bendylate, Compōz, Fenylhist, Nordryl, Nytol with DPH, Phen-Amin, SK-Diphenhydramine, Sominex Formula 2, Valdrene, Wehdryl)

Patient objectives	*Teaching plan content*
1 State the name of the medication, the dose prescribed, and the ordered frequency of administration.	This information should be obtained from the patient's physician.
2 Explain the use of diphenhydramine.	Diphenhydramine is used to treat parkinsonism and for nighttime sedation because of its ability to provide anesthesia by preventing initiation and transmission of nerve impulses.
3 Identify potential side effects of diphenhydramine.	Diphenhydramine has the following side effects: CNS: especially in the elderly—drowsiness, confusion, insomnia, headache, vertigo CV: palpitations EENT: photosensitivity, diplopia (double vision), nasal stuffiness GI: nausea, vomiting, diarrhea, dry mouth, constipation GU: dysuria (difficult urination) Skin: urticaria (hives), itching
4 Discuss guidelines to follow while taking diphenhydramine.	The patient should follow these guidelines while taking diphenhydramine: —Take only as directed. Do not adjust the dose or discontinue the drug without the physician's approval. —Do not drink alcoholic beverages without first consulting the physician. —Reduce GI distress by taking with food or milk. —Drink coffee or tea to reduce drowsiness. —Relieve dry mouth with sugarless gum, sour hard candy, or ice chips. —Do not drive or engage in hazardous activities until CNS response to drug is determined.

DIPHENOXYLATE WITH ATROPINE SULFATE (Lofene, Lomotil)

Patient objectives	Teaching plan content
1 State the name of the medication, the dose prescribed, and the ordered frequency of administration.	This information should be obtained from the patient's physician.
2 Explain the use of diphenoxylate with atropine sulfate.	Diphenoxylate with atropine sulfate is used to treat diarrhea because of its ability to diminish motility of the GI tract.
3 Identify potential side effects of diphenoxylate with atropine sulfate.	Diphenoxylate with atropine sulfate has the following side effects: CNS: sedation, dizziness, headache, drowsiness, lethargy, restlessness, depression, euphoria CV: tachycardia (increased heartbeat) GI: dry mouth, nausea, vomiting, abdominal discomfort or distention, anorexia, fluid retention in bowel GU: urinary retention Skin: pruritus, giant urticaria, rash Other: possible physical dependence in long-term use, respiratory depression
4 Discuss guidelines to follow while taking diphenoxylate with atropine sulfate.	The patient should follow these guidelines while taking diphenoxylate with atropine sulfate: —Take only as directed. Do not adjust the dose or discontinue the drug without the physician's approval. —Do not use for more than 2 days unless under a physician's guidance.

DIPIVEFRIN (Propine)

Patient objectives	Teaching plan content
1 State the name of the medication, the dose prescribed, and the ordered frequency of administration.	This information should be obtained from the patient's physician.
2 Explain the use of dipivefrin.	Dipivefrin is used to treat chronic open-angle glaucoma because of its ability to reduce intraocular pressure.

3 Identify potential side effects of dipivefrin.	Dipivefrin has the following side effects: Eye: burning, stinging CV: tachycardia, hypertension
4 Discuss guidelines to follow while using dipivefrin.	The patient should follow these guidelines while using dipivefrin: —Wash hands before and after administration. —Do not touch the dropper to the eye or to surrounding tissue. —Do not exceed recommended dosage.

DISULFIRAM (Antabuse)

Patient objectives	Teaching plan content
1 State the name of the medication, the dose prescribed, and the ordered frequency of administration.	This information should be obtained from the patient's physician.
2 Explain the use of disulfiram.	Disulfiram is used in the management of chronic alcoholism because it makes the patient extremely sensitive to alcohol. When alcohol is ingested, the patient becomes ill.
3 Identify potential side effects of disulfiram.	Disulfiram has the following side effects: CNS: drowsiness, headache, fatigue, delirium, depression, neuritis EENT: optic neuritis GI: metallic or garliclike aftertaste GU: impotence Skin: acneform or allergic dermatitis Other: disulfiram reaction, which may include flushing, throbbing headache, dyspnea, nausea, copious vomiting, sweating, thirst, chest pain, palpitations, hyperventilation, hypotension, syncope, anxiety, weakness, blurred vision, confusion. In severe reactions, respiratory depression, cardiovascular collapse, dysrhythmias, myocardial infarction, acute congestive heart failure, convulsions, unconsciousness, and even death can occur.
4 Discuss guidelines to follow when taking disulfiram.	The patient should follow these guidelines while taking disulfiram: —Avoid all foods and medicines that may contain alcohol, such as sauces and cough syrups. Even external

application of liniments, shaving lotion, or back-rub
preparations may precipitate disulfiram reaction.
—Wear a bracelet or carry a card supplied by the drug
manufacturer identifying yourself as a disulfiram user.
Cards may be obtained from Ayerst Laboratories, 685
Third Ave., New York, N.Y. 10017.
—Disulfiram-induced side effects, such as drowsiness,
fatigue, impotence, headache, peripheral neuritis, and
metallic or garliclike taste, subside after about 2 weeks
of therapy. Avoid activities that require alertness and
psychomotor coordination until the side effects have
subsided.

DOXEPIN (Sinequan)

Patient objectives	Teaching plan content
1 State the name of the medication, the dose prescribed, and the ordered frequency of administration.	This information should be obtained from the patient's physician.
2 Explain the use of doxepin.	Doxepin is used to treat depression because of its effects on the central nervous system.
3 Identify potential side effects of doxepin.	Doxepin has the following side effects: CNS: drowsiness, dizziness, excitation, tremors, weakness, confusion, headache, nervousness CV: orthostatic hypotension (light-headedness on rising), tachycardia, EKG changes, hypertension EENT: blurred vision, tinnitus (ringing in the ears), glossitis (inflammation of the tongue), mydriasis (pupil dilation) GI: dry mouth, constipation, nausea, vomiting, anorexia, paralytic ileus GU: urinary retention Skin: rash, urticaria (hives) Other: sweating, allergy After abrupt withdrawal of long-term therapy: nausea, headache, malaise. (These symptoms do not indicate addiction.)
4 Discuss guidelines to follow while taking doxepin.	The patient should follow these guidelines while taking doxepin: —Take only as directed. Do not adjust the dose or dis-

continue the drug without the physician's approval.
—Dilute oral concentrate with 120 ml of water, milk,
or juice (orange, grapefruit, tomato, prune, or pineapple). Avoid carbonated beverages.
—Increase fluids to lessen constipation. Inquire about a
stool softener, if needed.
—Avoid activities that require alertness and good psychomotor coordination until CNS response to drug is
determined.
—Relieve dry mouth with sugarless hard candy or
gum.
—Do not drink alcoholic beverages or take any other
drugs (over-the-counter or prescription) without first
consulting the physician.

DOXORUBICIN (Adriamycin)

Patient objectives	*Teaching plan content*
1 State the name of the medication, the dose prescribed, and the ordered frequency of administration.	This information should be obtained from the patient's physician.
2 Explain the use of doxorubicin.	Doxorubicin is used to treat bladder, breast, cervical, head, neck, liver, lung, ovarian, prostatic, stomach, testicular, and thyroid cancer; Hodgkin's disease; acute lymphoblastic and myeloblastic leukemia; Wilms' tumor; neuroblastomas; lymphomas; and sarcomas because of its ability to interfere with DNA synthesis of cells.
3 Identify potential side effects of doxorubicin.	Doxorubicin has the following side effects: Blood: leukopenia (reduction in leukocytes), especially agranulocytosis (decrease in granulocytes) during days 10 to 15, with recovery by day 21; thrombocytopenia (decrease in platelets) CV: cardiac depression, seen in such EKG changes as sinus tachycardia, T-wave flattening, ST segment depression, voltage reduction; dysrhythmias in 11% of patients; cardiomyopathy (sometimes with pulmonary edema) with mortality of 30% to 75% GI: nausea, vomiting, diarrhea, stomatitis (inflammation of the mouth), esophagitis (inflammation of the esophagus) GU: enhancement of cyclophosphamide-induced bladder injury Local: severe cellulitis (infection of the skin) or tissue

slough if drug extravasates
Skin: hyperpigmentation of the skin, especially in previously irradiated areas
Other: hyperpigmentation of nails and dermal creases, complete alopecia (hair loss) within 3 to 4 weeks; hair may regrow 2 to 5 months after drug is stopped

4 **Discuss guidelines to follow while taking doxorubicin.**	The patient should follow these guidelines while taking doxorubicin: —Be aware that urine will be red for 1 to 2 days and that alopecia will occur. —Notify the physician of any adverse effects.

ECHOTHIOPHATE IODIDE (Phospholine Iodide)

Patient objectives	Teaching plan content
1 **State the name of the medication, the dose prescribed, and the ordered frequency of administration.**	This information should be obtained from the patient's physician.
2 **Explain the use of echothiophate iodide.**	Echothiophate iodide is used to treat open-angle glaucoma and conditions obstructing aqueous outflow because of its ability to cause pupillary constriction and accommodation spasm.
3 **Identify potential side effects of echothiophate iodide.**	Echothiophate iodide has the following side effects: CNS: fatigue, muscle weakness, paresthesias, headache CV: bradycardia, hypotension Eye: ciliary spasm, ciliary or conjunctival infection, nonreversible cataract formation (time- and dose-related), reversible iris cysts, pupillary block, blurred or dimmed vision, eye or brow pain, lid twitching, hyperemia, photosensitivity, lens opacities, lacrimation, retinal detachment GI: diarrhea, nausea, vomiting, abdominal pain, intestinal cramps, salivation GU: frequent urination Other: flushing, sweating, bronchial constriction
4 **Discuss guidelines to follow while using echothiophate iodide.**	The patient should follow these guidelines while using echothiophate iodide: —Instill at bedtime, since this drug causes transient blurred vision. —Remain under constant medical supervision.

—Do not exceed recommended dosage. Take only as directed.
—Report salivation, diarrhea, profuse sweating, urinary incontinence, or muscle weakness.
—Do not touch the tip of the dropper to the eye or surrounding tissue.
—Apply light finger pressure on the lacrimal (tear) sac for 1 minute following instillation to minimize systemic absorption.
—Wash hands before and after administering medication.

EPINEPHRINE INHALANTS (Adrenalin, AsthmaHaler, Bronkaid Mist, Medihaler-Epi, Primatene Mist, Sus-Phrine)

Patient objectives	*Teaching plan content*
1 **State the name of the medication, the dose prescribed, and the ordered frequency of administration.**	This information should be obtained from the patient's physician.
2 **Explain the use of epinephrine.**	Epinephrine is used to treat bronchospasm, hypersensitivity reaction, and anaphylactic reaction (severe allergic response) due to exposure to allergens.
3 **Identify potential side effects of epinephrine.**	Epinephrine has the following side effects: CNS: nervousness, tremors, euphoria, anxiety, coldness of extremities, vertigo, headache, sweating, cerebral hemorrhage, disorientation, agitation. In patients with Parkinson's disease, the drug increases rigidity and tremor. CV: palpitations; widened pulse pressure; hypertension; tachycardia; ventricular fibrillation; cerebrovascular accident; anginal pain; EKG changes, including a decrease in T-wave amplitude Metabolic: hyperglycemia, glycosuria Other: pulmonary edema, dyspnea, pallor
4 **Discuss guidelines to follow while taking epinephrine.**	The patient should follow these guidelines while taking epinephrine: —Take only as directed. Do not adjust the dose without the physician's approval. —In acute hypersensitivity (allergic) reactions, administer the injectable form of the drug as instructed by the physician.

ERYTHROMYCIN (E-Mycin, Erythrocin, Ilosone, Ilotycin)

Patient objectives	*Teaching plan content*
1 State the name of the medication, the dose prescribed, and the ordered frequency of administration.	This information should be obtained from the patient's physician.
2 Explain the use of erythromycin.	Erythromycin is an antibiotic used to treat a wide variety of infections. It may also be used prophylactically to prevent endocarditis when dental procedures are done.
3 Identify potential side effects of erythromycin.	Erythromycin has the following side effects: Eye: slowed corneal wound healing Other: overgrowth of nonsusceptible organisms with long-term use; hypersensitivity, including itching and burning eyes, urticaria, dermatitis, angioedema
4 Discuss guidelines to follow while taking erythromycin.	The patient should follow these guidelines while taking erythromycin: —Take the medication for as long as prescribed, even if feeling better. —Take with a full glass of water 1 hour before or 2 hours after meals. If tablets are coated, they may be taken with meals. Do not drink fruit juice with erythromycin. Chewable erythromycin tablets should not be swallowed whole. —Watch for signs of other infections, such as vaginal, urinary, or respiratory discomfort, and report them to the physician. In addition, report any nausea, abdominal pain, or fever.

ETHAMBUTOL (Myambutol)

Patient objectives	*Teaching plan content*
1 State the name of the medication, the dose prescribed, and the ordered frequency of administration.	This information should be obtained from the patient's physician.
2 Explain the use of ethambutol.	Ethambutol is used to treat tuberculosis because of its ability to interfere with bacterial protein metabolism.

3 Identify potential side effects of ethambutol.	Ethambutol has the following side effects: CNS: headache, dizziness, mental confusion, possible hallucinations, peripheral neuritis (numbness and tingling of extremities) EENT: optic neuritis (vision loss and loss of color discrimination, especially of red and green) GI: anorexia, nausea, vomiting, abdominal pain Metabolic: elevated uric acid level Other: anaphylactic reactions, fever, malaise, bloody sputum
4 Discuss guidelines to follow while taking ethambutol.	The patient should follow these guidelines while taking ethambutol: —Take only as directed. Do not adjust the dose or discontinue the drug without the physician's approval. —Report any unusual adverse effects to the nurse or physician.

ETHIONAMIDE (Trecator-SC)

Patient objectives	*Teaching plan content*
1 State the name of the medication, the dose prescribed, and the ordered frequency of administration.	This information should be obtained from the patient's physician.
2 Explain the use of ethionamide.	Ethionamide is used to treat tuberculosis; how it works is not known.
3 Identify potential side effects of ethionamide.	Ethionamide has the following side effects: Blood: thrombocytopenia (decrease in platelets) CNS: peripheral neuritis, psychic disturbances (especially mental depression), drowsiness CV: postural hypotension GI: anorexia, metallic taste in mouth, nausea, vomiting, sialorrhea, epigastric distress, diarrhea, stomatitis, weight loss Hepatic: jaundice, hepatitis, elevated SGOT and SGPT levels Skin: rash Other: smell disturbances, acne, hair loss, increased breast size
4 Discuss guidelines to follow while taking ethionamide.	The patient should follow these guidelines while taking ethionamide: —Take only as directed. Do not adjust the dose or dis-

continue the drug without the physician's approval.
—Take with meals or antacids to minimize GI adverse effects.
—Avoid alcoholic beverages.

ETOPOSIDE (V.P.-16) (VePesid)

Patient objectives	Teaching plan content
1 State the name of the medication, the dose prescribed, and the ordered frequency of administration.	This information should be obtained from the patient's physician.
2 Explain the use of etoposide.	Etoposide is used to treat Kaposi's sarcoma because of its ability to block cell division of cancer cells.
3 Identify potential side effects of etoposide.	Etoposide has the following side effects: Blood: low blood cell count CV: hypotension from rapid infusion GI: nausea and vomiting Local: rarely, phlebitis Other: occasional headache and fever; reversible alopecia (hair loss); rarely, anaphylaxis (severe allergic response)
4 Discuss guidelines to follow while taking etoposide.	The patient should follow these guidelines while taking etoposide: —Any unusual adverse effects should be reported to the nurse or physician. —An infusion of this drug lasting less than 2 hours should be taken while lying down.

FLUCYTOSINE (Ancobon)

Patient objectives	Teaching plan content
1 State the name of the medication, the dose prescribed, and the ordered frequency of administration.	This information should be obtained from the patient's physician.
2 Explain the use of flucytosine.	Flucytosine is used to treat severe fungal infections caused by strains of *Candida albicans* because of its

	ability to penetrate fungal cells and antagonize their metabolic processes.
3 **Identify potential side effects of flucytosine.**	Flucytosine has the following side effects: Blood: anemia, leukopenia (reduction in the number of leukocytes), bone marrow depression, thrombocytopenia (decrease in the number of platelets) CNS: dizziness, drowsiness, confusion, headache GI: nausea, vomiting, diarrhea, abdominal bloating Hepatic: elevated SGOT and SGPT levels Metabolic: elevated serum alkaline phosphatase, blood urea nitrogen, and serum creatinine levels Skin: occasionally, rash
4 **Discuss guidelines to follow while taking flucytosine.**	The patient should follow these guidelines while taking flucytosine: —Take only as directed. Do not adjust the dose or discontinue the drug without the physician's approval. —Minimize nausea, vomiting, and stomach upset by taking the capsules over a 15-minute period.

FLUOROURACIL (5-FLUOROURACIL) (Adrucil, 5-FU)

Patient objectives	*Teaching plan content*
1 **State the name of the medication, the dose prescribed, and the ordered frequency of administration.**	This information should be obtained from the patient's physician.
2 **Explain the use of fluorouracil.**	Fluorouracil is used to treat colon, rectal, breast, ovarian, cervical, bladder, liver, and pancreatic cancers because of its ability to interfere with DNA synthesis.
3 **Identify potential side effects of fluorouracil.**	Fluorouracil has the following side effects: Blood: leukopenia (decrease in leukocytes), thrombocytopenia (decrease in platelets), anemia GI: stomatitis (inflammation of the mouth); GI ulcer, which precedes leukopenia, nausea, and vomiting in 30% to 50% of patients; diarrhea Skin: dermatitis; hyperpigmentation (increased color in skin), especially in blacks; nail changes; pigmented palmar creases Other: reversible alopecia (hair loss) in 5% to 20% of patients, weakness, malaise (general feeling of tiredness)

4 Discuss guidelines to follow while taking fluorouracil.	The patient should follow these guidelines while taking fluorouracil: —Use highly protective sun blockers to avoid inflammatory erythematous dermatitis. —Expect possible alopecia; it is reversible.

GLUTETHIMIDE (Doriden, Rolathimide)

Patient objectives	*Teaching plan content*
1 State the name of the medication, the dose prescribed, and the ordered frequency of administration.	This information should be obtained from the patient's physician.
2 Explain the use of glutethimide.	Glutethimide is used to treat insomnia, as a sedative, and as a preoperative medication.
3 Identify potential side effects of glutethimide.	Glutethimide has the following side effects: CNS: residual sedation, dizziness, ataxia, paradoxical excitation (variable excitation), headache, vertigo EENT: dry mouth, blurred vision GI: irritation, nausea, diarrhea GU: bladder atony (loss of bladder tone) Skin: rash, urticaria (hives)
4 Discuss guidelines to follow while taking glutethimide.	The patient should follow these guidelines while taking glutethimide: —Take only as directed. Do not adjust the dose or discontinue the drug without the physician's approval. —Do not drink alcoholic beverages or take other drugs (such as CNS depressants or narcotic analgesics) without first consulting a physician. —Avoid activities that require alertness.

GOLD (Myochrysine)

Patient objectives	*Teaching plan content*
1 State the name of the medication, the dose prescribed, and the ordered frequency of administration.	This information should be obtained from the patient's physician.

2 Explain the use of gold.	Gold is used to treat rheumatoid arthritis because of its ability to decrease inflammation.
3 Identify potential side effects of gold.	Gold has the following side effects: Blood: thrombocytopenia (decrease in platelets) with or without purpura, aplastic anemia, agranulocytosis (decrease in granulocytes), leukopenia (decrease in leukocytes) CNS: dizziness, syncope, sweating CV: bradycardia EENT: corneal gold deposition, corneal ulcers GI: metallic taste, stomatitis (inflammation of the mouth), difficulty swallowing, nausea, vomiting GU: albuminuria (albumin in the urine), proteinuria (protein in the urine), nephrotic syndrome, nephritis, acute tubular necrosis Hepatic: hepatitis, jaundice Skin: rash and dermatitis in 20% of patients. If drug is not stopped, it may lead to fatal exfoliative dermatitis (skin inflammation in which layers of skin peel off). Other: anaphylaxis (severe allergic reaction), angioneurotic edema
4 Discuss guidelines to follow while receiving gold salt therapy.	The patient should follow these guidelines while receiving gold salt therapy: —Be aware that most adverse effects are readily reversible if gold salt therapy is stopped immediately. —Lie down and remain recumbent for 10 to 20 minutes after injection. —Dermatitis is the most common adverse effect of gold salt therapy. Report any skin rashes or problems immediately. Pruritus (itching) often precedes dermatitis and should be considered a warning of impending skin reactions. Any pruritic skin eruption while receiving gold salt therapy should be considered a reaction until proven otherwise. Therapy will be stopped until the reaction subsides. —Stomatitis (inflammation of the mouth) is the second most common adverse effect of gold salt therapy and is often preceded by a metallic taste. Report this warning symptom to the physician immediately. —Expect urine to be analyzed for protein and sediment changes before each injection. —Close medical follow-up and frequent blood and urine tests during therapy are extremely important.

HALOPERIDOL (Haldol)

Patient objectives	*Teaching plan content*
1 State the name of the medication, the dose prescribed, and the ordered frequency of administration.	This information should be obtained from the patient's physician.
2 Explain the use of haloperidol.	Haloperidol is used to treat psychotic disorders because of its ability to block postsynaptic dopamine receptors in the brain.
3 Identify potential side effects of haloperidol.	Haloperidol has the following side effects: Blood: transient leukopenia (reduction in number of leukocytes) and leukocytosis (transient increase in number of leukocytes) CNS: high incidence of severe extrapyramidal reactions (tremors, choppy gait, trouble with coordination), low incidence of sedation CV: low incidence of cardiovascular effects with therapeutic dosages EENT: blurred vision, dry mouth GU: urinary retention, menstrual irregularities, gynecomastia (development of breasts and female attributes in the male) Skin: rash
4 Discuss guidelines to follow while taking haloperidol.	The patient should follow these guidelines while taking haloperidol: —Take only as directed. Do not adjust the dose or discontinue the drug without the physician's approval. —Do not mix with lithium, methyldopa, alcohol, or other depressants. —Avoid activities that require alertness or good psychomotor coordination until CNS response to drug is determined. —Protect medication from light. Slight yellowing of injection or concentrate is common and does not affect potency. Discard markedly discolored solutions. —Relieve dry mouth with sugarless gum, sour hard candy, or mouthwash.

HEPARIN

Patient objectives	*Teaching plan content*
1 State the name of the medication, the dose prescribed, and the ordered frequency of administration.	This information should be obtained from the patient's physician.
2 Explain the use of heparin.	Heparin is used in the treatment of pulmonary embolism and in the prevention and treatment of embolism and deep-vein thrombosis because of its ability to inactivate thrombin and prevent the conversion of fibrinogen to fibrin.
3 Identify potential side effects of heparin.	Heparin has the following side effects: Blood: hemorrhage with excessive dosage, overly prolonged clotting time, thrombocytopenia (decrease in platelets) Local: irritation, mild pain Other: hypersensitivity reactions, including chills, fever, pruritus (itching), rhinitis, burning of feet, conjunctivitis, lacrimation, arthralgia, urticaria (hives) Inform the nurse or physician if any of the above occurs.
4 Discuss procedures that will be followed when heparin is administered.	These procedures are followed when the patient is receiving heparin: —Frequent blood tests will be done to measure platelets and partial thromboplastin time. —He will be regularly inspected for bleeding gums, bruises on arms and legs, petechiae (pinpoint purplish dots caused by bleeding under the skin), nosebleeds, melena (dark stools stained with blood), tarry stools, hematuria (blood in urine), hematemesis (coughing up of blood). —The infusion or injection site will be checked frequently.

HYDROCORTISONE (INTRAARTICULAR INJECTION) (Cortef, Hydrocortone)

Patient objectives	*Teaching plan content*
1 State the name of the medication, the dose prescribed, and the ordered frequency of administration.	This information should be obtained from the patient's physician.

2 Explain the use of hydrocortisone by intraarticular injection.	Hydrocortisone is used to treat severe inflammation because of its ability to accelerate protein breakdown.
3 Identify potential side effects of hydrocortisone by intraarticular injection.	Hydrocortisone has the following side effects: Muscle and joint: increase in local joint pain and pain in surrounding tissues for 24 to 48 hours after intraarticular injection Other: fever, persistent increased pain, redness and swelling (These signs indicate septic arthritis.)
4 Discuss guidelines to follow after receiving hydrocortisone by intraarticular injection.	The patient should follow these guidelines after receiving hydrocortisone by intraarticular injection: —Avoid excessive use of the affected joint because it may mask pain. —Apply ice to the joint if permitted by the physician.

HYDROCORTISONE (OTIC)

Patient objectives	*Teaching plan content*
1 State the name of the medication, the dose prescribed, and the ordered frequency of administration.	This information should be obtained from the patient's physician.
2 Explain the use of hydrocortisone (otic).	Hydrocortisone (otic) is used to treat inflammation of the external ear canal because of its ability to control inflammation, edema, and pruritus (itching).
3 Identify potential side effects of hydrocortisone (otic).	Hydrocortisone (otic) has the following side effects: Systemic: adrenal suppression with long-term use Other: may mask or exacerbate underlying infection
4 Discuss guidelines to follow while using hydrocortisone (otic).	The patient should follow these guidelines while using hydrocortisone (otic): —Avoid touching the ear with the dropper. —Take only as directed.

HYDROMORPHONE (Dilaudid)

Patient objectives	*Teaching plan content*
1 State the name of the medication, the dose prescribed, and the ordered frequency of administration.	This information should be obtained from the patient's physician.
2 Explain the use of hydromorphone.	Hydromorphone is used to treat moderate-to-severe pain because of its ability to alter both the perception of and the emotional response to pain.
3 Identify potential side effects of hydromorphone.	Hydromorphone has the following side effects: CNS: sedation, somnolence (sleepiness), clouded sensorium, euphoria, convulsions with large doses CV: hypotension (low blood pressure), bradycardia (slow heartbeat) GI: nausea, vomiting, constipation, ileus GU: urinary retention Local: induration with repeated subcutaneous injection Other: respiratory depression, physical dependence
4 Discuss guidelines to follow while taking hydromorphone.	The patient should follow these guidelines while taking hydromorphone: —Take only as directed. Do not adjust the dose without the physician's approval. —Avoid drinking alcoholic beverages while taking this drug. —Avoid activities that require alertness. —Be aware that this drug may cause constipation.

HYDROXYCHLOROQUINE (Plaquenil)

Patient objectives	*Teaching plan content*
1 State the name of the medication, the dose prescribed, and the ordered frequency of administration.	This information should be obtained from the patient's physician.
2 Explain the use of hydroxychloroquine.	Hydroxychloroquine is used to treat rheumatoid arthritis. The exact mechanism of action is unknown.

3 Identify potential side effects of hydroxychloroquine.

Hydroxychloroquine has the following side effects:
Blood: agranulocytosis (decrease in granulocytes), leukopenia (decrease in leukocytes), thrombocytopenia (decrease in platelets), aplastic anemia
CNS: irritability, nightmares, ataxia (irregularity of muscle coordination), convulsions, psychic stimulation, toxic psychosis, vertigo, tinnitus (ringing in the ears), nystagmus (irregular movement of the eyes when they are horizontal or vertical), lassitude, fatigue, dizziness, hypoactive deep tendon reflexes, skeletal muscle weakness
EENT: visual disturbances (blurred vision; difficulty in focusing; reversible corneal changes; generally irreversible, sometimes progressive or delayed retinal changes—that is, narrowing of arterioles; macular lesions; pallor of optic disk; optic atrophy; visual field defects; patchy retinal pigmentation, often leading to blindness), ototoxicity (irreversible nerve deafness, tinnitus, labyrinthitis)
GI: anorexia, abdominal cramps, diarrhea, nausea, vomiting
Skin: pruritus (itching), lichen planus–like eruptions, skin and mucosal pigmentary changes
Other: weight loss, bleaching of hair

4 Discuss guidelines to follow while taking hydroxychloroquine.

The patient should follow these guidelines while taking hydroxychloroquine:
—This drug should be taken only as directed. Do not adjust the dose or discontinue the drug without the physician's approval.
—Complete blood counts and liver function studies should be made periodically during prolonged therapy.
—Baseline and periodic ophthalmologic examinations are needed. Report blurred vision, increased sensitivity to light, or muscle weakness.
—Audiometric examinations are recommended before, during, and after therapy, especially if long-term.

IBUPROFEN (Motrin, Rufen)

Patient objectives	*Teaching plan content*
1 State the name of the medication, the dose prescribed, and the ordered frequency of administration.	This information should be obtained from the patient's physician.

2 **Explain the use of ibuprofen.**	Ibuprofen is used to treat arthritis, dysmenorrhea, gout, and mild pain because of its ability to inhibit prostaglandin synthesis and therefore reduce inflammation.
3 **Identify potential side effects of ibuprofen.**	Ibuprofen has the following side effects: Blood: prolonged bleeding time CNS: headache, drowsiness, dizziness CV: peripheral edema EENT: visual disturbances, tinnitus GI: epigastric distress, nausea, occult blood loss GU: reversible renal failure Hepatic: elevated enzyme levels Skin: pruritus (itching), rash, urticaria (hives) Other: aseptic meningitis, bronchospasm, edema
4 **Discuss guidelines to follow while taking ibuprofen.**	The patient should follow these guidelines while taking ibuprofen: —Take only as directed. Do not adjust the dose or discontinue the drug without the physician's approval. —Report to the physician immediately any GI symptoms or signs of bleeding, visual disturbances, skin rashes, weight gain, or edema. —Take with meals to reduce GI adverse effects.

IMIPRAMINE (Janimine, Presamine, SK-Pramine, Tofranil)

Patient objectives	*Teaching plan content*
1 **State the name of the medication, the dose prescribed, and the ordered frequency of administration.**	This information should be obtained from the patient's physician.
2 **Explain the use of imipramine.**	Imipramine is used to treat depression because of its ability to increase the amount of norepinephrine and/or serotonin in the central nervous system.
3 **Identify potential side effects of imipramine.**	Imipramine has the following side effects: CNS: drowsiness, dizziness, excitation, tremors, weakness, confusion, headache, nervousness CV: orthostatic hypotension (light-headedness on rising), tachycardia, EKG changes, hypertension EENT: blurred vision, tinnitus, mydriasis GI: dry mouth, constipation, nausea, vomiting, anorexia, paralytic ileus

GU: urinary retention
Skin: rash, urticaria (hives)
Other: sweating, allergy
After abrupt withdrawal of long-term therapy: nausea, headache, malaise. (These symptoms do not indicate addiction.)

4 Discuss guidelines to follow while taking imipramine.	The patient should follow these guidelines while taking imipramine: —Take only as directed. Do not adjust the dose or discontinue the drug without the physician's approval. —Increase fluid intake to lessen constipation. Inquire about a stool softener, if needed. —Avoid activities that require alertness and good psychomotor coordination until response to drug is determined. —Relieve dry mouth with sugarless gum or hard candy. —Do not drink alcoholic beverages or take any other drugs without first consulting the physician.

IMMUNE SERUM GLOBULIN (Gamastan, Gamimune, Gammar, Immuglobin)

Patient objectives	*Teaching plan content*
1 State the name of the medication, the dose prescribed, and the ordered frequency of administration.	This information should be obtained from the patient's physician.
2 Explain the use of immune serum globulin.	Immune serum globulin is used to provide passive immunity against various infectious diseases or to suppress antibody formation. Immune serums contain preformed, protective substances (antibodies) from the serum of humans or animals that have been injected with the organisms or toxins of diseases. They are used as a prophylactic treatment in those persons who are immunodeficient or immunocompromised.
3 Identify potential side effects of immune serum globulin.	Immune serum globulin has the following side effects: Local: pain, erythema (redness), muscle stiffness Skin: urticaria (hives) Systemic: angioedema (temporary swelling of the skin

or mucous membranes), headache, malaise, fever, nephrotic syndrome (characterized by edema, protein in the urine, and a decrease in blood albumin level), anaphylaxis (severe allergic response)

4 **Discuss guidelines to follow while receiving immune serum globulin.**	The patient should follow these guidelines while receiving immune serum globulin: —Report any unusual reactions to the nurse or physician. —Give a full history of any allergies and reactions to immunizations *before* receiving immune serum globulin.

INDOMETHACIN (Indocin)

Patient objectives	*Teaching plan content*
1 **State the name of the medication, the dose prescribed, and the ordered frequency of administration.**	This information should be obtained from the patient's physician.
2 **Explain the use of indomethacin.**	Indomethacin is used primarily to treat arthritis and acute gouty arthritis because of its anti-inflammatory, analgesic, and antipyretic effects.
3 **Identify potential side effects of indomethacin.**	Indomethacin has the following side effects: Blood: hemolytic anemia, aplastic anemia, agranulocytosis (decrease in granulocytes), leukopenia (decrease in leukocytes), thrombocytopenic purpura (bruising from a decrease in platelets), iron deficiency anemia CNS: headache, dizziness, depression, drowsiness, confusion, peripheral neuropathy, convulsions, psychic disturbances, syncope, vertigo CV: hypertension, edema EENT: blurred vision, corneal and retinal damage, hearing loss, tinnitus GI: nausea, vomiting, anorexia, diarrhea, severe GI bleeding GU: hematuria (blood in urine), hyperkalemia (increased serum potassium level), acute renal failure Hepatic: elevated enzymes Skin: pruritus (itching), urticaria (hives) Other: hypersensitivity (shocklike symptoms, rash, respiratory distress, angioedema)

4 Discuss guidelines to follow while taking indomethacin.	The patient should follow these guidelines while taking indomethacin: —Take only as directed. Do not adjust the dose or discontinue the drug without the physician's approval. —Do not take any other drugs without first consulting the physician. —Notify the physician if headache or visual or hearing changes develop. —Take with meals.

INTERFERONS

Patient objectives	*Teaching plan content*
1 State the name of the medication, the dose prescribed, and the ordered frequency of administration.	This information should be obtained from the patient's physician.
2 Explain the use of interferons.	Interferons are proteins produced in human or animal cells following exposure chiefly to viruses. They are being used investigationally for cancer therapy because of their ability to alter cell growth and affect the immune system.
3 Identify potential side effects of interferons.	Interferons have the following side effects: Blood: myelosuppression with leukopenia and thrombocytopenia CNS: hypotension GI: anorexia, nausea, vomiting Skin: alopecia, erythema at injection site Other: fever, shivering, malaise, fatigue, pain at injection site
4 Discuss guidelines to follow while being given interferons.	The patient should follow these guidelines while being given interferons: —Report any unusual adverse effects to the nurse or physician. —Do not take aspirin or indomethacin; they might reduce interferon activity. —Come to a sitting position slowly when arising, to minimize hypotension.

INTERLEUKIN-2

Patient objectives	Teaching plan content
1 State the name of the medication, the dose prescribed, and the ordered frequency of administration.	This information should be obtained from the patient's physician.
2 Explain the use of interleukin-2.	Interleukin-2 is used investigationally to treat Kaposi's sarcoma in immunologically depressed patients.
3 Identify potential side effects of interleukin-2.	Interleukin-2 has the following side effects: GI: nausea, vomiting Muscular: mild aching Other: chills, fever
4 Discuss guidelines to follow while receiving interleukin-2.	The patient should follow these guidelines while receiving interleukin-2: —Report all unusual side effects to the nurse or physician.

ISOCARBOXAZID (Marplan)

Patient objectives	Teaching plan content
1 State the name of the medication, the dose prescribed, and the ordered frequency of administration.	This information should be obtained from the patient's physician.
2 Explain the use of isocarboxazid.	Isocarboxazid is used to treat depression because of its ability to block monoamine oxidase (MAO), causing a buildup of certain neurotransmitters (substances that carry impulses within the central nervous system) and resulting in an antidepressant action.
3 Identify potential side effects of isocarboxazid.	Isocarboxazid has the following side effects: CNS: dizziness, vertigo, weakness, headache, hyperactivity, hyperreflexia, tremors, muscle twitching, mania, insomnia, confusion, memory impairment, fatigue CV: orthostatic hypotension (light-headedness on rising), dysrhythmias, paradoxical hypertension (variable high blood pressure) EENT: blurred vision

GI: dry mouth, anorexia, nausea, diarrhea, constipation
GU: altered libido
Skin: rash
Other: peripheral edema, sweating, weight changes

4 Discuss guidelines to follow while taking isocarboxazid.	The patient should follow these guidelines while taking isocarboxazid: —Take only as directed. Do not adjust the dose or discontinue the drug without the physician's approval. —Do not drink alcoholic beverages or take any other drugs without the physician's permission. —Avoid foods high in the amino acids tyramine (such as cheeses, beer, wine, and beans) or tryptophan (such as meat and fish), large amounts of caffeine, and self-medication with over-the-counter cold, hay fever, or diet preparations. —Get out of bed slowly, sitting up first for 1 minute. This will help reduce orthostatic hypotension. —Continue precautions for 10 days after stopping the drug because of its long-lasting effects. —If symptoms of overdosage develop (palpitations, frequent headaches, or severe orthostatic hypotension), hold dose and notify the physician.

ISOFLUROPHATE (Floropryl)

Patient objectives	*Teaching plan content*
1 State the name of the medication, the dose prescribed, and the ordered frequency of administration.	This information should be obtained from the patient's physician.
2 Explain the use of isoflurophate.	Isoflurophate is used to treat glaucoma because of its ability to cause pupillary constriction and accommodation spasm.
3 Identify potential side effects of isoflurophate.	Isoflurophate has the following side effects: CNS: headache, muscle weakness Eye: moderate conjunctival hyperemia (increased collection of blood), eye pain, ciliary spasm causing discomfort, iris cysts, cataract formation, retinal detachment, paradoxical increase in intraocular pressure; precipitates attacks of acute narrow-angle glaucoma GI: diarrhea, salivation Other: sweating, bronchial constriction

| **4** Discuss guidelines to follow while using isoflurophate. | The patient should follow these guidelines while using isoflurophate:
—Use at bedtime if possible because of blurred vision and ciliary muscle spasm.
—Do not touch the tip of the tube to the eye, surrounding tissue, or moist surface.
—Apply light finger pressure on the lacrimal (tear) sac for 1 minute following instillation to minimize systemic absorption.
—Maintain close, constant medical supervision.
—Do not exceed prescribed dosage.
—Stop therapy at once and notify the physician if excessive salivation, diarrhea, sweating, or muscle weakness occurs.
—Store in refrigerator in a tightly closed container.
—Wash hands before and after administering medication. |

ISONIAZID (I.N.H.) (Laniazid, Teebaconin)

Patient objectives	*Teaching plan content*
1 State the name of the medication, the dose prescribed, and the ordered frequency of administration.	This information should be obtained from the patient's physician.
2 Explain the use of isoniazid.	Isoniazid is used to treat tuberculosis and *Mycobacterium avium intracellulare* because of its ability to inhibit bacterial cell wall synthesis.
3 Identify potential side effects of isoniazid.	Isoniazid has the following side effects: Blood: hemolytic anemia CNS: peripheral neuropathy, usually preceded by paresthesias (numbness and tingling) of hands and feet; psychosis GI: nausea, vomiting, epigastric distress, constipation, dryness of the mouth Hepatic: hepatitis, occasionally severe and sometimes fatal, especially in the elderly Local: irritation at injection site Metabolic: hyperglycemia, metabolic acidosis Other: hypersensitivity
4 Discuss guidelines to follow while taking isoniazid.	The patient should follow these guidelines while taking isoniazid: —Take only as directed. Do not adjust the dose or dis-

continue the drug without the physician's approval.
—Do not take with antacids or laxatives containing aluminum.
—Do not take with corticosteroids.
—Do not drink alcoholic beverages.
—Take pyridoxine, as ordered, to prevent peripheral neuropathy.
—Take this drug with food to decrease GI irritation.

ISOSORBIDE (Ismotic)

Patient objectives	Teaching plan content
1 State the name of the medication, the dose prescribed, and the ordered frequency of administration.	This information should be obtained from the patient's physician.
2 Explain the use of isosorbide.	Isosorbide is used for short-term reduction of intraocular pressure due to glaucoma because of its ability to redistribute water and promote diuresis (increased secretion of urine).
3 Identify potential side effects of isosorbide.	Isosorbide has the following side effects: CNS: vertigo, light-headedness, lethargy GI: gastric discomfort, diarrhea, anorexia Metabolic: hypernatremia, hyperosmolality
4 Discuss guidelines to follow while taking isosorbide.	The patient should follow these guidelines while taking isosorbide: —Pour over cracked ice for palatability. —Sip medication slowly.

ISOXSUPRINE (Vasodilan)

Patient objectives	Teaching plan content
1 State the name of the medication, the dose prescribed, and the ordered frequency of administration.	This information should be obtained from the patient's physician.
2 Explain the use of isoxsuprine.	Isoxsuprine is used to treat preterm labor because of its ability to stop uterine contractions through beta-receptor (adrenergic receptor tissue) stimulation.

3 Identify potential side effects of isoxsuprine.	Isoxsuprine has the following side effects: CNS: dizziness, nervousness, weakness, trembling, light-headedness CV: hypotension, tachycardia, transient palpitations GI: vomiting, abdominal distress, intestinal distention Skin: severe rash
4 Discuss guidelines to follow while taking isoxsuprine.	The patient should follow these guidelines while taking isoxsuprine: —Take only as directed. Do not adjust the dose or discontinue the drug without the physician's approval. —Discontinue the drug if a rash develops.

KAOLIN AND PECTIN MIXTURES (Kaopectate, Pecto Kay)

Patient objectives	*Teaching plan content*
1 State the name of the medication, the dose prescribed, and the ordered frequency of administration.	This information should be obtained from the patient's physician.
2 Explain the use of kaolin and pectin mixtures.	Kaolin and pectin mixtures are used for mild, nonspecific diarrhea because of their ability to decrease the stool's fluid content.
3 Identify potential side effects of kaolin and pectin mixtures.	Kaolin and pectin mixtures have the following side effects: GI: absorption of nutrients and enzymes; fecal impaction or ulceration in infants, the elderly, and the debilitated after chronic use; constipation
4 Discuss guidelines to follow while taking kaolin and pectin mixtures.	The patient should follow these guidelines while taking kaolin and pectin mixtures: —Take only as directed. Do not adjust the dose or discontinue the drug without the physician's approval. —Do not use for more than 2 days unless by a physician's order.

KETOCONAZOLE (Nizoral)

Patient objectives	Teaching plan content
1 State the name of the medication, the dose prescribed, and the ordered frequency of administration.	This information should be obtained from the patient's physician.
2 Explain the use of ketoconazole.	Ketoconazole is used to treat systemic candidiasis (a fungal infection) because of its ability to inhibit protein synthesis by the fungus, thereby making its cell walls fragile.
3 Identify potential side effects of ketoconazole.	Ketoconazole has the following side effects: CNS: headache, nervousness, dizziness GI: nausea, vomiting, abdominal pain, diarrhea, constipation Hepatic: elevated liver enzyme levels, fatal hepatotoxicity Skin: itching
4 Discuss guidelines to follow while taking ketoconazole.	The patient should follow these guidelines while taking ketoconazole: —Take only as directed. Do not adjust the dose or discontinue the drug without the physician's approval. —Continue treatment, as ordered, until all clinical and laboratory tests indicate that active fungal infection has subsided. —Do not take with antacids or cimetidine; they decrease absorption of this drug from the stomach. Wait at least 2 hours. —Anticipate nausea early in therapy; it will soon subside.

LEVAMISOLE

Patient objectives	Teaching plan content
1 State the name of the medication, the dose prescribed, and the ordered frequency of administration.	This information should be obtained from the patient's physician.

2 Explain the use of levamisole.	Levamisole is used as an adjunctive to chemotherapy in malignant disease because of its ability to prolong the disease-free period and increase survival time.
3 Identify potential side effects of levamisole.	Levamisole has the following side effects: Blood: neutropenia, thrombocytopenia, reversible agranulocytosis CNS: headache, confusion, insomnia, dizziness, hypotension CV: chest pain GI: nausea, vomiting, abdominal pain, taste disturbance Musculoskeletal: arthralgia, muscle pain, spastic contractions of muscles of the extremities, motor aphasia Renal: proteinuria Skin: rash, urticaria Other: influenza-like symptoms
4 Discuss guidelines to follow while taking levamisole.	The patient should follow these guidelines while taking levamisole: —Report any unusual adverse effects to the nurse or physician. —Conserve energy. —Take only as directed. Do not adjust the dose or discontinue the drug without the physician's approval.

LITHIUM (Cibalith-S, Eskalith, Eskalith CR, Lithane, Lithobid, Lithonate, Lithotabs)

Patient objectives	*Teaching plan content*
1 State the name of the medication, the dose prescribed, and the ordered frequency of administration.	This information should be obtained from the patient's physician.
2 Explain the use of lithium.	Lithium is used to treat acute manic or hypomanic episodes of manic-depressive disorders and to prevent their recurrence. Lithium is also being used investigationally to increase the white blood cell count during cancer chemotherapy.
3 Identify potential side effects of lithium.	Lithium has the following side effects: CNS: tremors, drowsiness, headache, confusion, restlessness, dizziness, stupor, lethargy, coma, seizures, impaired speech

CV: irregular heart rhythms, hypotension, ankle and wrist edema
EENT: tinnitus (ringing in the ears), blurred vision
GI: nausea, vomiting, anorexia, diarrhea, dry mouth, thirst, metallic taste
GU: increased urination
Metabolic: decreased serum sodium and blood glucose levels
Skin: rash, itching

4 Discuss guidelines to follow while taking lithium.	The patient should follow these guidelines while taking lithium: —Take only as directed. Do not adjust the dose or discontinue the drug without the physician's approval. —Take with plenty of water and after meals to minimize GI upset. —Do not mix with diuretics or any other prescription or over-the-counter drugs without the physician's guidance.

LOMUSTINE (C.C.N.U.) (CeeNU)

Patient objectives	*Teaching plan content*
1 State the name of the medication, the dose prescribed, and the ordered frequency of administration.	This information should be obtained from the patient's physician.
2 Explain the use of lomustine.	Lomustine is used to treat brain, colon, lung, and renal cell cancer; Hodgkin's disease; lymphomas; melanomas; and multiple myelomas because of its ability to cross-link strands of cellular DNA, causing an imbalance of growth that leads to cell death.
3 Identify potential side effects of lomustine.	Lomustine has the following side effects: Blood: leukopenia (decrease in leukocytes) delayed up to 6 weeks, lasting 1 to 2 weeks; thrombocytopenia (decrease in platelets) delayed up to 4 weeks, lasting 1 to 2 weeks GI: nausea and vomiting beginning within 4 to 5 hours, lasting 24 hours; stomatitis (inflammation of the mouth) GU: nephrotoxicity, progressive azotemia (retention of nitrogenous substances in the blood) Other: alopecia (hair loss)

4 Discuss guidelines to follow while taking lomustine.	The patient should follow these guidelines while taking lomustine: —Take only as directed. Do not adjust the dose or discontinue the drug without the physician's approval. —Take 2 to 4 hours after meals. Avoid nausea by taking an antiemetic beforehand, as ordered. —Expect possible alopecia; hair will grow back.

LOPERAMIDE (Imodium)

Patient objectives	*Teaching plan content*
1 State the name of the medication, the dose prescribed, and the ordered frequency of administration.	This information should be obtained from the patient's physician.
2 Explain the use of loperamide.	Loperamide is used for acute, nonspecific diarrhea because of its ability to decrease intestinal activity, prolonging the transit of intestinal contents.
3 Identify potential side effects of loperamide.	Loperamide has the following side effects: CNS: drowsiness, fatigue, dizziness GI: dry mouth; abdominal pain, distention, or discomfort; constipation; nausea; vomiting Skin: rash
4 Discuss guidelines to follow while taking loperamide.	The patient should follow these guidelines while taking loperamide: —Take only as directed. Do not adjust the dose or discontinue the drug without the physician's approval. —Report any unusual adverse effects to the nurse or physician.

MAGNESIUM SULFATE

Patient objectives	*Teaching plan content*
1 State the name of the medication, the dose prescribed, and the ordered frequency of administration.	This information should be obtained from the patient's physician.

2 Explain the use of magnesium sulfate.	Magnesium sulfate is used to prevent or control seizures in toxemia of pregnancy (preeclampsia or eclampsia) because of its anticonvulsant properties. The exact mechanism of action is unknown.
3 Identify potential side effects of magnesium sulfate.	Magnesium sulfate has the following side effects: CNS: sweating, drowsiness, depressed reflexes, flaccid paralysis, hypothermia CV: hypotension, flushing, circulatory collapse, depressed cardiac function, heart block Other: respiratory paralysis, hypocalcemia (decreased serum calcium level) Any side effect should be reported to the physician immediately.
4 Discuss procedures that will be followed while magnesium sulfate is administered.	These procedures are followed when the patient is receiving magnesium sulfate: —Magnesium sulfate can decrease the frequency and force of uterine contractions. Uterine contractions will be monitored closely. —Vital signs will be monitored every 15 minutes while the I.V. drug is being administered. —The patient must inform the nurse if respirations become slower and it becomes difficult to breathe. —Urinary output will be monitored closely by the nurse and the physician. —Deep tendon reflexes will be monitored periodically.

MAPROTILINE (Ludiomil)

Patient objectives	*Teaching plan content*
1 State the name of the medication, the dose prescribed, and the ordered frequency of administration.	This information should be obtained from the patient's physician.
2 Explain the use of maprotiline.	Maprotiline is used to treat the symptoms of depression because of its ability to increase the amount of norepinephrine and/or serotonin in the central nervous system.
3 Identify potential side effects of maprotiline.	Maprotiline has the following side effects: CNS: drowsiness, dizziness, excitation, seizures, tremors, weakness, confusion, headache, nervousness

CV: orthostatic hypotension (light-headedness on rising), tachycardia, EKG changes, hypertension
EENT: blurred vision, tinnitus (ringing in the ears), mydriasis (pupil dilation)
GI: dry mouth, constipation, nausea, vomiting, anorexia, paralytic ileus
GU: urinary retention
Skin: rash, urticaria (hives)
Other: sweating, allergy
After abrupt withdrawal of long-term therapy: nausea, headache, malaise. (These symptoms do not indicate addiction.)

4 Discuss guidelines to follow while taking maprotiline.	The patient should follow these guidelines while taking maprotiline: —Take only as directed. Do not adjust the dose or discontinue the drug without the physician's approval. —Do not take any other drugs without the physician's approval. —Increase fluids to lessen constipation. Inquire about a stool softener, if needed. —Avoid activities that require alertness and good psychomotor coordination until CNS response to drug is determined. Drowsiness and dizziness usually subside after a few weeks. —Relieve dry mouth with sugarless hard candy or gum.

MEPERIDINE (Demerol)

Patient objectives	*Teaching plan content*
1 State the name of the medication, the dose prescribed, and the ordered frequency of administration.	This information should be obtained from the patient's physician.
2 Explain the use of meperidine.	Meperidine is used to treat moderate-to-severe pain and to furnish preoperative sedation because of its ability to alter both the perception of and the emotional response to pain.
3 Identify potential side effects of meperidine.	Meperidine has the following side effects: CNS: sedation, somnolence (sleepiness), clouded sensorium, euphoria, convulsions with large doses CV: hypotension (low blood pressure), bradycardia (slow heartbeat)

GI: nausea, vomiting, constipation, ileus
GU: urinary retention
Local: pain at injection site, local tissue irritation and
induration after subcutaneous injection, phlebitis after
I.V. injection
Other: respiratory depression, physical dependence

4 **Discuss guidelines to follow while taking meperidine.**	The patient should follow these guidelines while taking meperidine: —Do not drink alcoholic beverages or take any other drugs (especially barbiturates) without the physician's approval. —Avoid activities that require alertness. —Take only as directed. Do not adjust the dose without the physician's approval. —Syrup has a local anesthetic effect: take with a full glass of water.

METHADONE (Dolophine, Methadone)

Patient objectives	*Teaching plan content*
1 **State the name of the medication, the dose prescribed, and the ordered frequency of administration.**	This information should be obtained from the patient's physician.
2 **Explain the use of methadone.**	Methadone is used to treat severe pain because of its ability to alter both the perception of and the emotional response to pain.
3 **Identify potential side effects of methadone.**	Methadone has the following side effects: CNS: sedation, somnolence (sleepiness), clouded sensorium, euphoria, convulsions with large doses CV: hypotension (low blood pressure), bradycardia (abnormally slow heartbeat) GI: nausea, vomiting, constipation, ileus GU: urinary retention Local: pain at injection site, tissue irritation, induration following subcutaneous injection Other: respiratory depression, physical dependence
4 **Discuss guidelines to follow while taking methadone.**	The patient should follow these guidelines while taking methadone via oral administration: —Take only as directed. Do not adjust the dose or discontinue the drug without the physician's approval.

— Do not drink alcoholic beverages or take any other drugs without the physician's approval.
—Avoid activities that require alertness.
—Constipation is often severe; inquire about a stool softener or laxative.

METHOTREXATE (Mexate)

Patient objectives	Teaching plan content
1 State the name of the medication, the dose prescribed, and the ordered frequency of administration.	This information should be obtained from the patient's physician.
2 Explain the use of methotrexate.	Methotrexate is used to treat acute leukemias, lymphosarcoma, trophoblastic tumors, meningeal leukemia, Burkitt's lymphoma, mycosis fungoides, and psoriasis because of its ability to prevent the breakdown of folic acid in the tumor cell, thereby interfering with cellular metabolism.
3 Identify potential side effects of methotrexate.	Methotrexate has the following side effects: Blood: anemia, leukopenia (decrease in leukocytes), thrombocytopenia (decrease in platelets)—all dose-related CNS: arachnoiditis (inflammation of the tissue surrounding the brain and spinal cord) within hours of intrathecal use; subacute neurotoxicity that may begin a few weeks later; necrotizing demyelinating leukoencephalopathy a few years later GI: stomatitis (inflammation of the mouth), diarrhea leading to hemorrhagic enteritis and intestinal perforation, nausea, vomiting GU: tubular necrosis Hepatic: hepatic dysfunction leading to cirrhosis or hepatic fibrosis Metabolic: hyperuricemia (an increase in serum uric acid) Skin: exposure to sun may aggravate psoriatic lesions, rash, photosensitivity Other: alopecia (hair loss); pulmonary interstitial infiltrates; osteoporosis (an increase in porousness of the bones) possible in children after long-term use
4 Discuss guidelines to follow while taking methotrexate.	The patient should follow these guidelines while taking methotrexate: —Take only as directed. Do not adjust the dose or dis-

continue the drug without the physician's approval.
—Do not drink alcoholic beverages or take any other drugs without the physician's approval.
—Avoid conception during and immediately after therapy because of possible abortion or congenital anomalies.
—Use highly protective sunscreening agents when exposed to sunlight.
—Watch for bleeding (especially GI) and infection.
—Take temperature daily, and watch for cough, dyspnea, or cyanosis.

METHYLPREDNISOLONE (OTIC) (Medrol)

Patient objectives	*Teaching plan content*
1 State the name of the medication, the dose prescribed, and the ordered frequency of administration.	This information should be obtained from the patient's physician.
2 Explain the use of methylprednisolone (otic).	Methylprednisolone (otic) is used to treat inflammation of the external ear canal because of its ability to control inflammation, edema, and pruritus (itching).
3 Identify potential side effects of methylprednisolone (otic).	Methylprednisolone (otic) has the following side effects: Systemic: adrenal suppression with long-term use Other: may mask or exacerbate underlying infection
4 Discuss guidelines to follow while using methylprednisolone (otic).	The patient should follow these guidelines while using methylprednisolone (otic): —Avoid touching the ear with the dropper. —Take only as directed.

MITOMYCIN (Mutamycin)

Patient objectives	*Teaching plan content*
1 State the name of the medication, the dose prescribed, and the ordered frequency of administration.	This information should be obtained from the patient's physician.
2 Explain the use of mitomycin.	Mitomycin is used to treat breast, colon, head, neck, lung, pancreatic, and stomach cancer and malignant

melanoma because of its ability to cross-link strands of DNA. This causes an imbalance of cell growth, leading to cell death.

3 Identify potential side effects of mitomycin.	Mitomycin has the following side effects: Blood: thrombocytopenia (decrease in platelets), leukopenia (decrease in leukocytes)—may be delayed up to 8 weeks and may be cumulative with successive doses CNS: paresthesias (numbness and tingling in extremities) GI: nausea, vomiting, anorexia, stomatitis (inflammation of the mouth) Local: desquamation, induration, pruritus (itching), pain at site of injection. Extravasation causes cellulitis, ulceration, and sloughing. Other: reversible alopecia (hair loss), purple nail beds, fever
4 Discuss guidelines to follow while taking mitomycin.	The patient should follow these guidelines while taking mitomycin: —Be aware that alopecia may occur but is reversible. —Watch for signs of unusual bleeding.

MORPHINE (RMS)

Patient objectives	*Teaching plan content*
1 State the name of the medication, the dose prescribed, and the ordered frequency of administration.	This information should be obtained from the patient's physician.
2 Explain the use of morphine.	Morphine is used for severe pain because of its ability to alter both the perception of and the emotional response to pain.
3 Identify potential side effects of morphine.	Morphine has the following side effects: CNS: sedation, somnolence (sleepiness), clouded sensorium, euphoria, convulsions with large doses CV: hypotension (low blood pressure), bradycardia (abnormally slow heartbeat) GI: nausea, vomiting, constipation, ileus GU: urinary retention Other: respiratory depression, physical dependence
4 Discuss guidelines to follow while taking morphine.	The patient should follow these guidelines while taking morphine via oral administration: —Take only as directed. Do not adjust the dose or dis-

continue the drug without the physician's approval.
—Do not drink alcoholic beverages or take any other
drugs without the physician's approval.
—Avoid activities that require alertness.
—Constipation is often severe; inquire about a stool
softener or laxative.

NAPHAZOLINE 0.012%, 0.02%, 0.1% (AK-Con Ophthalmic, Albalon Liquifilm Ophthalmic, Clear Eyes, Muro's Opcon, Naphcon, Naphcon Forte Ophthalmic, VasoClear, Vasocon Regular Ophthalmic)

Patient objectives	Teaching plan content
1 State the name of the medication, the dose prescribed, and the ordered frequency of administration.	This information should be obtained from the patient's physician.
2 Explain the use of naphazoline.	Naphazoline is used to treat ocular congestion, irritation, and itching because of its ability to produce vasoconstriction of the blood vessels of the conjunctiva.
3 Identify potential side effects of naphazoline.	Naphazoline has the following side effects: Eye: transient stinging, pupillary dilation, increased intraocular pressure, irritation
4 Discuss guidelines to follow while using naphazoline.	The patient should follow these guidelines while using naphazoline: —Report photophobia to the physician. —Do not exceed the recommended dosage. —Notify the physician if blurred vision, pain, or lid edema develops. —Store in a tightly closed container. —Do not touch the tip of the dropper to the eye or surrounding tissue.

NAPROXEN (Anaprox, Naprosyn)

Patient objectives	Teaching plan content
1 State the name of the medication, the dose prescribed, and the ordered frequency of administration.	This information should be obtained from the patient's physician.

2 Explain the use of naproxen.	Naproxen is used to treat arthritis and mild-to-moderate pain because of its ability to inhibit prostaglandin synthesis and to reduce inflammation.
3 Identify potential side effects of naproxen.	Naproxen has the following side effects: Blood: prolonged bleeding time CNS: headache, drowsiness, dizziness CV: peripheral edema GI: epigastric distress, occult blood loss, nausea GU: nephrotoxicity Hepatic: elevated enzyme levels Skin: pruritus (itching), rash, urticaria (hives)
4 Discuss guidelines to follow while taking naproxen.	The patient should follow these guidelines while taking naproxen: —Take only as directed. Do not adjust the dose or discontinue the drug without the physician's approval. —Report any GI upset to the physician immediately.

NEOMYCIN (OTIC)

Patient objectives	*Teaching plan content*
1 State the name of the medication, the dose prescribed, and the ordered frequency of administration.	This information should be obtained from the patient's physician.
2 Identify potential side effects of neomycin (otic).	Neomycin (otic) is used to treat external ear canal infections because of its ability to inhibit or destroy bacteria present in the ear canal.
3 Identify potential side effects of neomycin (otic).	Neomycin (otic) has the following side effects: Ear: ototoxicity (in patients undergoing tympanoplasty) Local: burning, erythema (redness), vesicular dermatitis, urticaria (hives) Other: overgrowth of nonsusceptible organisms
4 Discuss guidelines to follow while using neomycin (otic).	The patient should follow these guidelines while using neomycin (otic): —Watch for signs of superinfection (continued pain, inflammation, fever). —Avoid touching the ear with the dropper. —Use only as directed.

NORTRIPTYLINE (Aventyl, Pamelor)

Patient objectives	Teaching plan content
1 State the name of the medication, the dose prescribed, and the ordered frequency of administration.	This information should be obtained from the patient's physician.
2 Explain the use of nortriptyline.	Nortriptyline is used to treat the symptoms of depression because of its ability to increase the amount of norepinephrine and/or serotonin in the central nervous system.
3 Identify potential side effects of nortriptyline.	Nortriptyline has the following side effects: CNS: drowsiness, dizziness, excitation, seizures, tremors, weakness, confusion, headache, nervousness CV: tachycardia, EKG changes, hypertension (high blood pressure) EENT: blurred vision, tinnitus (ringing in the ears), mydriasis (pupil dilation) GI: dry mouth, constipation, nausea, vomiting, anorexia, paralytic ileus GU: urinary retention Skin: rash, urticaria (hives) Other: sweating, allergy After abrupt withdrawal of long-term therapy: nausea, headache, malaise. (These symptoms do not indicate addiction.)
4 Discuss guidelines to follow while taking nortriptyline.	The patient should follow these guidelines while taking nortriptyline: —Take only as directed. Do not adjust the dose or discontinue the drug without the physician's approval. —Avoid activities that require alertness and good psychomotor coordination until CNS response to this drug is determined. —Relieve dry mouth with sugarless hard candy or gum. —Do not drink alcoholic beverages or take any other drugs (prescription or over-the-counter) without first consulting the physician. —Increase fluids to lessen constipation. Inquire about a stool softener, if needed.

NYSTATIN (Mycostatin, Nilstat, O-V Statin)

Patient objectives	*Teaching plan content*
1 State the name of the medication, the dose prescribed, and the ordered frequency of administration.	This information should be obtained from the patient's physician.
2 Explain the use of nystatin.	Nystatin is used to treat infections caused by *Candida albicans* because of its ability to alter the cell membrane of the fungus.
3 Identify potential side effects of nystatin.	Nystatin has the following side effects: GI: transient nausea, vomiting, diarrhea (usually with large oral dose)
4 Discuss guidelines to follow while taking nystatin.	The patient should follow these guidelines while taking nystatin: —Take only as directed. Do not adjust the dose or discontinue the drug without the physician's approval. —For treatment of oral candidiasis (thrush): Be sure the mouth is clean of food debris before taking this drug. Hold the suspension in the mouth for several minutes before swallowing. —Avoid overuse of mouthwash or poorly fitting dentures; especially in older patients, these may alter flora and promote infection.

OXAZEPAM (Serax)

Patient objectives	*Teaching plan content*
1 State the name of the medication, the dose prescribed, and the ordered frequency of administration.	This information should be obtained from the patient's physician.
2 Explain the use of oxazepam.	Oxazepam is used to treat alcohol withdrawal, anxiety, and tension because of its ability to depress the central nervous system at the limbic (area associated with emotion and behavior) and subcortical levels of the brain, with sedative, relaxant, and anticonvulsant effects.

3 Identify potential side effects of oxazepam.	Oxazepam has the following side effects: CNS: drowsiness, lethargy, hangover, fainting CV: transient hypotension GI: nausea, vomiting, abdominal discomfort
4 Discuss guidelines to follow while taking oxazepam.	The patient should follow these guidelines while taking oxazepam: —Take only as directed. Do not adjust the dose or discontinue the drug without the physician's approval. —Do not drink alcoholic beverages or take other depressants. —Avoid activities that require alertness or good psychomotor coordination until response to this drug is determined. —Do not share medication with others.

OXYCODONE (Percocet, Percodan, Percodan-Demi, Tylox)

Patient objectives	*Teaching plan content*
1 State the name of the medication, the dose prescribed, and the ordered frequency of administration.	This information should be obtained from the patient's physician.
2 Explain the use of oxycodone.	Oxycodone is used to treat moderate-to-severe pain because of its ability to alter both the perception of and the emotional response to pain; the mechanism is unknown.
3 Identify potential side effects of oxycodone.	Oxycodone has the following side effects: CNS: sedation, somnolence (sleepiness), clouded sensorium, euphoria, convulsions with large doses CV: hypotension (low blood pressure), bradycardia (abnormally slow heartbeat) GI: nausea, vomiting, constipation, ileus GU: urinary retention Other: respiratory depression, physical dependence
4 Discuss guidelines to follow while taking oxycodone.	The patient should follow these guidelines while taking oxycodone: —Take only as directed. Do not adjust the dose or discontinue the drug without the physician's approval. —Do not drink alcoholic beverages or take other drugs (especially depressants and anticoagulants) without

the physician's approval.
—Avoid activities that require alertness.
—Take before pain is intense.
—Take after meals or with milk.

OXYTOCIN (Oxytocin, Pitocin, Syntocinon, Uteracon)

Patient objectives	*Teaching plan content*
1 State the name of the medication, the dose prescribed, and the ordered frequency of administration.	This information should be obtained from the patient's physician.
2 Explain the use of oxytocin.	Oxytocin is used for the induction and stimulation of labor, reduction of postpartum bleeding, and incomplete or inevitable abortion because of its ability to cause potent and selective stimulation of uterine smooth muscle.
3 Identify potential side effects of oxytocin.	Oxytocin has the following side effects: *Maternal:* Blood: afibrinogenemia (lack of fibrinogen)—may be related to increase in postpartum bleeding CNS: subarachnoid hemorrhage resulting from hypertension; convulsions or coma resulting from water intoxication CV: hypotension; increased heart rate, systemic venous return, and cardiac output; dysrhythmia GI: nausea, vomiting Other: hypersensitivity, tetanic contractions, abruptio placentae, impaired uterine blood flow, increased uterine motility *Fetal:* Blood: increased risk of hyperbilirubinemia CV: bradycardia, tachycardia, premature ventricular contractions Other: anoxia, asphyxia
4 Discuss guidelines to follow during administration of oxytocin.	The patient should follow these guidelines during administration of oxytocin: —Report any unusual feelings or adverse effects to the physician or nurse immediately. —Be aware that uterine contractions, maternal and fe-

tal heart rates, and maternal blood pressure are routinely monitored and recorded every 15 minutes.

PARA-AMINOSALICYLATE (P.A.S.)

Patient objectives	*Teaching plan content*
1 **State the name of the medication, the dose prescribed, and the ordered frequency of administration.**	This information should be obtained from the patient's physician.
2 **Explain the use of para-aminosalicylate.**	Para-aminosalicylate is used to treat tuberculosis because of its ability to inhibit bacterial enzyme production.
3 **Identify potential side effects of para-aminosalicylate.**	Para-aminosalicylate has the following side effects: Blood: hemolytic anemia CNS: encephalopathy CV: vasculitis (inflammation of blood vessels) GI: nausea, vomiting, diarrhea, abdominal pain GU: albuminuria (albumin in the urine), hematuria (blood in the urine), crystalluria (urate crystals in the urine) Hepatic: jaundice, hepatitis Metabolic: acidosis, hypokalemia (low serum potassium) Other: infectious mononucleosis–like symptoms, fever, lymphadenopathy
4 **Discuss guidelines to follow while taking para-aminosalicylate.**	The patient should follow these guidelines while taking para-aminosalicylate: —Take only as directed. Do not adjust the dose or discontinue the drug without the physician's approval. —Do not take other drugs (especially Benemid, Benadryl, or Rifadin) without the physician's approval. —Do not use if you are on a sodium-restricted diet. —Take this drug with meals or antacid to reduce GI distress. —Swallow enteric-coated tablets whole, and do not take them with antacids. —Protect this drug from water, heat, and sun; do not use if it turns brown or purple.

PENICILLIN G BENZATHINE (Bicillin L-A, Megacillin Suspension, Permapen)

Patient objectives	Teaching plan content
1 State the name of the medication, the dose prescribed, and the ordered frequency of administration.	This information should be obtained from the patient's physician.
2 Explain the use of penicillin G benzathine.	Penicillin G benzathine is an antibiotic used to treat syphilis and upper respiratory infections caused by a streptococcal agent. It may also be used as a prophylactic in poststreptococcal rheumatic fever.
3 Identify potential side effects of penicillin G benzathine.	Penicillin G benzathine has the following side effects: Blood: eosinophilia, hemolytic anemia, thrombocytopenia, leukopenia CNS: neuropathy, convulsions with high doses Local: pain and sterile abscess at injection site Other: hypersensitivity (maculopapular and exfoliative dermatitis, chills, fever, edema, anaphylaxis)
4 Discuss guidelines to follow while taking penicillin G benzathine.	The patient should follow these guidelines while taking penicillin G benzathine: —Tell the physician of any previous allergic reaction to this drug or any other penicillin. —Call the physician if rash, fever, or chills develop. —Be aware that a nurse or physician will administer this drug as an injection: in the buttocks in adults and in the thigh in infants and children.

PENICILLIN G POTASSIUM (Deltapen-VK, Falapen, M-Cillin B, Megacillin, P-50, Pentids, Pfizerpen)

Patient objectives	Teaching plan content
1 State the name of the medication, the dose prescribed, and the ordered frequency of administration.	This information should be obtained from the patient's physician.
2 Explain the use of penicillin G potassium.	Penicillin G potassium is used to treat a wide variety of infections.

3 Identify potential side effects of penicillin G potassium.	Penicillin G potassium has the following side effects: Blood: hemolytic anemia, leukopenia, thrombocytopenia CNS: neuropathy, convulsions with high doses Metabolic: possible severe potassium poisoning with high doses (hyperreflexia, convulsions, coma) Local: thrombophlebitis, pain at injection site Other: hypersensitivity (rash, urticaria, maculopapular eruptions, exfoliative dermatitis, chills, fever, edema, anaphylaxis), overgrowth of nonsusceptible organisms
4 Discuss guidelines to follow while taking penicillin G potassium.	The patient should follow these guidelines while taking penicillin G potassium: —Report any allergic reactions to penicillin to the physician before taking this drug. —Take the medication exactly as prescribed, even when feeling better. —Call the physician if rash, fever, or chills develop. —Take the medication 1 to 2 hours before meals or 2 to 3 hours after. —Never use leftover penicillin for a new illness or share penicillin with family and friends.

PENICILLIN G PROCAINE (Ayercillin, Crysticillin A.S., Duracillin A.S., Pfizerpen-AS, Wycillin)

Patient objectives	*Teaching plan content*
1 State the name of the medication, the dose prescribed, and the ordered frequency of administration.	This information should be obtained from the patient's physician.
2 Explain the use of penicillin G procaine.	Penicillin G procaine is an antibiotic used to treat a variety of moderate-to-severe infections. It is particularly effective in the treatment of uncomplicated gonorrhea and pneumococcal pneumonia.
3 Identify potential side effects of penicillin G procaine.	Penicillin G procaine has the following side effects: Blood: thrombocytopenia, hemolytic anemia, leukopenia CNS: arthralgia, convulsions Other: hypersensitivity (rash, urticaria, chills, fever, edema, prostration, anaphylaxis), overgrowth of nonsusceptible organisms

4 Discuss guidelines to follow while taking penicillin G procaine.	The patient should follow these guidelines while taking penicillin G procaine: —Tell the physician of any previous allergic reactions to this drug, or any other penicillin, before receiving the first dose. —Call the physician if rash, fever, or chills develop. —Be aware that a nurse or physician will administer this drug as an injection: in the buttocks in adults and in the thigh in infants and children. —With prolonged therapy, other infections may occur. Report any vaginal, urinary, or respiratory discomfort to the physician.

PENTAMIDINE ISETHIONATE (Pentam 300)

Patient objectives	*Teaching plan content*
1 State the name of the medication, the dose prescribed, and the ordered frequency of administration.	This information should be obtained from the patient's physician.
2 Explain the use of pentamidine isethionate.	Pentamidine isethionate is used to treat *Pneumocystis carinii.*
3 Identify potential side effects of pentamidine isethionate.	Pentamidine isethionate has the following side effects: Blood: impaired bone marrow function CV: irregular heart rhythm, hypotension GI: indigestion, nausea, vomiting Metabolic: decreased blood glucose level Other: impaired kidney and liver function, local abscess, flushing, weakness, rash
4 Discuss guidelines to follow while taking pentamidine isethionate.	The patient should follow these guidelines while taking pentamidine isethionate: —Report any unusual adverse effects to the physician or nurse.

PENTAZOCINE (Talwin, Talwin-Nx)

Patient objectives	*Teaching plan content*
1 State the name of the medication, the dose prescribed, and the ordered frequency of administration.	This information should be obtained from the patient's physician.

2 Explain the use of pentazocine.

Pentazocine is used to treat moderate-to-severe pain because of its ability to alter both the perception of and the emotional response to pain through an unknown mechanism.

3 Identify potential side effects of pentazocine.

Pentazocine has the following side effects:
CNS: sedation, visual disturbances, hallucinations, drowsiness, dizziness, light-headedness, confusion, euphoria, headache
GI: nausea, vomiting, dry mouth
GU: urinary retention
Local: induration, nodules, sloughing, and sclerosis of injection site
Other: respiratory depression, physical and psychological dependence

4 Discuss guidelines to follow while taking pentazocine.

The patient should follow these guidelines while taking pentazocine:
—Take only as directed. Do not adjust the dose or discontinue the drug without the physician's approval.
—Avoid activities that require alertness.

PENTOBARBITAL (Nembutal)

Patient objectives

Teaching plan content

1 State the name of the medication, the dose prescribed, and the ordered frequency of administration.

This information should be obtained from the patient's physician.

2 Explain the use of pentobarbital.

Pentobarbital is used for sedation and insomnia and as a preanesthetic because of its ability to interfere with transmission of impulses from the thalamus (relay center for sensory input) to the cortex (area associated with higher mental functions) of the brain.

3 Identify potential side effects of pentobarbital.

Pentobarbital has the following side effects:
CNS: drowsiness, lethargy, hangover, paradoxical (variable) excitement in the elderly
GI: nausea, vomiting
Skin: rash, urticaria (hives)

4 Discuss guidelines to follow while taking pentobarbital.

The patient should follow these guidelines while taking pentobarbital:
—Take only as directed. Do not adjust the dose with-

out the physician's approval.
—Do not drink alcoholic beverages or take any other drugs without first consulting the physician.
—Do not perform activities that require alertness or skill until response to this drug is determined.

PHENELZINE (Nardil)

Patient objectives	*Teaching plan content*
1 State the name of the medication, the dose prescribed, and the ordered frequency of administration.	This information should be obtained from the patient's physician.
2 Explain the use of phenelzine.	Phenelzine is used to treat depression because of its ability to promote accumulation of neurotransmitters by inhibiting MAO, resulting in an antidepressant action.
3 Identify potential side effects of phenelzine.	Phenelzine has the following side effects: CNS: dizziness, vertigo, headache, hyperactivity, hyperreflexia, tremors, muscle twitching, mania, jitters, insomnia, confusion, memory impairment, drowsiness, weakness, fatigue CV: paradoxical hypertension (variable high blood pressure), orthostatic hypotension (light-headedness on rising), dysrhythmias GI: dry mouth, anorexia, nausea, constipation Other: peripheral edema, sweating, weight changes
4 Discuss guidelines to follow while taking phenelzine.	The patient should follow these guidelines while taking phenelzine: —Take only as directed. Do not adjust the dose or discontinue the drug without the physician's approval. —Do not drink alcoholic beverages or take any other drugs without the physician's approval. —If symptoms of overdose (severe hypotension, palpitations, or frequent headaches) develop, hold dose and notify the physician. —Store the drug in a tight container, away from heat and light. —Avoid foods high in the amino acids tyramine (such as cheeses, beer, wine, and beans) or tryptophan (such

as meat and fish) and self-medication with over-the-counter cold, hay fever, or diet preparations.
—Expect possible orthostatic hypotension; its incidence with this drug is high.
—Continue precautions for 10 days after stopping this drug because of its long-lasting effects.

PHENOBARBITAL (Luminal)

Patient objectives	Teaching plan content
1 State the name of the medication, the dose prescribed, and the ordered frequency of administration.	This information should be obtained from the patient's physician.
2 Explain the use of phenobarbital.	Phenobarbital is used for sedation, preoperative sedation, and insomnia (inability to sleep) because of its ability to interfere with transmission of impulses from the thalamus (relay center for sensory input) to the cortex (area associated with higher mental functions) of the brain.
3 Identify potential side effects of phenobarbital.	Phenobarbital has the following side effects: CNS: drowsiness, lethargy, hangover, paradoxical (variable) excitement in the elderly GI: nausea, vomiting Local: pain, swelling, thrombophlebitis, necrosis, nerve injury Skin: rash, urticaria (hives)
4 Discuss guidelines to follow while taking phenobarbital.	The patient should follow these guidelines while taking phenobarbital: —Take only as directed. Do not adjust the dose or discontinue the drug without the physician's approval. —Do not drink alcoholic beverages or take any other drugs without the physician's approval. —Do not drive a vehicle, operate machinery, or perform activities requiring alertness or skill until response to this drug is determined. —Report any unusual signs or symptoms to your physician.

PHENYLBUTAZONE (Butazolidin)

Patient objectives	Teaching plan content
1 State the name of the medication, the dose prescribed, and the ordered frequency of administration.	This information should be obtained from the patient's physician.
2 Explain the use of phenylbutazone.	Phenylbutazone is used to treat pain and inflammation in arthritis, bursitis, and acute gouty arthritis.
3 Identify potential side effects of phenylbutazone.	Phenylbutazone has the following side effects: Blood: bone marrow depression (fatal aplastic anemia, agranulocytosis [decrease in granulocytes], thrombocytopenia [decrease in platelets]), hemolytic anemia, leukopenia CNS: agitation, confusion, lethargy CV: hypertension, edema, pericarditis, myocarditis, cardiac decompensation EENT: optic neuritis, blurred vision, retinal hemorrhage or detachment, hearing loss GI: nausea, vomiting, diarrhea, ulceration, occult blood loss GU: proteinuria (protein in urine), hematuria (blood in urine), glomerulonephritis, nephrotic syndrome, renal failure Hepatic: hepatitis Metabolic: hyperglycemia, toxic and nontoxic goiter, respiratory alkalosis, and metabolic acidosis Skin: petechiae (pinpoint purplish dots from bleeding under the skin), pruritus (itching), purpura (bruises), various dermatoses—from rash to toxic necrotizing epidermolysis
4 Discuss guidelines to follow while taking phenylbutazone.	The patient should follow these guidelines while taking phenylbutazone: —Take only as directed. Do not adjust the dose or discontinue the drug without the physician's approval. —Do not use with barbiturates, antidepressants, or cholestyramine unless under a physician's order. —Stop drug and notify the physician immediately if fever, sore throat, mouth ulcers, GI discomfort, tarry stools, bleeding, bruising, rash, or weight gain occurs. —Take with food, milk, or antacids. —Remain under close medical supervision and keep all physician and laboratory appointments.

PHENYLEPHRINE HYDROCHLORIDE (Alconefrin, Coricidin Nasal Mist, Neo-Synephrine, Sinarest Nasal, Sinophen, Vacon)

Patient objectives	*Teaching plan content*
1 State the name of the medication, the dose prescribed, and the ordered frequency of administration.	This information should be obtained from the patient's physician.
2 Explain the use of phenylephrine.	Phenylephrine reduces nasal congestion by constricting local arterioles.
3 Identify potential side effects of phenylephrine.	Phenylephrine has the following side effects: CNS: headache, tremors, dizziness, nervousness CV: palpitations, tachycardia, premature ventricular contractions, hypertension, pallor EENT: transient burning, stinging; dryness of nasal mucosa; possible rebound nasal congestion with continued use GI: nausea
4 Discuss guidelines to follow while taking phenylephrine.	The patient should follow these guidelines while taking phenylephrine: —Do not exceed the recommended dose. Use only as needed. —When applying the medication, keep head erect to minimize swallowing of medication. —Only one person should use dropper bottle or nasal spray.

PHENYLEPHRINE 0.12%, 2.5%, 10% (OPHTHALMIC) (AK-Dilate, Isopto Frin, Prefin)

Patient objectives	*Teaching plan content*
1 State the name of the medication, the dose prescribed, and the ordered frequency of administration.	This information should be obtained from the patient's physician.
2 Explain the use of phenylephrine (ophthalmic).	Phenylephrine (ophthalmic) is used to treat uveitis (inflammation of the iris, ciliary body, and choroid body of the eye), glaucoma, and minor eye irritations and as a decongestant. It produces vasoconstriction of the conjunctival blood vessels.

3 Identify potential side effects of phenylephrine (ophthalmic).	Phenylephrine (ophthalmic) has the following side effects: CNS: headache Eye: transient stinging, iris floaters (one or more spots that seem to float in front of the eye), narrow-angle glaucoma, blurred vision, reactive hyperemia, brow pain
4 Discuss guidelines to follow while using phenylephrine (ophthalmic).	The patient should follow these guidelines while using phenylephrine (ophthalmic): —Do not exceed the prescribed dose. —Do not use if solution is dark brown or contains precipitate. —Do not touch the tip of the dropper to the eye or surrounding tissue. —Keep container tightly sealed and away from light. —Do not share medication with others.

PILOCARPINE (Adsorbocarpine, Akarpine, Almocarpine, Isopto Carpine, Ocusert Pilo, Pilocar)

Patient objectives	*Teaching plan content*
1 State the name of the medication, the dose prescribed, and the ordered frequency of administration.	This information should be obtained from the patient's physician.
2 Explain the use of pilocarpine.	Pilocarpine is used to treat chronic open-angle glaucoma and before emergency surgery in acute narrow-angle glaucoma because of its ability to cause contraction of the sphincter muscles of the iris, resulting in miosis (constriction of the pupil).
3 Identify potential side effects of pilocarpine.	Pilocarpine has the following side effects: Eye: suborbital headache, myopia, ciliary spasm, blurred vision, conjunctival irritation, lacrimation, changes in visual field, brow pain GI: nausea, vomiting, abdominal cramps, diarrhea, salivation Other: bronchiolar spasm, pulmonary edema, hypersensitivity
4 Discuss guidelines to follow while taking pilocarpine.	The patient should follow these guidelines while taking pilocarpine: —Do not touch the dropper to the eye or to surrounding tissue.

—Apply light finger pressure on the lacrimal (tear) sac for 1 minute following instillation to minimize systemic absorption.
—Anticipate that vision will be temporarily blurred.

POLYMYXIN B SULFATE (OTIC)

Patient objectives	*Teaching plan content*
1 State the name of the medication, the dose prescribed, and the ordered frequency of administration.	This information should be obtained from the patient's physician.
2 Explain the use of polymyxin B sulfate (otic).	Polymyxin B sulfate (otic) is used to treat acute and chronic otitis media (inflammation of the middle ear), otitis externa (inflammation of the external ear), and otomycosis (fungal infection of the ear canal) because of its ability to inhibit and destroy bacteria present in the ear canal.
3 Identify potential side effects of polymyxin B sulfate (otic).	Polymyxin B sulfate (otic) has the following side effects: Ear: irritation, itching, urticaria (hives) Other: overgrowth of nonsusceptible organisms
4 Discuss guidelines to follow while using polymyxin B sulfate (otic).	The patient should follow these guidelines while using polymyxin B sulfate (otic): —Watch for signs of superinfection (continued pain, inflammation, fever). —Keep the container tightly closed and away from moisture. —Avoid touching the ear with the dropper. —Take only as directed.

PREDNISONE (Deltasone, Liquid Pred, Meticorten, Orasone, Prednicen-M, SK-Prednisone)

Patient objectives	*Teaching plan content*
1 State the name of the medication, the dose prescribed, and the ordered frequency of administration.	This information should be obtained from the patient's physician.

2 Explain the use of prednisone.	Prednisone is used to treat severe inflammation or immunosuppression because of its ability to influence protein metabolism by increasing protein catabolism (breakdown of protein molecules), decreasing use of amino acids for protein synthesis, and converting amino acids to glucose.
3 Identify potential side effects of prednisone.	Most adverse effects of corticosteroids are dose- or duration-dependent. Prednisone has the following side effects: CNS: euphoria, insomnia, psychotic behavior CV: congestive heart failure, hypertension, edema EENT: cataracts, glaucoma GI: peptic ulcer, gastrointestinal irritation, increased appetite Metabolic: possible hypokalemia (decreased serum potassium level), hyperglycemia (increased serum glucose level), and carbohydrate intolerance; growth suppression in children Skin: delayed wound healing, acne, various skin eruptions Other: muscle weakness, pancreatitis, hirsutism (manly hair growth in females), susceptibility to infections Acute adrenal insufficiency may occur with increased stress (infection, surgery, trauma) or abrupt withdrawal after long-term therapy. Withdrawal symptoms: rebound inflammation, fatigue, weakness, arthralgia, fever, dizziness, lethargy, depression, fainting, orthostatic hypotension, dyspnea, anorexia, hypoglycemia. Sudden withdrawal may be fatal.
4 Discuss guidelines to follow while taking prednisone.	The patient should follow these guidelines while taking prednisone: —Take only as directed. Do not adjust the dose or discontinue the drug without the physician's approval. —Do not take any other drugs without the physician's approval. —Weigh yourself daily; report sudden weight gain to the physician. —Report slow healing; it may mask or exacerbate infections. —Carry a card identifying your need for supplemental systemic glucocorticoids during stress. —Eat a salt-restricted diet rich in potassium and protein. A potassium supplement may be needed. —When possible, take P.O. dose with food to reduce GI irritation.

PROBENECID (Benemid, Probalan)

Patient objectives	*Teaching plan content*
1 State the name of the medication, the dose prescribed, and the ordered frequency of administration.	This information should be obtained from the patient's physician.
2 Explain the use of probenecid.	Probenecid is used to treat hyperuricemia (increased uric acid) of gout and gouty arthritis because of its ability to block renal tubular reabsorption of uric acid, increasing its excretion from the body.
3 Identify potential side effects of probenecid.	Probenecid has the following side effects: Blood: hemolytic anemia CNS: headache, dizziness CV: hypotension GI: anorexia, nausea, vomiting, gastric distress GU: urinary frequency Skin: dermatitis, pruritus (itching) Other: flushing, sore gums, fever
4 Discuss guidelines to follow while taking probenecid.	The patient should follow these guidelines while taking probenecid: —Take only as directed. Do not adjust the dose or discontinue the drug without the physician's approval. —Do not use together with aspirin or other salicylates. —Avoid alcohol; it increases the urate level. —Force fluids to maintain a minimum daily output of 2 to 3 liters. —Alkalinize urine with sodium bicarbonate or potassium citrate ordered by the physician. —Take with milk, food, or antacids to minimize GI distress. Continued disturbances might indicate the need to lower the dose. —Restrict foods high in purine: anchovies, liver, sardines, kidneys, sweetbreads, peas, lentils. —Take this drug regularly, as ordered, or gout attacks may result. —Visit the physician regularly so uric acid can be monitored and dosage adjusted if necessary.

PROCARBAZINE (Matulane)

Patient objectives	*Teaching plan content*
1 **State the name of the medication, the dose prescribed, and the ordered frequency of administration.**	This information should be obtained from the patient's physician.
2 **Explain the use of procarbazine.**	Procarbazine is used to treat lymphomas because of its ability to inhibit cancer cell reproduction by inhibiting DNA, RNA, and protein synthesis.
3 **Identify potential side effects of procarbazine.**	Procarbazine has the following side effects: Blood: bleeding tendency, anemia CNS: nervousness, depression, insomnia, nightmares, hallucinations, confusion EENT: retinal hemorrhage, photophobia GI: nausea, vomiting, anorexia, stomatitis (inflammation of the mucous membranes of the mouth), dry mouth, dysphagia (difficulty swallowing), diarrhea, constipation Skin: dermatitis Other: reversible alopecia
4 **Discuss guidelines to follow while taking procarbazine.**	The patient should follow these guidelines while taking procarbazine: —Take only as directed. Do not adjust the dose or discontinue the drug without the physician's approval. —Do not drink alcoholic beverages. —Watch for signs of unusual bleeding.

PROCHLORPERAZINE (Compazine)

Patient objectives	*Teaching plan content*
1 **State the name of the medication, the dose prescribed, and the ordered frequency of administration.**	This information should be obtained from the patient's physician.
2 **Explain the use of prochlorperazine.**	Prochlorperazine is used to treat severe nausea and vomiting because of its ability to inhibit or depress these symptoms.

3 Identify potential side effects of prochlorperazine.	Prochlorperazine has the following side effects: Blood: transient leukopenia (reduction in leukocytes), agranulocytosis (reduction in granulocytes) CNS: extrapyramidal reactions (tremors, choppy gait, problems with coordination—high incidence), sedation (low incidence), pseudoparkinsonism, EEG changes, dizziness CV: orthostatic hypotension (light-headedness on rising), tachycardia, EKG changes EENT: ocular changes, blurred vision GI: dry mouth, constipation GU: urinary retention, dark urine, menstrual irregularities, gynecomastia (development of enlarged breasts in the male), inhibited ejaculation Hepatic: cholestatic jaundice Metabolic: hyperprolactinemia Skin: mild photosensitivity, dermal allergic reactions, exfoliative dermatitis (inflammation in which the skin peels off in layers) Other: weight gain, increased appetite
4 Discuss guidelines to follow while taking prochlorperazine.	The patient should follow these guidelines while taking prochlorperazine: —Take only as directed. Do not adjust the dose without the physician's approval. —Dilute oral concentrate with tomato or fruit juice, milk, coffee, carbonated beverage, tea, water, soup, or pudding. —Use only when vomiting cannot be controlled by other measures or when only a few doses are required. If more than four doses are needed in a 24-hour period, notify the physician. —Keep oral concentrate out of direct light. Slight yellowing does not affect potency; discard very discolored solutions. —Avoid getting concentrate on hands or clothing to prevent contact dermatitis.

PROCYCLIDINE (Kemadrin)

Patient objectives	*Teaching plan content*
1 State the name of the medication, the dose prescribed, and the ordered frequency of administration.	This information should be obtained from the patient's physician.

2 Explain the use of procyclidine.	Procyclidine is used to treat parkinsonism and muscle rigidity because of its ability to inhibit the effects of acetylcholine (a neurotransmitter).
3 Identify potential side effects of procyclidine.	Procyclidine has the following side effects: CNS: light-headedness, giddiness EENT: blurred vision, mydriasis (pupil dilation) GI: constipation, dry mouth, nausea, vomiting, epigastric distress Skin: rash
4 Discuss guidelines to follow while taking procyclidine.	The patient should follow these guidelines while taking procyclidine: —Take only as directed. Do not adjust the dose or discontinue the drug without the physician's approval. —Take after meals to minimize GI distress. —Avoid activities that require alertness until response to this drug is determined. —Relieve dry mouth with cool drinks, ice chips, sugarless gum, or hard candy.

PROPOXYPHENE (Darvocet-N, Darvon, Darvon-N, Dolene)

Patient objectives	*Teaching plan content*
1 State the name of the medication, the dose prescribed, and the ordered frequency of administration.	This information should be obtained from the patient's physician.
2 Explain the use of propoxyphene.	Propoxyphene is used for mild-to-moderate pain because of its ability to alter both the perception of and the emotional response to pain through an unknown mechanism.
3 Identify potential side effects of propoxyphene.	Propoxyphene has the following side effects: CNS: dizziness, headache, sedation, euphoria, paradoxical (variable) excitement, insomnia GI: nausea, vomiting, constipation Other: psychological and physical dependence
4 Discuss guidelines to follow while taking propoxyphene.	The patient should follow these guidelines while taking propoxyphene: —Take only as directed. Do not adjust the dose without the physician's approval. —Avoid activities that require alertness. —Limit alcohol intake when taking this drug.

PROTRIPTYLINE (Vivactil)

Patient objectives	Teaching plan content
1 State the name of the medication, the dose prescribed, and the ordered frequency of administration.	This information should be obtained from the patient's physician.
2 Explain the use of protriptyline.	Protriptyline is used to treat the symptoms of depression because of its ability to increase the amount of norepinephrine and/or serotonin in the central nervous system.
3 Identify potential side effects of protriptyline.	Protriptyline has the following side effects: CNS: excitation, seizures, tremors, weakness, confusion, headache, nervousness CV: orthostatic hypotension (light-headedness on rising), tachycardia, EKG changes, hypertension EENT: blurred vision, tinnitus (ringing in the ears), mydriasis (pupil dilation) GI: dry mouth, constipation, nausea, vomiting, anorexia, paralytic ileus GU: urinary retention Skin: rash, urticaria (hives) Other: sweating, allergy After abrupt withdrawal of long-term therapy: nausea, headache, malaise. (These symptoms do not indicate addiction.)
4 Discuss guidelines to follow while taking protriptyline.	The patient should follow these guidelines while taking protriptyline: —Take only as directed. Do not adjust the dose or discontinue the drug without the physician's approval. —Increase fluids to lessen constipation. Inquire about a stool softener, if needed. —Avoid activities that require alertness and good psychomotor coordination until response to this drug is determined. Drowsiness and dizziness usually subside after a few weeks. —Relieve dry mouth with sugarless hard candy or gum. —Do not drink alcoholic beverages or use other drugs (prescription or over-the-counter) without first consulting the physician.

PSYLLIUM (Effersyllium Instant Mix, Hydrocil Instant, Hydrocil Plain, Konsyl, Metamucil Instant Mix, Metamucil Sugar-Free, Modane Bulk, Mucilose, Siblin, Syllact)

Patient objectives	Teaching plan content
1 State the name of the medication, the dose prescribed, and the ordered frequency of administration.	This information should be obtained from the patient's physician.
2 Explain the use of psyllium.	Psyllium is used to increase bulk in the intestine because of its ability to absorb water and expand to increase bulk and moisture content of the stool.
3 Identify potential side effects of psyllium.	Psyllium has the following side effects: GI: nausea, vomiting, diarrhea, all after excessive use; esophageal, gastric, small-intestinal, or colonic strictures when drug is taken in dry form; abdominal cramps, especially in severe constipation
4 Discuss guidelines to follow while taking psyllium.	The patient should follow these guidelines while taking psyllium: —Take only as directed. Do not adjust the dose or discontinue the drug without the physician's approval. —Psyllium may reduce appetite if taken before meals. —Mix with at least 8 oz of cold, pleasant tasting liquid, and stir only a few seconds. Drink immediately or mixture will congeal. Follow with an additional glass of liquid.

PYRIMETHAMINE (Daraprim)

Patient objectives	Teaching plan content
1 State the name of the medication, the dose prescribed, and the ordered frequency of administration.	This information should be obtained from the patient's physician.
2 Explain the use of pyrimethamine.	Pyrimethamine is used to treat toxoplasmosis because of its ability to inhibit enzyme activity of the causal organism.

3 **Identify potential side effects of pyrimethamine.**	Pyrimethamine has the following side effects: Blood: anemia CNS: stimulation and convulsions GI: anorexia, vomiting, diarrhea, tender tongue Skin: rashes, hair loss
4 **Discuss guidelines to follow while taking pyrimethamine.**	The patient should follow these guidelines while taking pyrimethamine: —Take only as directed. Do not adjust the dose or discontinue the drug without the physician's approval. —Take with meals to minimize GI upset.

Rh_o (D) IMMUNE GLOBULIN, HUMAN (Gamulin Rh, HypRho-D, MICRhoGAM, RhoGam)

Patient objectives	*Teaching plan content*
1 **State the name of the medication, the dose prescribed, and the ordered frequency of administration.**	This information should be obtained from the patient's physician.
2 **Explain the use of Rh_o (D) immune globulin.**	Rh_o (D) immune globulin is used to suppress the active antibody response in Rh-negative mothers exposed to Rh-positive fetuses (that is, it stops Rh-negative mothers from forming antibodies to their Rh-positive fetuses, which would ultimately cause rejection of the fetus by the mother's body and death of the fetus).
3 **Identify potential side effects of Rh_o (D) immune globulin.**	Rh_o (D) immune globulin has the following side effects: Local: discomfort at injection site Other: slight fever
4 **Discuss guidelines to follow after receiving an injection of Rh_o (D) immune globulin.**	The patient should follow these guidelines after receiving an injection of Rh_o (D) immune globulin: —Report any unusual reactions to the physician. —Report any decrease or change in fetal movement.

RIFAMPIN (Rifadin, Rimactane)

Patient objectives	Teaching plan content
1 State the name of the medication, the dose prescribed, and the ordered frequency of administration.	This information should be obtained from the patient's physician.
2 Explain the use of rifampin.	Rifampin is used to treat tuberculosis because of its ability to inhibit bacterial RNA synthesis.
3 Identify potential side effects of rifampin.	Rifampin has the following side effects: Blood: hemolytic anemia CNS: headache, fatigue, drowsiness, ataxia, dizziness, mental confusion, generalized numbness GI: epigastric distress, anorexia, nausea, vomiting, abdominal pain, diarrhea, flatulence, sore mouth and tongue Metabolic: hyperuricemia (increased serum uric acid) Hepatic: serious hepatotoxicity as well as transient abnormalities in liver function tests Skin: pruritus (itching), urticaria (hives), rash Other: flulike symptoms
4 Discuss guidelines to follow while taking rifampin.	The patient should follow these guidelines while taking rifampin: —Take only as directed. Do not adjust the dose or discontinue the drug without the physician's approval. —Do not mix with para-aminosalicylate or probenecid. —Anticipate the possibility of red-orange discoloration of urine, feces, saliva, sweat, sputum, and tears. Soft contact lenses may be permanently stained. —Avoid alcoholic beverages. —Take 1 hour before or 2 hours after meals; if GI upset occurs, take with meals.

RITODRINE (Yutopar)

Patient objectives	Teaching plan content
1 State the name of the medication, the dose prescribed, and the ordered frequency of administration.	This information should be obtained from the patient's physician.

2 Explain the use of ritodrine.	Ritodrine is used in the management of preterm labor because of its ability to inhibit uterine smooth muscle contractility.
3 Identify potential side effects of ritodrine.	Ritodrine has the following side effects: *Intravenous:* CNS: nervousness, anxiety, headache CV: dose-related alterations in blood pressure, palpitations, pulmonary edema, tachycardia, EKG changes GI: nausea, vomiting Other: erythema (excess blood collection) *Oral:* CNS: tremors, nervousness CV: palpitations GI: nausea, vomiting Skin: rash
4 Discuss guidelines to follow while taking ritodrine.	The patient should follow these guidelines while taking ritodrine: —Take only as directed. Do not adjust the dose or discontinue the drug without the physician's approval. —Do not take with steroids or drugs labeled as beta blockers. —Keep *all* appointments with the physician for close follow-up on patient and fetal condition.

SCOPOLAMINE (INJECTION)

Patient objectives	*Teaching plan content*
1 State the name of the medication, the dose prescribed, and the ordered frequency of administration.	This information should be obtained from the patient's physician.
2 Explain the preoperative use of scopolamine.	Scopolamine is used preoperatively to reduce secretions in the nasopharynx and mouth, which prevents aspiration and its consequences.
3 Identify potential side effects of scopolamine.	Scopolamine has the following side effects: CNS: disorientation, restlessness, irritability, incoherence, headache CV: palpitations, tachycardia, paradoxical bradycardia (variable, abnormally slow heartbeat) EENT: dilated pupils, blurred vision, photophobia, increased intraocular pressure, difficulty swallowing

GI: constipation, mouth dryness, nausea, vomiting, epigastric distress
GU: urinary hesitancy or retention
Skin: flushing, dryness
Other: bronchial plugging, fever, depressed respirations. Adverse effects may be due to pending atropine-like toxicity and are dose-related. Individual tolerance varies greatly.

4 Discuss guidelines to follow when receiving scopolamine injection.	The patient should follow these guidelines when receiving scopolamine: —Avoid any activity that requires alertness. —Empty the bladder before administration of scopolamine. —Remain in bed after administration of scopolamine.

SCOPOLAMINE (OPHTHALMIC) (Isopto Hyoscine)

Patient objectives	*Teaching plan content*
1 State the name of the medication, the dose prescribed, and the ordered frequency of administration.	This information should be obtained from the patient's physician.
2 Explain the use of scopolamine (ophthalmic).	Scopolamine (ophthalmic) is used for cycloplegic refraction (paralysis of ciliary muscle of the eye) as well as to treat iritis and uveitis (inflammation of the iris, ciliary body, and choroid body of the eye). This is because of its ability to dilate the pupil of the eye.
3 Identify potential side effects of scopolamine (ophthalmic).	Scopolamine (ophthalmic) has the following side effects: Eye: ocular congestion with prolonged use, conjunctivitis, blurred vision, eye dryness, increased intraocular pressure, photophobia, contact dermatitis Systemic: flushing, fever, dry skin and mouth, tachycardia, hallucinations, ataxia (loss of coordination), irritability, confusion, delirium, somnolence (sleepiness), acute psychotic reactions
4 Discuss guidelines to follow while using scopolamine (ophthalmic).	The patient should follow these guidelines while using scopolamine (ophthalmic): —Wear dark glasses to ease discomfort of photophobia. —Do not touch the dropper to the eye or to surrounding tissue. —Apply light finger pressure on the lacrimal (tear) sac for 1 minute following instillation to minimize systemic absorption.

—Wash hands before and after administration.
—Expect that vision will be temporarily blurred; do not drive a car or operate machinery until the effect wears off.

SECOBARBITAL (Seconal)

Patient objectives	Teaching plan content
1 State the name of the medication, the dose prescribed, and the ordered frequency of administration.	This information should be obtained from the patient's physician.
2 Explain the use of secobarbital.	Secobarbital is used to treat insomnia and psychotic agitation and for preoperative sedation because of its ability to interfere with transmission of impulses from the thalamus (relay center for sensory input) to the cortex (area associated with higher mental functions) of the brain.
3 Identify potential side effects of secobarbital.	Secobarbital has the following side effects: CNS: drowsiness, lethargy, hangover, paradoxical (variable) excitement in the elderly GI: nausea, vomiting Skin: rash, urticaria (hives)
4 Discuss guidelines to follow while taking secobarbital.	The patient should follow these guidelines while taking secobarbital: —Take only as directed. Do not adjust the dose without the physician's approval. —Do not drink alcoholic beverages or take any other drugs without the physician's approval. —Do not perform activities requiring alertness or skill until response to this drug is determined.

SODIUM CHLORIDE, HYPERTONIC (Adsorbonac Ophthalmic, Hypersal 5%, Muro Ointment, Sodium Chloride Ointment 5%)

Patient objectives	Teaching plan content
1 State the name of the medication, the dose prescribed, and the ordered frequency of administration.	This information should be obtained from the patient's physician.

2 Explain the use of hypertonic sodium chloride.	Hypertonic sodium chloride is used postoperatively for corneal edema and in trauma and bullous keratopathy (a noninflammatory, vesicle-forming disease of the cornea) because of its ability to remove excess fluid from the cornea of the eye.
3 Identify potential side effects of hypertonic sodium chloride.	Hypertonic sodium chloride has the following side effects: Eye: slight stinging Other: hypersensitivity
4 Discuss guidelines to follow while using hypertonic sodium chloride.	The patient should follow these guidelines while using hypertonic sodium chloride: —Store in a tightly closed container. —Do not touch the tip of the dropper or tube to the eye or surrounding tissue. —Do not operate machinery or drive a car while using ointment; it may cause blurred vision.

SPIRAMYCIN (Rovamycine)

Patient objectives	*Teaching plan content*
1 State the name of the medication, the dose prescribed, and the ordered frequency of administration.	This information should be obtained from the patient's physician.
2 Explain the use of spiramycin.	Spiramycin is used to treat bacterial infections because of its ability to inhibit bacterial protein synthesis.
3 Identify potential side effects of spiramycin.	Spiramycin has the following side effects: GI: vomiting and epigastric pain, diarrhea CNS: paresthesias (numbness, tingling) Other: sweating, giddiness
4 Discuss guidelines to follow while taking spiramycin.	The patient should follow these guidelines while taking spiramycin: —Take only as directed. Do not adjust the dose or discontinue the drug without the physician's approval. —Spiramycin is not commercially available in the United States and must be obtained through the physician. —Do not share this medication with anyone. —Notify the physician if any unusual side effects occur.

STREPTOMYCIN

Patient objectives	*Teaching plan content*
1 State the name of the medication, the dose prescribed, and the ordered frequency of administration.	This information should be obtained from the patient's physician.
2 Explain the use of streptomycin.	Streptomycin is used to treat tuberculosis because of its ability to inhibit bacterial protein synthesis.
3 Identify potential side effects of streptomycin.	Streptomycin has the following side effects: CNS: transient paresthesias (numbness and tingling), muscle weakness EENT: hearing loss, ringing in the ears, vertigo, nausea and vomiting, ataxia, blurred vision Local: pain and irritation at the injection site Other: decreased serum potassium level, impaired kidney function
4 Discuss guidelines to follow while taking streptomycin.	The patient should follow these guidelines while taking streptomycin: —Increase fluid intake during therapy. —Do not mix with ethacrynic acid, furosemide, or dimenhydrinate.

SULFADIAZINE (Microsulfon)

Patient objectives	*Teaching plan content*
1 State the name of the medication, the dose prescribed, and the ordered frequency of administration.	This information should be obtained from the patient's physician.
2 Explain the use of sulfadiazine.	Sulfadiazine is used as an adjunct to treat toxoplasmosis because of its ability to interrupt the life cycle of the causative organism (a protozoan).
3 Identify potential side effects of sulfadiazine.	Sulfadiazine has the following side effects: Blood: agranulocytosis (decrease in number of granulocytes), aplastic anemia, thrombocytopenia (decrease in platelets), leukopenia (decrease in leukocytes), hemolytic anemia

CNS: headache, mental depression, convulsions, hallucinations
GI: nausea, vomiting, diarrhea, abdominal pain, anorexia, stomatitis (inflammation of the mouth)
GU: toxic nephrosis with oliguria (scanty urine production) and anuria (no urine production); crystalluria (urate crystals in the urine); hematuria (blood in the urine)
Hepatic: jaundice
Skin: generalized skin eruption, epidermal necrolysis, exfoliative dermatitis, photosensitivity, urticaria (hives), pruritus (itching)
Local: irritation, extravasation
Other: hypersensitivity, serum sickness, drug fever, anaphylaxis (severe allergic reaction)

---

4 Discuss guidelines to follow while taking sulfadiazine.

The patient should follow these guidelines while taking sulfadiazine:
—Do not take with ammonium chloride or ascorbic acid.
—Take only as directed. Do not adjust the dose or discontinue the drug without the physician's approval.
—Drink a full glass of water with each dose, and drink plenty of water throughout the day to prevent crystalluria.
—Take sulfadiazine for as long as prescribed, even if you feel better.
—Avoid direct sunlight and ultraviolet light to prevent photosensitivity reaction.
—Promptly report skin rash, sore throat, fever, or mouth sores.

SULFINPYRAZONE (Anturane)

Patient objectives	Teaching plan content
1 State the name of the medication, the dose prescribed, and the ordered frequency of administration.	This information should be obtained from the patient's physician.
2 Explain the use of sulfinpyrazone.	Sulfinpyrazone is used as maintenance therapy for common gout and for reduction and prevention of joint changes and tophi (deposits of urate crystals under the skin) formation because of its ability to increase excretion of uric acid through the kidneys.

3 Identify potential side effects of sulfinpyrazone.

Sulfinpyrazone has the following side effects:
GI: nausea, dyspepsia (indigestion), epigastric pain, blood loss, reactivation of peptic ulcers
Skin: rash

4 Discuss guidelines to follow while taking sulfinpyrazone.

The patient should follow these guidelines while taking sulfinpyrazone:
—Take only as directed. Do not adjust the dose or discontinue the drug without the physician's approval.
—Do not use with aspirin or salicylate-containing medications.
—Force fluids to maintain a minimum daily output of 2 to 3 liters. Alkalinize urine with sodium bicarbonate or other agent ordered by the physician.
—Take with milk, food, or antacids to minimize GI disturbances.
—Restrict foods high in purine: anchovies, liver, sardines, kidneys, sweetbreads, peas, lentils.
—Take this drug regularly, as ordered, or gout attacks may result.
—Visit the physician regularly so blood levels can be monitored and dosage adjusted if necessary.

SULFISOXAZOLE (Gantrisen, Novosoxazole)

Patient objectives	*Teaching plan content*
1 State the name of the medication, the dose prescribed, and the ordered frequency of administration.	This information should be obtained from the patient's physician.
2 Explain the use of sulfisoxazole.	Sulfisoxazole is an antibiotic used to treat urinary tract and other infections because of its ability to decrease bacterial folic acid synthesis.
3 Identify potential side effects of sulfisoxazole.	Sulfisoxazole has the following side effects: Blood: agranulocytosis, aplastic anemia, megaloblastic anemia, thrombocytopenia, leukopenia, hemolytic anemia CNS: headache, mental depression, convulsions, hallucinations GI: nausea, vomiting, diarrhea, abdominal pain, anorexia, stomatitis GU: toxic nephrosis with oliguria and anuria, crystalluria, hematuria Hepatic: jaundice

Skin: erythema multiforme (Stevens-Johnson syndrome), generalized skin eruption, epidermal necrolysis, exfoliative dermatitis, photosensitivity, urticaria, pruritus
Other: hypersensitivity, serum sickness, drug fever, anaphylaxis

4 Discuss guidelines to follow while taking sulfisoxazole.	The patient should follow these guidelines while taking sulfisoxazole: —Drink a full glass of water with each dose, and drink plenty of water throughout the day to prevent crystalluria. —Take the medication for as long as prescribed, even after you feel better. —Avoid direct sunlight and ultraviolet light to prevent a photosensitivity reaction. —Report early signs of blood dyscrasias (sore throat, fever, pallor) immediately to physician.

TAMOXIFEN (Nolvadex)

Patient objectives	*Teaching plan content*
1 State the name of the medication, the dose prescribed, and the ordered frequency of administration.	This information should be obtained from the patient's physician.
2 Explain the use of tamoxifen.	Tamoxifen is used to treat advanced premenopausal and postmenopausal breast cancer because of its ability to act as an estrogen antagonist and decrease DNA synthesis in tumor cells.
3 Identify potential side effects of tamoxifen.	Tamoxifen has the following side effects: Blood: transient fall in white blood cells or platelets GI: nausea in 10% of patients, vomiting, anorexia GU: vaginal discharge and bleeding Skin: rash Other: temporary bone or tumor pain, hot flashes in 7% of patients. Brief exacerbation of pain from osseous metastases.
4 Discuss guidelines to follow while taking tamoxifen.	The patient should follow these guidelines while taking tamoxifen: —Take only as directed. Do not adjust the dose or discontinue the drug without the physician's approval. —Use an analgesic to relieve pain. —Be aware that acute exacerbation of bone pain dur-

ing tamoxifen therapy usually indicates that the drug will produce a good response.
—Short-term therapy induces ovulation in premenopausal women. In these cases, *mechanical* contraception is recommended.

TERBUTALINE (Brethine)

Patient objectives	*Teaching plan content*
1 State the name of the medication, the dose prescribed, and the ordered frequency of administration.	This information should be obtained from the patient's physician.
2 Explain the use of terbutaline.	Terbutaline is used to treat preterm labor because of its ability to stop uterine contractions.
3 Identify potential side effects of terbutaline.	Terbutaline has the following side effects: CNS: nervousness, tremors, headache, drowsiness, sweating CV: palpitations, increased heart rate GI: vomiting, nausea
4 Discuss guidelines to follow while taking terbutaline.	The patient should follow these guidelines while taking terbutaline: —Take only as directed. Do not adjust the dose or discontinue the drug without the physician's approval. —Do not take any other drugs without the physician's approval.

TETRAHYDROZOLINE (Murine Plus, Optigene 3, Soothe, Visine)

Patient objectives	*Teaching plan content*
1 State the name of the medication, the dose prescribed, and the ordered frequency of administration.	This information should be obtained from the patient's physician.
2 Explain the use of tetrahydrozoline.	Tetrahydrozoline is used to treat ocular congestion, irritation, and allergic conditions because of its ability to produce vasoconstriction of the blood vessels of the conjunctiva.

3 Identify potential side effects of tetrahydrozoline.	Tetrahydrozoline has the following side effects: Eye: transient stinging, pupillary dilation, increased intraocular pressure, irritation, iris floaters (one or more spots that seem to drift in front of the eye) in the elderly Systemic: drowsiness, depression, cardiac irregularities, headache, dizziness, tremors, insomnia
4 Discuss guidelines to follow while using tetrahydrozoline.	The patient should follow these guidelines while using tetrahydrozoline: —Do not exceed the recommended dosage. —Do not touch the dropper to the eye or to surrounding tissue. —Do not share medication with others.

TIMOLOL (Timoptic Solution)

Patient objectives	Teaching plan content
1 State the name of the medication, the dose prescribed, and the ordered frequency of administration.	This information should be obtained from the patient's physician.
2 Explain the use of timolol.	Timolol is used to treat open-angle glaucoma, secondary glaucoma, and aphakic (absence of the lens of the eye) glaucoma because it has the ability to reduce aqueous formation and possibly increase aqueous outflow.
3 Identify potential side effects of timolol.	Timolol has the following side effects: CNS: headache, depression, fatigue CV: slight reduction in resting heart rate Eye: minor irritation; long-term use may decrease corneal sensitivity GI: anorexia Other: apnea in infants, evidence of hypotension, bradycardia, syncope, exacerbation of asthma, and congestive heart failure
4 Discuss guidelines to follow while taking timolol.	The patient should follow these guidelines while taking timolol: —Sometimes a few weeks may be required to stabilize pressure-lowering response. The patient will need to return to the physician after 4 weeks to have his intraocular pressure checked.

—Do not touch the dropper to the eye or surrounding tissue.
—This drug can be used safely by persons with glaucoma who wear conventional hard contact lenses.
—Lightly depress the lacrimal (tear) sac with a finger after drug administration to decrease the chance of systemic absorption.

TRANYLCYPROMINE (Parnate)

Patient objectives	*Teaching plan content*
1 State the name of the medication, the dose prescribed, and the ordered frequency of administration.	This information should be obtained from the patient's physician.
2 Explain the use of tranylcypromine.	Tranylcypromine is used to treat depression because of its ability to block MAO, causing certain neurotransmitters to build up, resulting in an antidepressant action.
3 Identify potential side effects of tranylcypromine.	Tranylcypromine has the following side effects: CNS: dizziness, vertigo, headache, hyperactivity, hyperreflexia, tremors, muscle twitching, mania, jitters, confusion, memory impairment, fatigue CV: orthostatic hypotension (light-headedness on rising), dysrhythmias, paradoxical (variable) hypertension EENT: blurred vision GI: dry mouth, anorexia, nausea, diarrhea, constipation, abdominal pain GU: changed libido, impotence Skin: rash Other: peripheral edema, sweating, weight changes, chills
4 Discuss guidelines to follow while taking tranylcypromine.	The patient should follow these guidelines while taking tranylcypromine: —Take only as directed. Do not adjust the dose or discontinue the drug without the physician's approval. —Avoid foods high in the amino acids tyramine (such as cheeses, beer, wine, and beans) or tryptophan (such as meat and fish) and self-medication with over-the-counter cold, hay fever, or weight loss preparations. —Do not drink alcoholic beverages or take any other drugs (prescription or nonprescription) without the physician's approval.

—Get out of bed slowly, sitting up first for 1 minute.

TRIHEXYPHENIDYL (Artane, Tremin, Trihexane, Trihexidyl)

Patient objectives	Teaching plan content
1 State the name of the medication, the dose prescribed, and the ordered frequency of administration.	This information should be obtained from the patient's physician.
2 Explain the use of trihexyphenidyl.	Trihexyphenidyl is used to treat drug-induced parkinsonism because of its ability to inhibit the effects of acetylcholine (a neurotransmitter).
3 Identify potential side effects of trihexyphenidyl.	Trihexyphenidyl has the following side effects: CNS: disorientation, restlessness, irritability, incoherence, headache CV: palpitations, tachycardia, paradoxical bradycardia (variable, slow heartbeat) EENT: dilated pupils, blurred vision, photophobia, increased intraocular pressure, difficulty swallowing GI: constipation, mouth dryness, nausea, vomiting, epigastric distress GU: urinary hesitancy or retention Skin: flushing, dryness Other: bronchial plugging, fever, depressed respirations Adverse effects may be due to pending atropine-like toxicity and are dose-related. Individual tolerance varies greatly.
4 Discuss guidelines to follow while taking trihexyphenidyl.	The patient should follow these guidelines while taking trihexyphenidyl: —Take only as directed. Do not adjust the dose or discontinue the drug without the physician's approval. —Avoid activities requiring alertness until response to this drug is determined. —Do not take with amantadine. —Relieve dry mouth with cool drinks, ice chips, sugarless gum, or hard candy.

TRIMIPRAMINE (Surmontil)

Patient objectives	*Teaching plan content*
1 State the name of the medication, the dose prescribed, and the ordered frequency of administration.	This information should be obtained from the patient's physician.
2 Explain the use of trimipramine.	Trimipramine is used to treat the symptoms of depression because of its ability to increase the amount of norepinephrine and/or serotonin in the central nervous system.
3 Identify potential side effects of trimipramine.	Trimipramine has the following side effects: CNS: drowsiness, dizziness, excitation, seizures, tremors, weakness, confusion, headache, nervousness CV: orthostatic hypotension (light-headedness on rising), tachycardia, EKG changes, hypertension EENT: blurred vision, tinnitus, mydriasis GI: dry mouth, constipation, nausea, vomiting, anorexia, paralytic ileus GU: urinary retention Skin: rash, urticaria (hives) Other: sweating, allergy After abrupt withdrawal of long-term therapy: nausea, headache, malaise. (These symptoms do not indicate addiction.)
4 Discuss guidelines to follow while taking trimipramine.	The patient should follow these guidelines while taking trimipramine: —Take only as directed. Do not adjust the dose or discontinue the drug without the physician's approval. —Increase fluids to reduce constipation. Inquire about a stool softener, if needed. —Avoid activities that require alertness and good psychomotor coordination until response to this drug is determined. —Relieve dry mouth with sugarless gum or hard candy. —Do not drink alcoholic beverages or take any other drugs without first consulting the physician.

VINBLASTINE (Velban)

Patient objectives	Teaching plan content
1 State the name of the medication, the dose prescribed, and the ordered frequency of administration.	This information should be obtained from the patient's physician.
2 Explain the use of vinblastine.	Vinblastine is used to treat breast or testicular cancer, Hodgkin's disease, non-Hodgkin's lymphoma, choriocarcinoma, lymphosarcoma, neuroblastoma, mycosis fungoides, and histiocytosis because of its ability to arrest cell division.
3 Identify potential side effects of vinblastine.	Vinblastine has the following side effects: Blood: leukopenia (reduction in leukocytes), thrombocytopenia (decrease in platelets) CNS: depression, paresthesias (numbness and tingling in extremities), peripheral neuropathy and neuritis, numbness, loss of deep tendon reflexes, muscle pain and weakness EENT: pharyngitis GI: nausea, vomiting, stomatitis (inflammation of the mouth), ulcer and bleeding, constipation, ileus, anorexia, weight loss, abdominal pain GU: oligospermia, aspermia, urinary retention Skin: dermatitis, vesiculation Local: irritation, phlebitis, cellulitis (skin inflammation), necrosis if I.V. infiltrates Other: reversible alopecia (hair loss) in 5% to 10% of patients, pain in tumor site, low fever
4 Discuss guidelines to follow while taking vinblastine.	The patient should follow these guidelines while taking vinblastine: —Take laxatives and stool softeners as needed if physician approves. —Take antiemetics as ordered before administration of vinblastine to reduce nausea.

VINCRISTINE (Oncovin)

Patient objectives	*Teaching plan content*
1 **State the name of the medication, the dose prescribed, and the ordered frequency of administration.**	This information should be obtained from the patient's physician.
2 **Explain the use of vincristine.**	Vincristine is used to treat acute lymphoblastic and other leukemias, Hodgkin's disease, lymphosarcoma, reticulum cell sarcoma, neuroblastoma, rhabdomyosarcoma, Wilms' tumor, osteogenic and other sarcomas, and lung and breast cancer because of its ability to arrest cell division.
3 **Identify potential side effects of vincristine.**	Vincristine has the following side effects: Blood: rapidly reversible mild anemia and leukopenia (reduction in leukocytes) CNS: peripheral neuropathy, sensory loss, deep tendon reflex loss, paresthesias, wristdrop and footdrop, ataxia, cranial nerve palsies (headache, jaw pain, hoarseness, vocal cord paralysis, visual disturbances), muscle weakness and cramps, depression, agitation, insomnia. Neurotoxicities may be permanent. EENT: diplopia (double vision), optic and extraocular neuropathy, ptosis (drooping eyelids) GI: constipation, cramps, ileus that mimics surgical abdomen, nausea, vomiting, anorexia, stomatitis (inflammation of the mouth), weight loss, dysphagia GU: urinary retention Local: severe local reaction when extravasated, phlebitis, cellulitis (inflammation of the skin) Other: reversible alopecia (hair loss) in up to 71% of patients
4 **Discuss guidelines to follow while taking vincristine.**	The patient should follow these guidelines while taking vincristine: —Expect possible alopecia; it is reversible. —Take a stool softener, a laxative, or water before vincristine dose.

ZINC SULFATE (Eye-Sed Ophthalmic, Op-Thal-Zin)

Patient objectives	Teaching plan content
1 State the name of the medication, the dose prescribed, and the ordered frequency of administration.	This information should be obtained from the patient's physician.
2 Explain the use of zinc sulfate.	Zinc sulfate is used to treat ocular congestion and irritation because of its astringent (contractive) action on the conjunctiva of the eye.
3 Identify potential side effects of zinc sulfate.	Zinc sulfate has the following side effects: Eye: irritation
4 Discuss guidelines to follow while using zinc sulfate.	The patient should follow these guidelines while using zinc sulfate: —Store in a tightly closed container. —Do not touch the dropper tip to the eye or surrounding tissue.

Patient-Teaching Aid

DEALING WITH CONSTIPATION

Dear Patient:

If you are taking a narcotic medication, it may make you constipated. Here are some guidelines to help:

• Eat more high-fiber foods, including raw fruits and vegetables, whole grain breads and cereals, dried fruits, and nuts. Choose high-fiber snack foods such as date-nut bread, oatmeal cookies, or granola. Add 1 to 2 tbs of bran to your cereal or eggs.

• Drink warm or hot beverages to stimulate bowel activity.

• Avoid hard cheeses and refined grain products, such as rice and macaroni.

• Get more exercise (for example, walking) if you can.

Patient-Teaching Aid

TAKING YOUR MEDICATION

Dear Patient:

Your physician has ordered the following medication for you: _____

_____

_____

_____

This medication will help treat your: _____

_____

_____

_____

_____

Take the medication at these times: _____

_____

_____

_____

_____

Follow these instructions: _____

_____

_____

_____

_____

_____

_____

_____

_____

Call the physician if you notice any of the following:

_____

_____

_____

_____

_____

_____

_____

_____

Patient-Teaching Aid

YOUR MEDICATION: WHAT YOU SHOULD KNOW

Dear Patient:

The medication you are taking is _____

_____.

The physician has prescribed it because _____

_____.

Take this medication exactly as the label directs. Pay particular attention to these directions:

_____

_____.

Avoid these foods or liquids while you are taking this medication:

_____.

Tell the physician at once if you notice:

_____.

Store your medication as follows:

_____.

IMPORTANT: Whenever you take any medication, remember these guidelines:

• Follow the directions for taking medication exactly. Do not try to make it last longer than the physician intended.

• Try to take your medication at the same time each day. You will be less likely to forget it.

• Do not permit others to take your medication, and do not try any of theirs. The physician's prescription is intended for your specific needs.

• If your medication is a liquid, use a measuring spoon to ensure an accurate dose. Do not use a regular eating spoon.

• Periodically check the expiration date on the label of your medication. Throw away any outdated medication, as well as medication that is more than several years old.

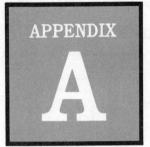

Educational Resources

The following educational resources have been compiled for the use of both the health care professional and the patient. Some materials may be provided free; others may involve a charge. Inclusion in this list does not necessarily constitute the publisher's endorsement of any of the materials or organizations.

A

Al-Anon (Family Group Headquarters, Inc.)
One Park Ave.
New York, N.Y. 10016
Multimedia on life with an alcoholic, including braille and tape

Alcoholics Anonymous World Services, Inc.
P.O. Box 459
Grand Central Station
New York, N.Y. 10163
Multimedia on alcoholism for patients, their families, friends, and employees

American Academy of Family Physicians
1740 West 92nd St.
Kansas City, Mo. 64114
Information on cancer

American Academy of Ophthalmology
P.O. Box 7424
1833 Filmore St.
San Francisco, Calif. 94120
Information on ophthalmology

American Academy of Otolaryngology— Head and Neck Surgery
1101 Vermont Ave., N.W.
Suite 302
Washington, D.C. 20005
Information on otolaryngology

American Association for Cancer Education
University of Nebraska Medical Center
Department of Medicine
42nd and Dewey Aves.
Omaha, Neb. 68105
Teaching and training programs on cancer

American Association for Health, Physical Education, Recreation, and Dance
1900 Association Drive
Reston, Va. 22091
Materials on nutrition and weight control

American Association for Maternal and Child Health
c/o Harold J. Fishbein
233 Prospect, P-204
La Jolla, Calif. 92037
Materials on gynecology/obstetrics

American Association of Sex Educators, Counselors, and Therapists
11 Dupont Circle, N.W.
Suite 220
Washington, D.C. 20036
Information on sex education

American Bakers Association
1111 14th St., N.W.
Suite 300
Washington, D.C. 20005
Materials on nutrition and weight control

American Cancer Society
777 Third Ave.
New York, N.Y. 10017
Multimedia on cancer

American College of Obstetrics and Gynecology
600 Maryland Ave., S.W.
Suite 300
Washington, D.C. 20024
Information on cancer, obstetrics, and gynecology

American Council on Alcohol Problems
2908 Patricia Drive
Des Moines, Iowa 50322
Booklets on alcoholism

American Dietetic Association
430 North Michigan Ave.
Chicago, Ill. 60611
Publications and materials on special diets, weight control, and allergies; information for both the professional and the public

American Dry Milk Institute
130 North Franklin St.
Chicago, Ill. 60606
Booklets on nutrition and weight control

American Egg Board
1460 Renaissance Drive
Park Ridge, Ill. 60068
Booklets on nutrition and weight control

American Foundation for the Blind
15 West 16th St.
New York, N.Y. 10011
Multimedia on braille, guide dogs, rehabilitation, and employment

American Hospital Association
840 North Lake Shore Drive
Chicago, Ill. 60611
Multiple publications for the professional concerning patient education

American Institute of Baking
Consumer Service Department
1213 Bakers Way
Manhattan, Kan. 66502
Booklets on nutrition

American Meat Institute
P.O. Box 3556
Washington, D.C. 20007
Booklets on nutrition

American Medical Association
535 North Dearborn St.
Chicago, Ill. 60610
Information on topics such as drug abuse, alcoholism, physical fitness, mental health, and nutrition; posters and teaching kits on some topics

American Nurses' Association
2420 Pershing Rd.
Kansas City, Mo. 64108
Publications for the nurse on patient education

American Occupational Therapy Association
1383 Piccard Drive
Suite 301
Rockville, Md. 20850
Materials on occupational therapy and rehabilitation

American Optometric Association
243 North Lindbergh Blvd.
St. Louis, Mo. 63141
Printed materials and posters on eyesight

American Physical Therapy Association
1111 North Fairfax St.
Alexandria, Va. 22314
Booklets on rehabilitation

American Podiatric Medical Association
20 Chevy Chase Circle, N.W.
Washington, D.C. 20015
Films and publications on foot care

American Psychiatric Association
1700 K St., N.W.
Washington, D.C. 20009
Printed materials on mental health

American Public Health Association
1015 15th St., N.W.
Washington, D.C. 20036
Education materials for health workers

American Red Cross
17th and D Sts., N.W.
Washington, D.C. 20006
Materials on health and safety

American Social Health Association
260 Sheridan Ave.
Suite 307
Palo Alto, Calif. 94306
Information on venereal disease and drug
abuse

**American Society for Psychoprophylaxis
in Obstetrics**
1840 Wilson Blvd.
Suite 204
Arlington, Va. 22201
Multimedia on childbirth

Armour Food Company
Consumer Services Department
Greyhound Towers
Phoenix, Ariz. 85013
Materials on nutrition and weight control

The Arthritis Foundation
1314 Spring St., N.W.
Atlanta, Ga. 30309
Written materials on arthritis, nutrition,
and weight control

Ayerst Laboratories
(Division of American Home Products
Corporation)
685 Third Ave.
New York, N.Y. 10017
Information on obstetrics

B

Beecham Laboratories
101 Possumtown Rd.
Piscataway, N.J. 08854
Printed materials on obstetrics and
gynecology

Best Foods
Consumer Service Department
(Division of CPC International, Inc.)
International Plaza
Englewood Cliffs, N.J. 07632
Multimedia on nutrition and weight control

Channing L. Bete Company, Inc.
200 State Rd.
South Deerfield, Mass. 01373
Printed materials on arthritis, cancer, drug
abuse, obstetrics, gynecology, and other
topics

Better Vision Institute
230 Park Ave.
New York, N.Y. 10169
Materials on eye care and blindness

Blue Cross and Blue Shield Association
676 North Saint Clair St.
Chicago, Ill. 60611
Printed materials on nutrition, weight
control, obstetrics, and gynecology

The Borden Company
Marketing Services
180 East Broad St.
Columbus, Ohio 43215
Materials on nutrition and weight control

Bureau of Audiovisual Instruction
University of Wisconsin
1327 University Ave.
Madison, Wis. 53701
Audiovisual information on obstetrics and
gynecology

C

California Prune Advisory Board
103 World Trade Center
San Francisco, Calif. 94111
Information on nutrition and weight control

Campbell Soup Company
Food Service Products Division
Campbell Place
Camden, N.J. 08101
Information on nutrition and weight control

Cancer Information Service
1825 Connecticut Ave., N.W.
Suite 218
Washington, D.C. 20009
Professional and public information on cancer

Carnation Company
Medical Marketing Department
5045 Wilshire Blvd.
Los Angeles, Calif. 90036
Information on nutrition

Centers for Disease Control
1600 Clifton Rd., N.E.
Atlanta, Ga. 30333
National AIDS Hotline—(800) 342-AIDS

Chicago Dietetic Supply, Inc.
405 East Shawnut Ave.
La Grange, Ill. 60525
Information on nutrition and weight control

Churchill Films
662 North Robertson Blvd.
Los Angeles, Calif. 90069
Multimedia on obstetrics

Consumer and Foods Economic Institute
Federal Building, Room 325-A
Hyattsville, Md. 20782
Information on nutrition and weight control

Core Communications in Health, Inc.
1916-38 Park Ave.
New York, N.Y. 10037
Multimedia on arthritis, obstetrics, and cancer

D

Del Monte Kitchens
P.O. Box 3575
San Francisco, Calif. 94105
Written materials on nutrition and weight control

Department of Agriculture
Office of Information
14th St. and Independence Ave., S.W.
Washington, D.C. 20250
Information on nutrition and home safety

Department of Health and Human Services
Centers for Disease Control—Bureau of Health Education
1600 Clifton Rd., N.E.
Atlanta, Ga. 30333
Materials on accident prevention and disease control

Diabetes and Arthritis Program
National Institutes of Health
9000 Rockville Pike
Building 10, Room 9N-222
Bethesda, Md. 20205
Information on arthritis and diabetes

Division of Long-Term Care
Health Standards and Quality Bureau
Dogwood East Building
1849 Gwynn Oak Ave.
Baltimore, Md. 21207
Materials on nutrition and weight control

E

The Equitable Life Assurance Society of the United States
1285 Avenue of the Americas
New York, N.Y. 10019
Information on nutrition and weight control

F

Film-Com Audience Planners
108 West Grand
Chicago, Ill. 60610
Multimedia on eye care and blindness

Fleischmann's Margarine
625 Madison Ave.
New York, N.Y. 10022
Information on nutrition and weight control

Food Council of America
1750 Pennsylvania Ave., N.W.
Washington, D.C. 20005
Materials on nutrition and weight control

Food and Drug Administration
Parklawn Building
5600 Fishers Lane
Rockville, Md. 20857
Information on safety and accident prevention

The Food and Nutrition Information and Educational Materials Center
National Agricultural Library
Beltsville, Md. 20705
Information on nutrition and weight control

G

General Foods Corporation
Consumer Service Department
250 North St.
White Plains, N.Y. 10605
Information on nutrition

Gerber Products Company
445 State St.
Freemont, Mich. 49412
Materials on nutrition and weight control

The Godfather Fund—c/o The Tavern Guild
P.O. Box 11309
San Francisco, Calif. 94101
Provides personal care items to people with AIDS and AIDS-related conditions

Good Food
1864 East Washington
Pasadena, Calif. 91103
Materials on nutrition and weight control

Good Housekeeping Bulletin Service
959 Eighth Ave.
New York, N.Y. 10019
Materials on nutrition and weight control

Green Giant Company
Home Services Department
Hazeltine Gates
Chaska, Minn. 55318
Information on nutrition and weight control

H

Health Films Library
One West Wilson St.
P.O. Box 309
Madison, Wis. 53701
Information on cancer

Health Insurance Association of America
150 K St., N.W.
Washington, D.C. 20006
Booklets on general health

H. J. Heinz
Consumer Relations
1062 Progress St.
Pittsburgh, Pa. 15212
Printed materials on nutrition

I

International AIDS Prospective Epidemiology Network
259 East Erie, Room 101C
Chicago, Ill. 60611
(312) 943-6600
Information on AIDS and pre-AIDS conditions

International Apple Institute
Public Relations
P.O. Box 1137
6707 Old Dominion Drive
McLean, Va. 22101
Information on nutrition and weight control

International Council of Guilds for Infant Survival
P.O. Box 3841
Davenport, Iowa 52808
Materials on parenting

J

Johnson & Johnson
Health Care Division
501 George St.
New Brunswick, N.J. 08903
Multimedia on parenting

K

Kaiser Permanente Medical Center
280 West MacArthur Blvd.
Oakland, Calif. 94611
Multimedia on arthritis, obstetrics, and gynecology

Kellogg Company
Department of Home Economic Services
235 Porter St.
Battle Creek, Mich. 49017
Information on nutrition and weight control

Kimberly-Clark Corporation
Life Cycle Center—Box 2001
Neenah, Wis. 54956
Printed materials on obstetric topics

Knox Gelatin, Inc.
(Subsidiary of Thomas J. Lipton)
Route 523
Flemington, N.J. 08822
Information on nutrition and weight control

Kraft Foods
Kraft Court
Chicago, Ill. 60025
Information on nutrition and weight control

L

La Leche League International
9616 Minneapolis Ave.
Franklin Park, Ill. 60131
Printed materials on prenatal care,
childbirth, breast-feeding, and family
nutrition

Learning Resources Facility
Institute of Rehabilitation Medicine
400 East 34th St.
New York, N.Y. 10016
Information on arthritis

Lee Creative Communications, Inc.
P.O. Box 1367
Rochester, N.Y. 14618
Information on arthritis

Leukemia Society of America
733 Third Ave.
New York, N.Y. 10017
Patient, professional, and public service and
information on leukemia

Libby, McNeil, and Libby
200 South Michigan Ave.
Chicago, Ill. 60604
Information on nutrition

M

Make Today Count (MTC)
P.O. Box 222
Osage Beach, Mo. 65065
Support group for cancer patients and their
immediate families

**Martland Hospital Health Education
Project**
College of Medicine and Dentistry
of New Jersey
100 Bergen St.
Newark, N.J. 07103
Audiovisual materials on health subjects

Maternity Center Association
48 East 92nd St.
New York, N.Y. 10128
Multimedia, including teaching aids, on
maternity care, drugs, nutrition, and
childbearing

Mead Johnson and Company
Pharmaceutical Division
2404 West Pennsylvania St.
Evansville, Ind. 47712
Information on parenting, obstetrics,
nutrition, and weight control

Medfact, Incorporated
1112 Andrew Ave., N.E.
Massilon, Ohio 44646
Multimedia on parenting, eye care, and
obstetrics

Mental Health Materials Center
30 East 29th St.
New York, N.Y. 10016
Information on mental health and the
family

Merck Sharp & Dohme
(Division of Merck and Company, Inc.)
West Point, Pa. 19486
Information on nutrition and weight control

Metropolitan Life Insurance Company
Health and Welfare Division
One Madison Ave.
New York, N.Y. 10010
Materials on parenting

N

**National AIDS Research and Education
Foundation**
54 Tenth St.
San Francisco, Calif. 94013
(415) 626-8784
Information on AIDS

National Association of the Deaf
814 Thayer Ave.
Silver Spring, Md. 20910
Materials on hearing and hearing loss

National Association for Hearing and Speech Action
10801 Rockville Pike
Rockville, Md. 20852
Materials on hearing and speech problems

National Association for Visually Handicapped
305 East 24th St.
New York, N.Y. 10010
Large-print materials for the partially sighted

National Cancer Institute
Office of Cancer Communications
9000 Rockville Pike
Building 31, Room 10A-29
Bethesda, Md. 20205
Materials on cancer

National Clearinghouse for Alcohol Information
P.O. Box 2345
Rockville, Md. 20857
Variety of printed materials on alcohol, alcohol abuse, drinking, and alcoholism

National Clearinghouse for Drug Abuse Information
5600 Fishers Lane
Room 10A-J3
Rockville, Md. 20857
Materials on drug abuse and drug addiction

National Clearinghouse for Mental Health Information
5600 Fishers Lane
Rockville, Md. 20857
Materials on aspects of mental health problems for the public and the professional

National Council on Aging
600 Maryland Ave., S.W.
Washington, D.C. 20024
Professional materials on the elderly

National Council on Alcoholism
12 West 21st St.
New York, N.Y. 10010
Materials on alcoholism

National Dairy Council
6300 North River Rd.
Rosemont, Ill. 60018
Materials on nutrition and weight control

National Easter Seal Society
2023 West Ogden Ave.
Chicago, Ill. 60612
Information on speech disorders, stroke rehabilitation, and orthopedic conditions

National Eye Institute
9000 Rockville Pike
Building 31, Room 6A-03
Bethesda, Md. 20205
Printed materials on eyesight

National Hemophilia Foundation
19 West 34th St.
Room 1204
New York, N.Y. 10001
Information for hemophiliacs on AIDS

National Institute on Alcohol Abuse and Alcoholism
5600 Fishers Lane
Rockville, Md. 20857
Printed materials on alcoholism

National Institute of Allergy and Infectious Diseases
9000 Rockville Pike
Building 31, Room 7A-03
Bethesda, Md. 20205
Printed materials on allergies and infectious diseases

National Institute of Arthritis, Metabolic, and Digestive Diseases
9000 Rockville Pike
Building 31, Room 9A-52
Bethesda, Md. 20205
Booklets on arthritis and metabolic diseases

National League for Nursing
Ten Columbus Circle
New York, N.Y. 10019
Information for the nurse on patient education

National Mental Health Association
1021 Prince St.
Arlington, Va. 22314
Materials on mental illness

National People with AIDS Projects
c/o AID Atlanta
1801 Piedmont Rd.
Suite 208
Atlanta, Ga. 30324
Support material for people with AIDS

National Retired Teachers Association
American Association of Retired Persons
1909 K St., N.W.
Washington, D.C. 20049
Multimedia on chronic diseases

National Society to Prevent Blindness
79 Madison Ave.
New York, N.Y. 10016
Multimedia on eye care and blindness
prevention

Nutrition Foundation
888 17th St., N.W.
Washington, D.C. 20006
Booklets on nutrition

O

**Occupational Safety and Health
Administration**
Department of Labor
200 Constitution Ave., N.W.
Washington, D.C. 20210
Information on occupational safety

Office of Consumer Affairs
621 Reporters Building
300 Seventh Ave., S.W.
Washington, D.C. 20201
Written materials on general health

Ortho Pharmaceutical Corporation
Route 202
Raritan, N.J. 08869
Information on obstetrics

P

Pennwalt Pharmaceutical Division
755 Jefferson Rd.
Rochester, N.Y. 14623
Information on nutrition and weight control

Perennial Education, Inc.
477 Roger Williams
P.O. Box 855 Ravinia
Highland Park, Ill. 60035
Information on obstetric topics

Pet Incorporated
Office of Consumer Affairs
400 South Fourth St.
St. Louis, Mo. 63102
Information on nutrition and weight control

**Pharmaceutical Manufacturers
Association**
1100 15th St., N.W.
Washington, D.C. 20005
Catalog of materials available for patients
and professionals from member drug
companies

**Planned Parenthood Federation of
America**
810 Seventh Ave.
New York, N.Y. 10019
Multimedia on contraception, childbirth,
and human reproduction

Professional Research, Inc.
660 South Bonnie Brae St.
Los Angeles, Calif. 90057
Multimedia on eye care and obstetrics

Prudential Insurance Company of America
P.O. Box 388
Fort Washington, Pa. 19034
Materials on nutrition and weight control

Public Affairs Committee
381 Park Ave. South
New York, N.Y. 10016
Booklets on obstetrics and gynecology

Public Health Service
200 Independence Ave., S.W.
Washington, D.C. 20201
Printed material on foot care, eye care,
blindness, nutrition, and weight control

Public Television Library
475 L'Enfant Plaza, S.W.
Washington, D.C. 20024
Videotapes on many topics

Q

Quaker Oats Company
Consumer Services
West Merchandise Mart Plaza
Chicago, Ill. 60654
Information on nutrition and weight control

R

Ralston Purina Company
Nutrition Service
Checkerboard Square
835 South Eighth St.
St. Louis, Mo. 63101
Information on nutrition and weight control

Rice Council of America
P.O. Box 140123
Houston, Tex. 77271
Information on nutrition

Roche Laboratories
(Division of Hoffman-LaRoche, Inc.)
340 Kingsland St.
Nutley, N.J. 07110
Information on nutrition and weight control

Ross Laboratories
(Division of Abbott Laboratories)
Creative Services and Information
Department
625 Cleveland Ave.
Columbus, Ohio 43216
Multimedia on obstetrics, eye care,
nutrition, weight control, and parenting

S

The San Francisco AIDS Fund
1547 California St.
San Francisco, Calif. 94109
Limited direct cash assistance to people
with AIDS to assist with financial
emergencies

**Sex Information and Education Council of
the United States**
80 Fifth Ave.
Suite 801
New York, N.Y. 10011
Printed materials on sex education, family
planning, sexual problems of the
handicapped and elderly, obstetrics, and
gynecology

Society for Nutrition Education
1736 Franklin St.
Oakland, Calif. 94612
Materials on food, pregnancy, nutrition,
diets, and weight control

Society for Public Health Education, Inc.
703 Market St.
Suite 535
San Francisco, Calif. 94103
Professional materials on health education

Standard Brands Food Division
625 Madison Ave.
New York, N.Y. 10022
Information on nutrition

Stokely-Van Camp, Inc.
Home Economics Department
941 North Meridian St.
Indianapolis, Ind. 46204
Nutritional information

Sunkist Growers, Inc.
Consumer Services
14130 Riverside Drive
Sherman Oaks, Calif. 91423
Materials on nutrition and weight control

Swift and Company
Public Relations Department
115 West Jackson Blvd.
Chicago, Ill. 60604
Information on nutrition and weight control

U

**United Fresh Fruit and Vegetable
Association**
P.O. Box 1417 E35
Alexandria, Va. 22313
Information on nutrition and weight control

United States Pharmacopeial Convention
Publication Department
12601 Twinbrook Pkwy.
Rockville, Md. 20852
Patient-education materials on drugs and
drug therapy

United Way
701 North Fairfax St.
Alexandria, Va. 22314
General information

University of Illinois Medical Center
Public Information Office
1740 West Taylor St.
Chicago, Ill. 60612
Videotapes on health information

University of Kansas
College of Health Sciences and Hospital
39th St. and Rainbow Blvd.
Kansas City, Kan. 66103
Videotapes on health topics

**University of North Carolina
at Chapel Hill**
Institute of Nutrition
Allied Health Sciences Building
311 Pittsboro St.
Chapel Hill, N.C. 27514
Multimedia on nutrition and weight control

University of Toronto
Division of Instructional Media Services
Toronto, Ontario, Canada M5S-1A8
Videotapes on health topics

Upjohn Company
7000 Portage Rd.
Kalamazoo, Mich. 49001
Information on nutrition, weight control,
and preventive health

V

Vitamin Information Bureau, Inc.
664 North Michigan Ave.
Chicago, Ill. 60611
Multimedia on nutrition and weight control

W

Wheat Flour Institute
Home Economics Department
600 Maryland Ave., S.W.
West Wing, Suite 305
Washington, D.C. 20024
Nutritional information

Winthrop Laboratories
90 Park Ave.
New York, N.Y. 10016
Materials on parenting

Women's AIDS Network
707 San Bruno Ave.
San Francisco, Calif. 94117
Information network for women about AIDS,
and for women working with AIDS patients

Wyeth Laboratories
Division of American Home Products
Corporation
177 King of Prussia Rd.
Radnor, Pa. 19087
Materials on obstetrics and parenting

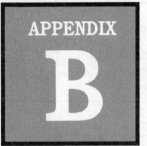

Preoperative & Postoperative Teaching

PREOPERATIVE TEACHING

Before any type of surgery or invasive procedure is performed, a patient must be informed of the nature of the procedure, its risks and benefits, what is expected of him before and after the procedure, and any options he might have. In most cases, a permit must be signed by the patient before the procedure is performed. This legal document is the responsibility of the physician; the nurse's responsibility is to teach the patient what he needs to know in order to make informed choices concerning the proposed procedure(s).

Prior to initiating teaching with the patient, it is helpful if the nurse contacts the physician to find out what procedure is planned and what special modifications, if any, will be made (for example, the use of a local versus a general anesthetic). When the nurse approaches the patient, she should begin by asking him what procedure the physician told him would be performed. His answer may reveal inaccuracies in his understanding or at least give her an idea of where to begin her teaching.

One of the roles of nurses is to encourage patients to be their own health care advocates and to question health care providers about the care being received. The nurse can encourage a patient to seek answers to his questions from physicians and nurses; to seek a second opinion, if he so desires; and to obtain the information necessary for him to make informed decisions concerning appropriate treatment.

Preoperative teaching includes both physical *and* psychological preparation. In addition to being taught about his specific treatment, a patient must be given the time and the media to express himself. He should be provided with paper and pencil to write down his questions, thoughts, or concerns and encouraged to express his fears and hopes about the procedure. Only misperceptions should be corrected.

Preoperative teaching includes information about what will happen before, during, and after the procedure. Communicating this information can be accomplished by discussion, demonstration, the use of pictures, or even having the patient talk to another patient who had the same procedure. Topics to be discussed include the following:

Topic	Considerations
1 Preoperative medications	—When will medication(s) be given, and by what route? —What is the purpose of the medication(s), and what restrictions will be placed on the patient after administration?
2 Nutrition restrictions	—Will the patient be NPO; if so, starting when? —May the patient have water?
3 Preoperative treatments	—GI (enemas or special mixtures to clean out the system): How much time and inconvenience will be involved in bowel evacuation? How much discomfort will be involved? Why is it necessary? —Skin preparation: What is the rationale for this? Where will it be performed, when, by whom, and what will it entail? How much of the body will be prepped? Is a shower required? —Starting an I.V.: When will this be done and by whom? How long will the I.V. be necessary? How often might it have to be changed? —Insertion of a urinary catheter: When will this be done and by whom? How much discomfort will be involved? How long will the catheter remain in place?
4 Anesthesia	—What kind of anesthetic will the patient get? How does it work? What precautions will be taken before and after its administration? Will he be awake for the procedure? Will he feel anything?
5 Room change	—If the patient will be recovering in a special room, such as an ICU, inform him of this, and, if possible, take him to see the unit before the procedure. Make sure he is aware of the routine noises and sights in that unit.

6 Preparation for post-operative treatment	—This is the time to prepare the patient for the skills he will be required to use after the surgical procedure. The patient should be taught the use of incentive spirometry, deep breathing, and supported coughing (chest splinting) as well as how to turn in bed or use a trapeze while he is free of pain. —Also, prepare the patient at this time for the various routine tasks that will be performed and the equipment (such as tubes) that will be present after the procedure so that he will know that they are normal; for example, frequent monitoring of vital signs, function and nursing responsibility for various tubes and catheters, I.V.'s, and dietary restrictions. Include a discussion of the various consequences of the procedure that may be expected, such as bloody urine.
7 Personal business and psychological support	—Some patients need to write a will or discuss with you what they would like to happen "just in case something goes wrong." Listen without being judgmental, and then bring the discussion back to their preparation for the procedure. —Assure the patient that he will not be alone before or during the procedure. Also assure him that his privacy will be respected and that he will be covered except for the operative site.
8 Significant others	—Can significant others stay at the hospital the night before the procedure? Can they visit the morning before the procedure? Can they accompany the patient to the procedure site? Where can they wait while the procedure is in progress, and will the physician come to talk to them immediately after the procedure? How can they assist in the preoperative and postoperative management of their loved one?
9 Valuables	—Discuss arrangements for valuables and/or prostheses. Does the patient understand why prostheses must be removed?
10 Hospital dress code for procedures	—Can nail polish be worn? Does the patient need to wear a hospital gown and/or surgical hat, and why?
11 Transportation	—How will the patient get to the procedure? Does he have a choice?

POSTOPERATIVE TEACHING

Because patients are often uncomfortable immediately after surgery, postoperative teaching should be short and to the point. Because of the anesthetic and medications in the patient's system, teaching may need to be repeated and reinforced many times. Teaching should include the following:

Topic	*Considerations*
1 Termination of the test or procedure	—Explain to the patient that the test or procedure is over. This may have to be repeated as the patient awakens.
2 Pain medication	—Explain the availability of pain medication, if applicable, and how often it can be administered. Develop a scale for measuring pain, such as 1 = mild pain and 10 = severe pain. This gives the patient some control in assessing his pain and determining his need for pain medication.
3 Reinforcement of information	—Once the physician has informed the patient what was done and the results of the procedure, the nurse should ensure that the patient understands what was done and its implications.
4 Psychological support	—The patient may project anger toward the health care providers for the pain, disfigurement, and grieving that he has gone through. This release is important for the patient's mental health, and the nurse can incorporate measures to enhance its expression in her nursing plan.

Patient Checklist Chart

This Patient-Teaching Checklist will assist you in your role as teacher. It has a fourfold purpose designed to help you:
- organize your teaching sessions
- record the content
- evaluate the effectiveness
- save time.

Copy it and use it to focus on specific learning objectives on a daily basis.

With this information at your fingertips, you can save much of your valuable time and be more effective in helping the patient maintain or regain good health.

PATIENT-TEACHING CHECKLIST FOR _____

PATIENT OBJECTIVES	PRE-TEST RESULTS	SESSION I CONTENT	SESSION II CONTENT	POST-TEST RESULTS
	Date: _____	Date: _____	Date: _____	Date: _____
	Date: _____	Date: _____	Date: _____	Date: _____
	Date: _____	Date: _____	Date: _____	Date: _____

PATIENT-TEACHING CHECKLIST FOR _____

PATIENT OBJECTIVES	PRE-TEST RESULTS	SESSION I CONTENT	SESSION II CONTENT	POST-TEST RESULTS
	Date: _____	Date: _____	Date: _____	Date: _____
	Date: _____	Date: _____	Date: _____	Date: _____
	Date: _____	Date: _____	Date: _____	Date: _____

Selected References

Abraham, Suzanne, and Jones, Derek. *Eating Disorders: The Facts.* New York: Oxford University Press, 1984.

Attending Ob/Gyn Patients. Nursing Photobook Series. Springhouse, Pa.: Springhouse Corp., 1982.

Barber, Triphy, and Langfitt, Dot E., *Teaching the Medical-Surgical Patient: Diagnostics and Procedures.* East Norwalk, Conn.: Appleton & Lange, 1983.

Barnhart, Edward R., ed. *Physicians' Desk Reference,* 41st ed. Oradell, N.J.: Medical Economics Books, 1987.

Beare, P., et al. *Nursing Implications of Diagnostic Tests,* 2nd ed. Philadelphia: J.B. Lippincott Co., 1985.

Bille, D.A. *Practical Approaches to Patient Teaching.* Boston: Little, Brown & Co., 1981.

Bloom, B., et al. *Taxonomy of Educational Objectives. Handbook I: Cognitive Domain.* White Plains, N.Y.: Longman Inc., 1977.

Bobak, Irene M., and Jensen, Margaret D. *Essentials of Maternity Nursing.* St. Louis: C.V. Mosby Company, 1984.

Brunner, Lillian, and Suddarth, Doris. *Textbook of Medical-Surgical Nursing,* 5th ed. Philadelphia: J.B. Lippincott Co., 1984.

Carpenito, L.J. *Nursing Diagnosis: Application to Clinical Practice.* Philadelphia: J.B. Lippincott Co., 1983.

Clark, Carolyn C. *Classroom Skills for Nurse Educators,* vol. 4. New York: Springer Publishing Co., 1978.

Cushing, Maureen. "Legal Lessons on Patient Teaching," *American Journal of Nursing* 84(6):721-22, June 1984.

DeVita, V., et al. *AIDS: Etiology, Diagnosis, Treatment, and Prevention.* Philadelphia: J.B. Lippincott Co., 1985.

Diagnostics, 2nd ed. Springhouse, Pa.: Springhouse Corp., 1986.

Diseases, 2nd ed. Springhouse, Pa.: Springhouse Corp., 1987.

D'Onofrio, C.N. "Evaluating Patient Education: Purposes, Politics, and a Proposal for Practitioners," in *Patient Education—An Inquiry into the State of the Art.* Edited by Squyres, W.D. New York: Springer Publishing Co., 1980.

Donovan, Marilee, and Richardson, S.G., eds. *Cancer Care Nursing.* East Norwalk, Conn.: Appleton & Lange, 1984.

DSM III—*Diagnostic and Statistical Manual of Mental Disorders,* 3rd ed. Washington, D.C.: American Psychiatric Association, 1980.

DuBrey, Rita. *Promoting Wellness in Nursing Practice: A Step-by-Step Approach in Patient Education.* St. Louis: C.V. Mosby Co., 1982.

Emmett, S.W., ed. *Theory and Treatment of Anorexia Nervosa and Bulimia: Biomedical, Sociocultural, and Psychological Perspectives.* New York: Brunner-Mazel, Inc., 1985.

Freedman, Carol. *Teaching Patients.* San Diego: Courseware, Inc., 1978.

Garfinkel, P.E., and Garner, D.M. *Anorexia Nervosa: A Multidimensional Perspective.* New York: Brunner-Mazel, Inc., 1982.

Griffith, H. Winter. *Instructions for Patients,* 3rd ed. Philadelphia: W.B. Saunders Co., 1982.

Gross, Meir. *Anorexia Nervosa: A Comprehensive Approach.* Lexington, Mass.: D.C. Heath Co., 1982.

Haber, J., et al. *Comprehensive Psychiatric Nursing,* 2nd ed. New York: McGraw-Hill Book Co., 1982.

Howes, A.C. "Nursing Diagnoses and Care Plans for Ambulatory Care Patients with AIDS," *Topics in Clinical Nursing* 6(2):61-66, July 1984.

Isselbacher, Kurt, et al. *Harrison's Principles of Internal Medicine: Update Two,* 9th ed. New York: McGraw-Hill Book Co., 1982.

Juneau, Patricia. *Essentials of Maternity Nursing.* Philadelphia: F.A. Davis Co., 1985.

Kernaghan, Salvinija. "Preadmission Preoperative Teaching: A Promising Option, but Easier Said than Done," *Promoting Health* 6(2):6-8, March/April, 1985.

Lego, Suzanne. *American Handbook of Psychiatric Nursing.* Philadelphia: J.B. Lippincott Co., 1984.

Lewis, S., and Collier, I. *Medical-Surgical Nursing: Assessment and Management of Clinical Problems.* New York: McGraw-Hill Book Co., 1983.

Lillard, J., Lotspeich, P., Gurich, J., Hesse, J. (1984). "Acquired Immunodeficiency Syndrome in Home Care: Maximizing Helpfulness and Minimizing Hysteria," *Home Healthcare Nurse* 2(5), 11-14.

Luckmann, Joan, and Sorenson, Karen. *Medical-Surgical Nursing: A Psychophysiologic Approach, 2nd ed.* Philadelphia: W.B. Saunders Co., 1980.

Madnick, Myra E., ed. *Consumer Health Education: A Guide to Hospital-Based Programs.* Rockville, Md.: Aspen Systems Corp., 1980.

Malasanos, L., et al. *Health Assessment.* St. Louis: C.V. Mosby Co., 1985.

Martin, J. (1985, October). *Physical Assessment Guideline for Nurses.* San Francisco: VNA of San Francisco, AIDS Home Care and Hospice Program.

Martin, J. (1986). Sustaining Care of Persons with AIDS. *The Person With AIDS: Nursing Perspectives.* Chicago: Springer Publishing Company.

Monograph: *Biopsychiatric Insights in Depression;* Chairman and moderator—Solomon H. Synder, MD
Ire Extein—*The Role of Thyroid Function Tests*
Bernard J. Carroll—*The Role of the Dexamethasone Suppression Test (DST)*
Frederick Goodwin—*The Role of Urine MHPG*

Nathan, Peter E., and Harris, Sandra L. *Psychopathology and Society,* 2nd ed. New York: McGraw-Hill Book Co., 1980.

Nursing87 Drug Handbook. Springhouse, Pa.: Springhouse Corp., 1987.

Olds, Sally B., et al. *Maternal-Newborn Nursing, A Family-Centered Approach,* 2nd ed. Reading, Mass.: Addison-Wesley Publishing Co., 1984.

Paparella, Michael M., and Shumrick, Donald A. *Otolaryngology*, 3 vols, 2nd ed. Edited by Meyerhoff, William L., and Seid, Allan B. Philadelphia: W.B. Saunders Co., 1980.

Pasquali, E.A., et al. *Mental Health Nursing: A Holistic Approach*, 2nd ed. St. Louis: C.V. Mosby Co., 1985.

Pillitteri, Adele. *Maternal-Newborn Nursing: Care of the Growing Family*, 3rd ed. Boston: Little, Brown & Co., 1985.

Rankin, Sally, and Duffy, Karen L. *Patient Education: Issues, Principles and Guidelines*. Philadelphia: J.B. Lippincott Co., 1983.

Redman, Barbara K. *The Process of Patient Teaching in Nursing*, 5th ed. St. Louis: C.V. Mosby Co., 1983.

Rivlin, Michel, et al. *Manual of Clinical Problems in Obstetrics and Gynecology with Annotated Key References*. Boston: Little, Brown & Co., 1982.

Scheie, Harold G., and Alert, Daniel M. *Textbook of Ophthalmology*, 9th ed. Philadelphia: W.B. Saunders Co., 1977.

Schultz, J., and Dark, S.L. *Manual of Psychiatric Nursing Care Plans*, 2nd ed. Boston: Little, Brown & Co., 1986.

Shamansky, Sherry L., et al. *Primary Health Care Handbook: Guidelines for Patient Education*. Boston: Little, Brown & Co., 1984.

Smith, Elizabeth. *Maternity Care: A Guide for Patient Education*. East Norwalk, Conn.: Appleton & Lange, 1981.

Storlie, Frances. *Patient Teaching in Critical Care*. East Norwalk, Conn.: Appleton & Lange, 1975.

Stuart, G.W., and Sundeen, S.J. *Principles and Practice of Psychiatric Nursing*, 2nd ed. St. Louis: C.V. Mosby Co., 1983.

Surr, Claire White. "Teaching Patients to Use the New Blood-Glucose Monitoring Products, Part 1," *Nursing83* 13(1):42-45, January 1983.

Twycross, R., Lack, S. (1984). *Oral Morphine in Advanced Cancer*. Beaconsfield, England: Beaconsfield Publishers Ltd.

Veenker, C.H., "Evaluating Health Practice and Understanding," *Health Education* 16(2):80-82, February 1985.

Viele, C.S., et al. "Caring for Acquired Immune Deficiency Syndrome Patients...Experiences of One AIDS Nursing Unit," *Oncology Nursing Forum* 11(3):56-60, May/June 1984.

Wilson, H.S., and Kneisl, C.R. *Psychiatric Nursing*, 2nd ed. Menlo Park, Calif.: Addison-Wesley Publishing Co., 1983.

Woldum, Karyl, et al. *Patient Education: Foundations of Practice*. Rockville, Md.: Aspen Systems Corp., 1984.

Wolman, Benjamin B. *Psychological Aspects of Obesity: A Handbook*. New York: Van Nostrand Reinhold Co., 1981.

Ziegel, Erna, and Cranley, Mecca. *Obstetric Nursing*, 7th ed. New York: Macmillan Publishing Co., 1978.

Index

A

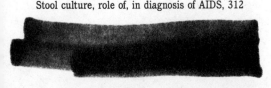